Endometriosis Research: From Bench to Bedside

Endometriosis Research: From Bench to Bedside

Editors

Antonio Simone Laganà
Valentina Lucia La Rosa

MDPI • Basel • Beijing • Wuhan • Barcelona • Belgrade • Manchester • Tokyo • Cluj • Tianjin

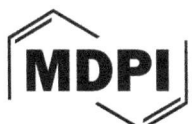

Editors
Antonio Simone Laganà
Department of Obstetrics
and Gynecology
"Filippo Del Ponte" Hospital
University of Insubria
Varese
Italy

Valentina Lucia La Rosa
Department of Educational
Sciences
University of Catania
Catania
Italy

Editorial Office
MDPI
St. Alban-Anlage 66
4052 Basel, Switzerland

This is a reprint of articles from the Special Issue published online in the open access journal *International Journal of Molecular Sciences* (ISSN 1422-0067) (available at: www.mdpi.com/journal/ijms/special_issues/endometriosis_research).

For citation purposes, cite each article independently as indicated on the article page online and as indicated below:

LastName, A.A.; LastName, B.B.; LastName, C.C. Article Title. *Journal Name* **Year**, *Volume Number*, Page Range.

ISBN 978-3-0365-2799-4 (Hbk)
ISBN 978-3-0365-2798-7 (PDF)

© 2021 by the authors. Articles in this book are Open Access and distributed under the Creative Commons Attribution (CC BY) license, which allows users to download, copy and build upon published articles, as long as the author and publisher are properly credited, which ensures maximum dissemination and a wider impact of our publications.

The book as a whole is distributed by MDPI under the terms and conditions of the Creative Commons license CC BY-NC-ND.

Contents

About the Editors vii

Antonio Simone Laganà, Simone Garzon, Martin Götte, Paola Viganò, Massimo Franchi, Fabio Ghezzi and Dan C. Martin
The Pathogenesis of Endometriosis: Molecular and Cell Biology Insights
Reprinted from: *Int. J. Mol. Sci.* **2019**, *20*, 5615, doi:10.3390/ijms20225615 1

Costin Vlad Anastasiu, Marius Alexandru Moga, Andrea Elena Neculau, Andreea Bălan, Ioan Scârneciu, Roxana Maria Dragomir, Ana-Maria Dull and Liana-Maria Chicea
Biomarkers for the Noninvasive Diagnosis of Endometriosis: State of the Art and Future Perspectives
Reprinted from: *Int. J. Mol. Sci.* **2020**, *21*, 1750, doi:10.3390/ijms21051750 43

Stefano Angioni, Maurizio Nicola D'Alterio, Alessandra Coiana, Franco Anni, Stefano Gessa and Danilo Deiana
Genetic Characterization of Endometriosis Patients: Review of the Literature and a Prospective Cohort Study on a Mediterranean Population
Reprinted from: *Int. J. Mol. Sci.* **2020**, *21*, 1765, doi:10.3390/ijms21051765 67

Jieliang Zhou, Bernard Su Min Chern, Peter Barton-Smith, Jessie Wai Leng Phoon, Tse Yeun Tan, Veronique Viardot-Foucault, Chee Wai Ku, Heng Hao Tan, Jerry Kok Yen Chan and Yie Hou Lee
Peritoneal Fluid Cytokines Reveal New Insights of Endometriosis Subphenotypes
Reprinted from: *Int. J. Mol. Sci.* **2020**, *21*, 3515, doi:10.3390/ijms21103515 91

Gaetano Riemma, Antonio Simone Laganà, Antonio Schiattarella, Simone Garzon, Luigi Cobellis, Raffaele Autiero, Federico Licciardi, Luigi Della Corte, Marco La Verde and Pasquale De Franciscis
Ion Channels in The Pathogenesis of Endometriosis: A Cutting-Edge Point of View
Reprinted from: *Int. J. Mol. Sci.* **2020**, *21*, 1114, doi:10.3390/ijms21031114 107

Carla Trapero, August Vidal, Maria Eulàlia Fernández-Montolí, Buenaventura Coroleu, Francesc Tresserra, Pere Barri, Inmaculada Gómez de Aranda, Jean Sévigny, Jordi Ponce, Xavier Matias-Guiu and Mireia Martín-Satué
Impaired Expression of Ectonucleotidases in Ectopic and Eutopic Endometrial Tissue Is in Favor of ATP Accumulation in the Tissue Microenvironment in Endometriosis
Reprinted from: *Int. J. Mol. Sci.* **2019**, *20*, 5532, doi:10.3390/ijms20225532 119

Jeong Sook Kim, Young Sik Choi, Ji Hyun Park, Jisun Yun, Soohyun Kim, Jae Hoon Lee, Bo Hyon Yun, Joo Hyun Park, Seok Kyo Seo, SiHyun Cho, Hyun-Soo Kim and Byung Seok Lee
Role of B-Cell Translocation Gene 1 in the Pathogenesis of Endometriosis
Reprinted from: *Int. J. Mol. Sci.* **2019**, *20*, 3372, doi:10.3390/ijms20133372 139

About the Editors

Antonio Simone Laganà

Medical Doctor at the Department of Obstetrics and Gynecology, "Filippo Del Ponte" Hospital, University of Insubria, Varese, Italy.

Antonio Simone Laganà is Deputy of the Special Interest Group for Endometriosis & Endometrial Disorders (SIGEED) of the European Society of Human Reproduction and Embryology (ESHRE) and Ambassador of the World Endometriosis Society (WES).

His research interests include endometriosis, reproductive immunology, infertility, gynaecological endocrinology, laparoscopy, and hysteroscopy. He is the author of more than 300 papers published in PubMed-indexed international peer-reviewed journals, and his presence is often requested as an invited speaker at international congresses. He is currently an editor of high-impact journals, including Scientific Reports, PLOS One, Journal of Minimally Invasive Gynecology, Journal of Ovarian Research, Gynecologic and Obstetric Investigation, and many others.

He is habilitated as Associate Professor in Italy for Gynecology and Obstetrics.

Valentina Lucia La Rosa

Valentina Lucia La Rosa is a psychologist and is specialized in Psychotherapy. She is a Ph.D. student at the Department of Educational Sciences of the University of Catania. She is a member of several prestigious scientific societies including Italian Association of Psychology (AIP); Lacanian School of Psychoanalysis (SLP); World Association of Psychoanalysis (WAP); European Society of Human Reproduction and Embryology (ESHRE); Italian Society of Human Reproduction (SIRU); and Italian Society of Andrology and Sexual Medicine (SIAMS). Her main research interests are currently trauma and psychological well-being at different stages of development and during the COVID-19 pandemic.

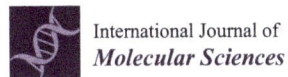

Review

The Pathogenesis of Endometriosis: Molecular and Cell Biology Insights

Antonio Simone Laganà [1,*,†], Simone Garzon [1,†], Martin Götte [2], Paola Viganò [3], Massimo Franchi [4], Fabio Ghezzi [1] and Dan C. Martin [5,6]

1. Department of Obstetrics and Gynecology, "Filippo Del Ponte" Hospital, University of Insubria, Piazza Biroldi 1, 21100 Varese, Italy; simone.garzon@univr.it (S.G.); fabio.ghezzi@uninsubria.it (F.G.)
2. Department of Gynecology and Obstetrics, Münster University Hospital, D-48149 Münster, Germany; mgotte@uni-muenster.de
3. Reproductive Sciences Laboratory, Division of Genetics and Cell Biology, San Raffaele Scientific Institute, Via Olgettina 60, 20136 Milan, Italy; vigano.paola@hsr.it
4. Department of Obstetrics and Gynecology, AOUI Verona, University of Verona, Piazzale Aristide Stefani 1, 37126 Verona, Italy; massimo.franchi@univr.it
5. School of Medicine, University of Tennessee Health Science Center, 910 Madison Ave, Memphis, TN 38163, USA; danmartin46@gmail.com
6. Virginia Commonwealth University, 907 Floyd Ave, Richmond, VA 23284, USA
* Correspondence: antoniosimone.lagana@uninsubria.it; Tel.: +1-39-0332-278111
† Equal contributions (joint first authors).

Received: 2 October 2019; Accepted: 7 November 2019; Published: 10 November 2019

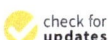

Abstract: The etiopathogenesis of endometriosis is a multifactorial process resulting in a heterogeneous disease. Considering that endometriosis etiology and pathogenesis are still far from being fully elucidated, the current review aims to offer a comprehensive summary of the available evidence. We performed a narrative review synthesizing the findings of the English literature retrieved from computerized databases from inception to June 2019, using the Medical Subject Headings (MeSH) unique ID term "Endometriosis" (ID:D004715) with "Etiology" (ID:Q000209), "Immunology" (ID:Q000276), "Genetics" (ID:D005823) and "Epigenesis, Genetic" (ID:D044127). Endometriosis may origin from Müllerian or non-Müllerian stem cells including those from the endometrial basal layer, Müllerian remnants, bone marrow, or the peritoneum. The innate ability of endometrial stem cells to regenerate cyclically seems to play a key role, as well as the dysregulated hormonal pathways. The presence of such cells in the peritoneal cavity and what leads to the development of endometriosis is a complex process with a large number of interconnected factors, potentially both inherited and acquired. Genetic predisposition is complex and related to the combined action of several genes with limited influence. The epigenetic mechanisms control many of the processes involved in the immunologic, immunohistochemical, histological, and biological aberrations that characterize the eutopic and ectopic endometrium in affected patients. However, what triggers such alterations is not clear and may be both genetically and epigenetically inherited, or it may be acquired by the particular combination of several elements such as the persistent peritoneal menstrual reflux as well as exogenous factors. The heterogeneity of endometriosis and the different contexts in which it develops suggest that a single etiopathogenetic model is not sufficient to explain its complex pathobiology.

Keywords: endometriosis; pathogenesis; genetics; epigenetics; immunology

1. Introduction

The etiopathogenesis of endometriosis is a multifactorial process resulting in a heterogeneous disease [1]. Its origin may be from Müllerian or non-Müllerian stem cells. These could include stem cells of the endometrial basal layer, Müllerian remnants, bone marrow, or the peritoneum. Furthermore, the innate ability of endometrial stem cells to regenerate cyclically under the influence of estrogen followed by estrogen/progesterone stimulation and then hormonal withdrawal seems to play a key role. The presence of such cells in the peritoneal cavity and what leads to the development of endometriosis is a complex process with a large number of interconnected factors potentially both inherited and acquired [2]. Genetic studies have confirmed a complex genetic nature [3]. At the same time, the epigenetic mechanisms underlying endometriosis support the processes that promote the acquisition and maintenance of immunologic, immunohistochemical, histological, and biological aberrations that characterize both the eutopic and ectopic endometrium in patients affected by endometriosis. This may be related to the particular combination of factors linked menstrual reflux into the peritoneal cavity as well as exogenous factors [4]. Once started, the process is variable and can lead to the development of endometriosis or can reach a limit to its growth and then stabilize or regress. As a result, the heterogeneity of endometriosis and the different phenotypes suggest that a single etiopathogenetic explaining model is not sufficient.

What is Endometriosis?

Endometriosis is a common, benign, inflammatory, generally gynecologic disease that includes the presence and growth of dysfunctional endometrial-like glands and stroma often with reactive fibrosis and muscular metaplasia outside the uterus [5]. It is associated with pelvic pain and subfertility in reproductive age women and can severely compromise the quality of life of affected women [6–11] and require extensive surgery when more conservative treatment options fail [12,13]. The prevalence rate of symptomatic endometriosis is estimated to be 10% with an incidence of about 2-7/1000 women per year and a further 11% of undiagnosed cases, although there are only a few studies with well-estimated prevalence and incidence of endometriosis in the general population [14–16] and some suggesting that many, if not all, women have endometriosis as a transient phenomenon [17,18].

Since the introduction of the term "endometriosis" and its pathogenesis theories by Sampson [19–21], extensive basic and clinical research concerning the etiopathogenesis of endometriosis has been carried out. However, the exact origin and mechanism of endometriosis development remain theoretical. The growing body of evidence confirms the multifactorial nature of endometriosis that is the result of the combined contribution of anatomical, hormonal, immunological, reactive, estrogenic, genetic, epigenetic, and environmental factors in affected women [7]. These multiple interconnected factors may explain the complex and heterogeneous presentations of the disease with different locations, appearances, developments, and hormone responsiveness. The heterogeneity and differences among the three main classes of endometriosis presentation (peritoneal, ovarian, and deep infiltrating endometriosis) are such as to suggest different pathogenetic pathways [22,23]. Moreover, a generally accepted hypothesis is that endometriosis is a phenomenon that may occur intermittently in all women during menstrual cycles, but that develops in a disabling disease only in a subset of women [17,18,24,25]. Understanding the multiple pathogenetic pathways underlining the development of endometriosis is of paramount importance, as they may have implications in the prevention, diagnosis, treatment, and prognosis of the disease [6].

2. Theories on the Origin of Endometriosis

The first question about the pathogenesis of endometriosis was about the origin of the endometrial-like glands and stroma that constitute the disease. Several hypotheses have been proposed since 1870 [26], some of only historical interest and some that are now considered the most plausible; nevertheless, none is able to completely explain the pathogenesis of endometriosis and all the different presentations of the disease [27]. Overall, all the proposed hypotheses for the cell origin can be categorized into two main theories: the in-situ theory and the transplantation theory.

2.1. The in Situ Theory

All the hypotheses belonging to this category are based on the concept that stroma and glands of endometrial-like tissue of endometriosis originate in-situ from the local tissues by metaplasia or by embryological origin. This hypothesis was proposed by Waldeyer in 1870 [26], who suggested that endometriosis develops from the germinal epithelium of the ovary by "metaplasia". Later, Von Recklinghausen in 1895 and Russell in 1899 introduced the concept of embryological origin from mesonephric/Wolffian remnants and Müllerian remnants, respectively [27].

The terms metaplasia and differentiation, whether these refer to the endometrium, to endometriotic cells, or pluripotent stem cells to endometriotic cells [28], are both used in this manuscript based on the original source document. We do not attempt to distinguish the differences between those two terms with overlapping meanings.

The Müllerian remnants hypothesis explains endometrial-like tissue as having developed from differentiation and proliferation of embryonic cell rests that are constituted by misplaced cells of primitive endometrial tissue along the migratory pathway of Müllerian ducts [29,30]. The cells spread across the posterior pelvic floor due to aberrant migration and differentiation during organogenesis of the female genital tract. Based on this hypothesis, "Müllerianosis" and "Secondary Müllerian system" theories were proposed as theoretical explanations of cell origin and dissemination of Müllerian-type epithelium outside the expected area of Müllerian duct development, including endometriosis, adenomyosis, endosalpingiosis, and endocervicosis [29,30]. However, embryological studies support the presence of Müllerian rests near the normal deep cul-de-sac area and not in other sites such as the ovary, sigmoid colon, appendix, or more distal sites such as the diaphragm and pleura [31].

The "Müllerianosis" hypothesis might explain that endometriosis is often found in the cul-de-sac, uterosacral ligaments, and medial broad ligaments; that peritoneal pockets with and without endometriosis have been associated with congenital tract malformations; and that endometriosis seems to have higher prevalence even in women with non-obstructive Müllerian abnormalities [32]. Moreover, this hypothesis is supported by the fact that is able to explain the presence of endometriosis in women with Mayer–Rokitansky–Küster–Hauser syndrome, in adolescents before or shortly after menarche, and in human female fetuses; where organoid structures outside uterine cavity resembling primitive endometrium were reported [31,33–35]. As previously noted, Signorile et al. [31] found CD10 positive remnants in the deep cul-de-sac only. Finally, Müllerian remnants or coelomic metaplasia in prostate and utricle may explain rare cases of endometriosis reported in males, after long-term high doses of estrogens for prostate carcinoma [36,37]. Immunohistochemical studies in men support both Müllerianosis and metaplasia theories [37].

Coelomic metaplasia or the stem cell differentiation hypothesis is based on the fact that, in the embryonic phase, the coelomic epithelium gives rise to both mesothelium of serosae and the epithelium lining of the cavity of Müllerian ducts, which forms the endometrium in the uterine body. This hypothesis explains endometriosis as developing from the metaplastic transformation of germinal ovarian epithelium and/or peritoneum serosa [38,39]. These metaplastic changes are supposed to occur secondary to hormonal influences [40,41], inflammatory processes [42,43], or the action of one or several endogenous biochemical or immunological factors derived from eutopic endometrium, based on the "induction" theory [44,45]. The induction theory is based on animal model studies suggesting that specific cell-free endometrial products were capable of inducing the metaplasia of undifferentiated mesenchyme into endometrial epithelium and glands, although no endometrial stroma was found. On that basis, it was supposed that these substances, released by uterine endometrium, may diffuse into the lymphatic and bloodstream and induce the formation of endometriosis in distant parts of the body [44,45]. The coelomic metaplasia hypothesis and the Müllerian remnants hypothesis may explain endometriosis in the absence of menstruation; and, additionally, it may explain the presence of endometriosis outside the pelvis such as in the chest, diaphragm, pleura, and lungs [36,46], although direct infiltration through the diaphragm or dissemination through diaphragmatic fenestrations or perforations are retrograde possibilities.

The main strength of in-situ theories is that they are able to explain endometriosis in women without menses or endometrium. Nevertheless, several factors are against in-situ theories. If peritoneal cells can easily undergo metaplastic transformation, endometriosis should be observed more frequently in men, in the thoracic cavity, and with a uniform distribution in the peritoneum. Moreover, if coelomic metaplasia resembles common metaplasia, the incidence of endometriosis should increase with advancing age. Finally, although some evidence suggests that endometriosis has a higher prevalence even in women with non-obstructive Müllerian abnormalities [32], other studies reported endometriosis to be more frequent in patients with Müllerian anomalies and outflow obstruction, and not in Müllerian anomalies as a whole [47,48].

2.2. The Transplantation Theory

In this category, the hypotheses are based on the concept that the stroma and glands of endometriosis originate from the eutopic endometrium. Endometriosis is proposed as benign metastasis of eutopic endometrium, which is displaced from the uterine cavity to another location inside the body through different routes. Hematogenous, lymphatic, and iatrogenic (mechanical) spread of endometrial or endometriotic cells can explain all uncommon extraperitoneal locations [49]. However, the most popular theory was introduced by Sampson in 1927 based on clinical and anatomical observations. Sampson proposed the retrograde menstruation theory that concludes that most endometriosis derives from the reflux of eutopic endometrial fragments through the fallopian tubes during menstruation, with subsequent implantation, transition from endometrium to endometriosis, and growth on and into the peritoneum and the ovary [19–21]. In addition, Sampson recognized that retrograde menstruation could not explain all forms of endometriosis and suggested venous dissemination or metaplasia as alternate theories [19,20].

Over the years, a growing body of evidence has supported the "retrograde menstruation" theory, and it is now the most accepted hypothesis for most forms of endometriosis. The most important step was the demonstration that the tubal reflux of menstrual tissue is a common event in women with patent fallopian tubes documented in 76-90% of women [6]. Blood was found in peritoneal fluid by laparoscopy in 90% of women with patent tubes and only in 15% with occluded tubes during the peri-menstrual period [50], and endometrial epithelial cells have been isolated in the peritoneal fluid of women during the early proliferative phase [51]. The second step was the identification of viable endometrium, single cells, and glandular structures in the shed menstrual tissue [52]. The demonstration that reflux of viable endometrium in the peritoneal cavity is a common event in fertile age women was essential to consider the "retrograde menstruation" theory plausible.

Moreover, the anatomical distribution of endometriosis in the pelvis with higher prevalence in the left side than in the right side, that is compatible with anatomical differences between the right and left hemipelvis [53], and the distribution in the abdomen with higher prevalence in the right diaphragm than in the left following the counter-clockwise distribution of peritoneal fluid [54], further supports the "retrograde menstruation" theory [53–55].

However, the transplantation theories are unable to explain endometriosis in women with Mayer–Rokitansky–Küster–Hauser syndrome, in adolescents before or shortly after menarche, and in males [19,31,33–35,37]. Moreover, available evidence suggests that endometriosis is not simply a transplanted normal endometrium. Numerous differences in hormone receptor levels, as well as histological, morphological, and biological characteristics, were reported when comparing endometriosis with eutopic endometrium, with only limited similarities. Although Sampson recognized that endometriosis was different from endometrium "both in structure and in function" and noted a transition from one to the other [19,20], his 1920s observations of a transition do not include all of the inflammatory, chemical, immunologic, epigenetic and genetic changes that have been discovered the last 40 years. Those changes require additional understanding of the transformation of any Müllerian (endometrial or rest) or non-Müllerian cell to endometriosis. Furthermore, eutopic endometrium of affected women is reported to have similar alterations of endometriotic lesions, that are not found in the eutopic endometrium of healthy women. This supports the hypothesis that the primary defect might be rooted in eutopic endometrium of women with endometriosis, although the gap between the incidence of refluxed menstruation and the incidence of endometriosis highlights the presence of further mechanisms [2].

3. Behind the Origins of Endometriosis

Although the origin of endometrial-like tissue that constitutes endometriosis is theoretical and debated, it is generally agreed that endometriosis is a phenomenon that may occur in all women during reproductive age, close laparoscopic examination of otherwise healthy peritoneum and microscopic examination of resected bowel can reveal almost microscopic or minimal peritoneal lesions [56–58], and many, if not most, of the small lesions tend to resolve or become inactive spontaneously. Therefore, only a subset of women with endometriosis develops a disabling disease regardless of the tissue origin [17,18,24,25]. To understand the origin of endometriosis and the mechanisms that explain the development of endometriosis as a disabling disease instead of spontaneous resolution, in vitro and in vivo studies and immunohistochemical, genetic, and epigenetic analysis were conducted [59–61]. Some studies, typically based on in vitro and in vivo models, were developed to investigate the stepwise formation of endometriotic lesions in order to test different specific hypotheses of the origin of endometriosis and to identify mechanisms that allow endometriotic lesion development [59,60]. Conversely, other studies, typically immunohistochemical, genetic, and epigenetic analysis, focused the investigation on the identification of prerequisites for the development of the disease instead of spontaneous resolution, comparing ectopic with eutopic endometrium in affected women or comparing parameters between affected and unaffected women [54,62–64]. Overall, this growing body of evidence suggests that endometriosis is not simply ectopic endometrium, with many reported differences between the endometrial-like tissue of endometriosis and eutopic endometrium in affected women [65]. However, this data has not clarified when replanted endometrium or Müllerian remnants begin the transition from ectopic Müllerian tissue to endometriosis, or when non-Müllerian stem cells are committed to differentiate into endometriosis. At the same time, when women with symptomatic endometriosis are compared with women without or minimal disease, the differences were reported not only at the level of endometriosis implants but even at the level of eutopic endometrium [66], uterus [67], and peritoneal environment [68].

3.1. Comprehensive Models on the Origin of Endometriosis

The induction theory was tested by in vivo studies on rabbit models. Endometrium was implanted in the abdominal cavity, and tissue was histologically evaluated for seven days [44]. Endometrial implants degenerated during the first four days, and cysts and endometrium-like differentiation were observed in the next three days in the surrounding connective tissue. If the tissue was dissociated before implantation, better results were obtained. These findings were further confirmed in a study in which viable and ischemic endometrial tissue was implanted intraperitoneally in rabbits within Millipore filters, that allowed only chemical substances to pass due to the small pore size [45]. Endometrium-like epithelium and glands were observed in the connective tissue adjacent to the implants. Although these changes did not include stroma, these observations support the hypothesis that endometrial tissue liberates specific substances inducing undifferentiated mesenchyme to develop into endometrial tissue.

Conversely, investigating the possibility that retrograde menstruation of shed endometrium is the origin of endometriosis, a chicken chorioallantoic membrane (CAM) model, an in vitro model that uses the membrane covering the chicken embryo, was used to study the stepwise endometriotic lesion formation involved in this process [69]. Tissue can be transplanted onto CAM and interventions can be carried out, allowing the behavior of the tissue and the consequences of interventions to be observed. In order to visualize the different steps of "retrograde menstruation" theory, human menstrual endometrial fragments were collected and were transplanted onto the CAM. After 24, 48, and 72 hours, cross-sections of the CAMs were cut and immunohistochemically stained. After 24 hours, direct contact was present between menstrual tissue fragments and the CAM mesenchyme. After 48 h, the menstrual endometrium was reorganized inside the CAM mesenchyme, and after 72 hours, a complete endometrium with glands and stroma was present in the CAM mesenchyme. Moreover, blood vessels attracted from the CAM were present inside the endometrium fragment. This model showed that viable endometrium is necessary to form an endometriotic lesion, and that stroma and glands of shed menstrual endometrium are able to adhere to and degrade the matrix and to induce neo-angiogenesis in order to survive [70].

3.2. Role of Hormones

Why a transplanted or congenital ectopic endometrium develops into endometriosis is the source of much research. The causes of this development include research on the role of estrogen and estrogen receptors (ERs), the estrogen-dependent physiologic and molecular changes [71], the local levels of estrogen [71,72], the role of estrogen in macrophage-nerve interaction [72], the effects of environmental toxicants on estrogen signaling [73], and the intracellular estrogen production related to aromatase activity. In addition, the normal control of cyclic estrogen and progesterone requires activation and crosstalk of cAMP and progesterone mediated signaling pathways [74].

Intracellular production of estrogens has a key role in the pathogenesis of endometriosis, particularly in post-menopausal women [75], as well as of other benign and malignant diseases of the female reproductive tract. Aromatase P450 catalyzes the conversion of androgens to estrogens and is physiologically expressed in different human tissues, including ovaries and adipose tissue, but usually not in the endometrium [76,77].

In women with endometriosis, this enzyme has been found in both endometriotic tissue and eutopic endometrium [77,78]. Moreover, in endometriosis the protective action of 17β-hydroxysteroid dehydrogenase (17β-HSD) type 2 is lost due to enzymatic deficiency. 17β-HSD lowers the level of the strong 17β-estradiol, converting it into the weak estrone, modulating the exposure to estrogens action [79]. The local production of estrogens and the loss of protective mechanisms determine a higher estradiol level that characterizes both endometriosis and eutopic endometrium of affected women, as demonstrated by the higher estradiol level of menstrual effluent in women with endometriosis as compared to controls [80]. Moreover, the increased estrogen production in endometriotic lesions and eutopic endometrium determines a positive feedback loop resulting in further estrogen production through the induction of cyclo-oxygenase type 2 (COX-2) enzyme. The subsequently elevated levels of prostaglandin E2 further stimulates the aromatase activity [78,81].

Of interest, the local production of estrogen was reported as a result of the activation of tissue injury and repair (TIAR) mechanisms induced by microtrauma at the level of basal endometrial layer. The basal endometrial layer has stem cell characteristics and exhibits the potential for dislocation and proliferation, that was reported enhanced in women with endometriosis [82,83]. The fragments of basal endometrium dislocated into the peritoneal cavity may induce chronic inflammation and TIAR mechanisms, that activate local production of estrogen, proliferation, and infiltrative growth resulting in endometriosis [67,84].

The estrogenic microenvironment was reported able to activate macrophages into peritoneum with the consequent secretion of pro-inflammatory cytokines such as tumor necrosis factor-α (TNF-α) and interleukin-1β (IL-1β) that stimulate the activation of NFkB. Moreover, these mechanisms induce vascular endothelial growth factor (VEGF) expression, cell cycle activation, and activation of the anti-apoptotic gene Bcl-2 [7,85] (Figure 1).

The key role of estrogens in endometriotic tissue survival and development is mediated by ERs. Endometriotic tissue development was reported suppressed by ER-selective modulators inhibiting estrogen receptor alfa (ERα) or beta (ERβ) [86], as well as ectopic implants did not develop normally in ERα- or ERβ-knockout mice [87,88]. ERs have similar affinity for estrogens and are transcriptional factors for similar subset of genes. Nevertheless, the differences between target genes, estrogen affinity, and tissue distribution of ERα and ERβ homodimers as well as ERα/ERβ heterodimer explain the reciprocal inhibitory and regulatory functions, as well as the different roles [89]. Although ERα was historical investigated due to his higher prevalence in the uterus and the supposed inhibitory effect of ERβ in the eutopic endometrium [90], in the endometriotic tissue ERα was reported having a normal expression level as compared to normal endometrium. Conversely, ERβ was reported overexpressed, determining an inversion of ERβ to ERα ratio as compared to eutopic endometrium [91]. On that basis, it was supposed that both the high estrogens concentration and the overexpression of ERβ are involved in the estrogen-based ectopic tissue survival and development. At the cytoplasmatic level, ERβ was reported involved in the inhibition and disruption of TNF-α-induced apoptosis signaling [88]. At nuclear level, ERβ was identified involved in the direct activation of the NFkB pathway and the radical oxygen species detoxification system, that are able to improve cell survival and cell escaping from immune clearance [92]. At the same time, ERβ was related to the upregulation of hypoxia-induced signaling, epithelial mesenchymal transition signaling, and cytoskeleton components, that are all involved in the invasion and progression of endometriotic implants [92].

The synergistic counterpart of estrogen overproduction and ERs overexpression is the progesterone resistance in endometriotic tissue, that impedes to modulate genes involved in the decidualization, cell cycle regulation, and estrogen response inhibition [93]. The progesterone resistance is a characteristic of the endometriotic tissue as compared to the eutopic endometrium, although it was identified in the eutopic endometrium of affected women as compared to controls [94].

The main mechanism involved in the progesterone resistance is the downregulation of progesterone receptor (PR) in the ectopic tissue, that determines a variation in the expression of progesterone target genes, such as the gene coding the 17β-HSD [93,95].

The pathways potentially underlining the PR suppression are multiple. The concentration of pro-inflammatory cytokines, such as TNF-α and IL-1β involved in the chronic inflammation and TIAR mechanisms, is reported directly correlated with PR expression [96]. The activation of NFkB pathway by inflammation signaling determines a direct interaction with PR thorough an antagonist effect [97]. Similarly, the persistent phosphorylation of AKT determined by inflammation is involved in the inhibition of PR expression [98].

These mechanisms explain the progesterone resistance as an acquired characteristic of the endometriotic tissue versus an individual predisposition. This is further supported by the inconsistent results provided by genetic studies [99] and the involvement of epigenetic mechanisms, such as the methylation of the gene and related promoter coding for the PR [100], and the higher expression of miRNAs blocking the estrogen-dependent PR expression [101].

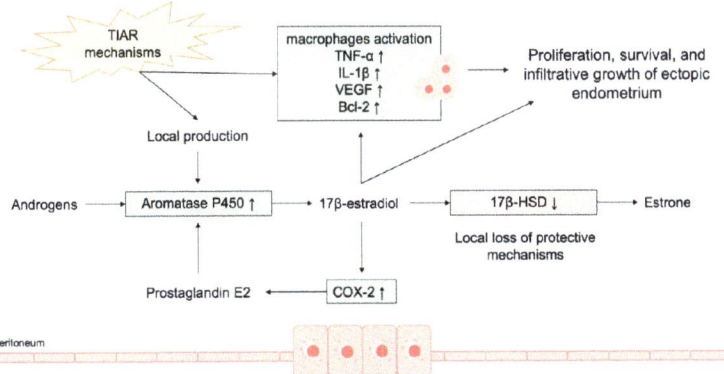

Figure 1. Summary of the mechanisms underlining the key role of estrogens in the pathogenesis of endometriosis. Tissue injury and repair (TIAR); Tumor necrosis factor (TNF); Interleukins (IL); Vascular endothelial growth factor (VEGF); Antiapoptotic protein B cell lymphoma 2 (Bcl-2); 17β-hydroxysteroid dehydrogenase (17β-HSD).

3.3. The Peritoneal Microenvironment and the Role of Immune Surveillance

The peritoneal fluid is produced by peritoneal and, mainly, ovarian exudation. It is a microenvironment that contains different cells, such as immune cells, endometrial cells, and red blood cells, which produce and secrete growth factors, angiogenic factors, and cytokines, that are able to affect processes in the abdominal cavity [102]. Of note, studies reported shed endometrial cells differing from eutopic cells; this may be explained by the different environments of bloodstream as compared to the peritoneal fluid [2]. In the abdominal cavity, the menstrual effluent determines an inflammatory response, of which physiological role is to clear the ectopic cells and tissue. Neutrophils, phagocytic leukocytes, and chemotactic leukocytes are attracted from the circulation, where an increased influx of bone marrow-derived cells is physiologically observed before the menstruation onset. Approximately 70-80% are macrophages CD14+, 20% are natural killer cells (NK cells) CD56+, and 10% are T-cells CD3+. This system is suggested to be overwhelmed or insufficient in women with endometriosis [103–105]. Shorter intervals and longer menstrual periods with heavy blood flow, that are often reported in women with endometriosis, may result in larger amounts of endometrial tissue collected in the abdominal cavity that overwhelms this system of cleansing [106,107]. Larger endometrial tissue fragments may provide protection from enzymatic and phagocytic activity to cells residing inside, that continue to produce angiogenic factors due to continued hypoxia. Moreover, the overwhelmed capacity to clean the peritoneum due to excessive refluxed endometrium may explain the higher prevalence of some anatomical defects reported in women with endometriosis, such as uterine malformations that prevent or disturb normal antegrade menstruation or that determine dysfunctional retrograde contractions [47,48,108,109].

Moreover, in women with endometriosis, endometrial cells were more resistant to the cytolytic action of autologous peritoneal macrophages than in healthy controls [110]. The cytotoxicity of NK cells against endometrial cells was reported as decreased with an inverse correlation with the stage of the disease [111]. Protection against the cytotoxicity of peritoneal NK cells seems to be provided by an altered antigenicity due to the overexpression of human leukocyte antigen class I [62,112]. Additionally, the eutopic endometrium of women with endometriosis releases higher levels of the soluble form of intercellular adhesion molecule-1 (sICAM-1) than those of women without endometriosis; and the ectopic endometrial cells express higher levels of sICAM-1 when compared to their eutopic endometrium. sICAM-1 modulates the cytotoxic activity of NK and CD8+ cells competing with ICAM-1 to bind leukocyte function antigen-1 (LFA-1). Binding of sICAM-1 to LFA-1 impedes leukocytes to bind ICAM-1 on the surface of target cells, preventing leukocyte activation [113–115]. The inflammatory response in endometriosis is further accentuated by the increased expression and activity of COX- 2, interleukins, and oxidative stress that act through the mitogen-activated protein kinase (MAPK) pathways. The subsequent dysregulation of MAPK signaling pathways increases inflammation, thereby recruiting immune cells and amplifying the inflammatory response. Moreover, MAPK signaling increases expression of growth factors, determines the development of pain and hypersensitivity to pain, and induces antiapoptotic signals. Of note, the dysregulation of apoptotic pathways and subsequent resistance to apoptosis contribute to the failure of immune clearance [116,117].

The failure to remove fragments of menstrual effluent from the abdominal cavity induces excessive local inflammation with further and persistent activation of macrophages, which may secrete an altered pattern of cytokines and chemokines. Evidence suggests that the number and activity level of peritoneal macrophages are higher in women with endometriosis, but their cytotoxic power is reduced [118–120]. Compared to physiology, macrophages in the peritoneum of affected women are not destroyed after completing their functions due to overexpression of the antiapoptotic protein Bcl-2, which protects them from apoptosis [121]. Peritoneal macrophages imbalance in M1 and M2 macrophages was reported in both eutopic and ectopic endometrium with upregulation of M2 type as compared to M1 type. Compared to M1 macrophages, which produce inflammatory cytokines and eliminate microorganisms and defective cells, the M2 macrophages modulate adaptive immune response, scavenge cellular debris, induce tissue repair, and induce angiogenesis. On that basis and experiments with macrophage depletion, M2 macrophages are supposed to have a key role in endometriosis development [116,122]. Moreover, smaller amounts of pro-inflammatory cytokines modulating the activation of macrophages (IL-6, IL-13, and IL-10 family) were produced and liberated in the eutopic endometrium of women with endometriosis as compared to the endometrium of healthy controls, reducing their cytotoxic capacity in the endometrium [120,123]. Production of IL-6 and MAPK activation in endometriotic cells are furthermore regulated by the proteoglycan Syndecan-1 (CD138), which also acts as a modulator of leukocyte and dendritic cell recruitment in mouse models of inflammation [124–126]. Studies reported that pro-inflammatory cytokines of Th1 profile are prevalent in the early stages, while these change to a Th2 profile in late stages, exerting an immunosuppressive effect and activating tissue injury-repair mechanisms [127]. This is consistent with data reporting reduced activity of cytotoxic T cells, a relative reduction of Th1 cell numbers, and a higher CD4/CD8 ratio in women affected by endometriosis as compared to healthy controls. Moreover, women with endometriosis were reported with both increased number and activation of B cells with an associated higher production of antibodies and higher numbers of regulatory T cells [116,128,129]. It is supposed that this altered inflammatory response may favor survival and implantation of ectopic endometrium with extracellular matrix (ECM) remodeling and angiogenesis as well as may cause metaplasia of the peritoneum or the development of Müllerian remnants, particularly overexpression of IL-1, IL-8, TNF-α [6,7]. Of interest, it is still unclear whether this altered peritoneal microenvironment is a cause or a consequence of endometriosis. Moreover, the presence of this altered inflammatory microenvironment could favor the implantation and development of endometriosis from refluxed endometrium or induce coelomic metaplasia of in situ mesothelium [20].

3.4. Apoptosis Defects

Cell turnover in human endometrium is regulated by apoptosis, which eliminates senescent cells from the functional layer during menses. Although apoptosis is regulated by several genes with variable expression during the menstrual cycle (bax, c-myc, and P53 induce it, while sentrin, B-cell lymphoma/leukemia-xL, and Bcl-2 inhibit it), the variation of endometrial apoptosis in the menstrual cycle seems to be primarily modulated by ovarian steroids through the up- and downregulation of Bcl-2 and bax expression, from the expression level of bax depends on the Bcl-2 action. Bcl-2 maximum expression was reported during the proliferative phase when the estrogens production and the expression of receptors in glandular cells is greatest [85,130–132].

In women with endometriosis, the eutopic endometrium is reported to exhibit significantly reduced apoptosis compared to women without endometriosis, particularly in the late secretory, menstrual, and early proliferative cycle phases. This may explain a reduced percentage of apoptotic cells and a greater number of surviving cells entering the peritoneal cavity, which is a prerequisite for the development of endometriosis [85,133–135]. The resistance to apoptosis could be related to different mechanisms. Inappropriate signal transduction was related to the dysregulated expression of proteins involved in the modulation of apoptosis, such as the increased expression of Bcl-2, that along with bax represent the key proteins of apoptosis regulation in endometriosis [85]. Compared to the cyclical activity of mTOR in eutopic endometrium, mTOR in endometriosis is constantly activated with persistent inhibition of cell autophagy and apoptosis [136]. Further studies identified the altered and excessive expression of the soluble-FasL in women with endometriosis, with subsequent dysregulated interaction between Fas and FasL that represent a possible cause of apoptosis resistance in endometriotic cells, in addition to immunoescaping. Of note, concomitant induced expression of FasL in stromal cells seems to mediate apoptosis of activated immune cells [116,137]. A constant source of TNF-α that initiates and modulates apoptosis during menses, and the absence of apoptosis induced by signals from adhesion receptors in cells that do not adhere to the peritoneal mesothelium, such as the E-cadherin suppression, are further mechanisms reported related to escape from apoptosis in endometriosis [131,135]. Of note, accumulating evidence suggests that apoptotic resistance has a key role in the "immunoescaping" of endometriotic cells from immune homeostasis of the peritoneal microenvironment [136] (Figure 2).

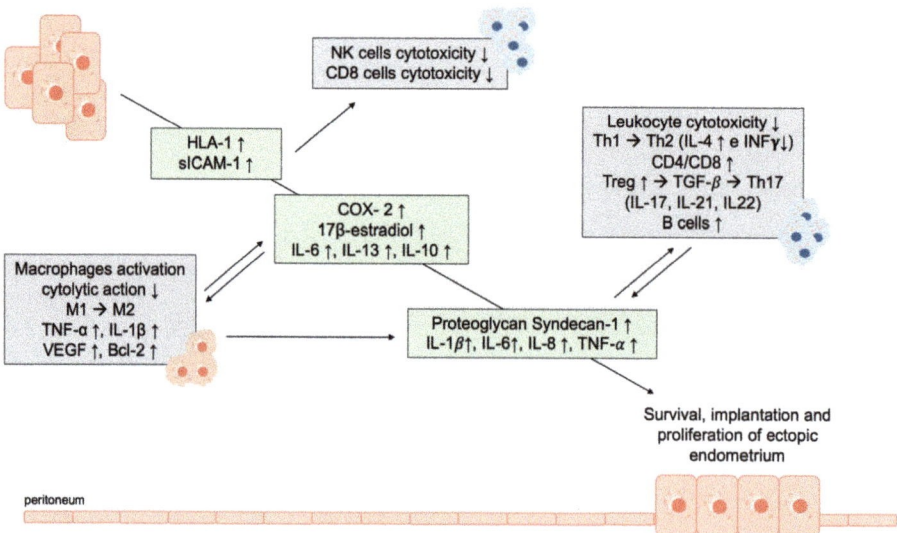

Figure 2. Immunoescaping mechanisms involved in the etiopathogenesis of endometriosis. Human leukocyte antigen class I (HLA-1); Intercellular adhesion molecule-1 (sICAM-1); Natural killer (NK); Cyclo-oxygenase type 2 (COX-2); Interleukins (IL); Tumor necrosis factor (TNF); Vascular endothelial growth factor (VEGF); Antiapoptotic protein B cell lymphoma 2 (Bcl-2); Interferon (INF); transforming growth factor-β (TGF-β).

3.5. Cell-Matrix and Cell-Cell Adhesion

Dysregulated cell-cell and cell-matrix adhesion has a role in the development of endometriosis [138]. Endometrial cells derived from proliferative and secretory endometrial fragments, as well as menstrual endometrial fragments, are able to adhere to where the peritoneal mesothelium is damaged and the basement membrane or the interstitial ECM are exposed. Although an intact mesothelial lining may prevent adhesion and implantation of menstrual endometrial fragments, mesothelium can easily be damaged by surgery, inflammatory cells, and menstrual endometrium [139–142]. Some studies reported that isolated cells from menstrual endometrial fragments as well as non-cellular medium prepared from menstrual effluent are able to induce morphological alterations in the mesothelium, from an epithelial to a mesenchymal phenotype, and to damage it, creating its own adhesion sites at the mesothelial lining [143–147].

Adhesion of retrograde menstrual endometrium to the peritoneum is mediated by adhesion molecules that modulate cell-matrix and cell-cell attachments and are expressed by endometrial cells, including cadherins, integrins, proteoglycans such as syndecans, laminin-binding proteins, the immunoglobulin superfamily, and CD44. Integrins, syndecans, cadherins, CD44, and CD44's binding partner hyaluronan have been studied extensively in endometrium and in endometriosis [138].

The integrins are transmembrane glycoproteins that modulate cell-matrix attachment and are involved in cell motility and invasion. The endometrial expression of integrins changes during the menstrual cycle under hormonal regulation. Altered patterns of expression that have been associated with endometriosis are able to express or to not express certain integrins independently of the hormones without cyclical modifications. Endometriosis is reported to have an overall highly variable and aberrant integrin expression as compared with eutopic endometrium. Fibronectin receptors were identified in glands of endometriosis implants but not in eutopic endometrial glands, suggesting that fibronectin receptors may contribute to the adhesion of endometriotic cells during menstruation [148–152].

Moreover, differences were observed between the eutopic endometrium of affected women and healthy women. The αvβ3 integrin is expressed in the endometrium at the time of implantation from 19-20 days of the menstrual cycle, and its absence suggests out of phase endometrium. In women with endometriosis, αvβ3 integrin is constantly absent in the eutopic endometrium although in the presence of in-phase histological features. This defect was associated with nulliparity and inversely related to the stage of disease [152,153].

Another family of ECM receptors is formed by the syndecans, four transmembrane-anchored proteoglycans that are expressed in the endometrium in a menstrual cycle-dependent manner [154]. Notably, the most ubiquitous member of the family, syndecan-4, was shown to be upregulated in the eutopic endometrium of endometriosis patients compared to an IVF control collective, and functional studies in an endometriotic cell line revealed that experimental syndecan-4 downregulation resulted in reduced invasiveness in vitro, and reduced expression of the cytoskeletal modulator Rac1, the transcription factor ATF-2, and MMP3 [155]. In addition, functional studies revealed a similar invasion-modulating role for the epithelial member of the syndecans family, syndecan-1: siRNA knockdown of this proteoglycan in endometriotic cells resulted in a substantial inhibition of Matrigel invasiveness, which was accompanied by a reduction of IL-6 secretion, MMP9 expression and MMP2 activity, and upregulation of plasminogen activator inhibitor-1 protein [124]. Overall, these data suggest that syndecans dysregulation in endometriosis contributes mechanistically to proteolytic remodeling, alterations in cell motility, and the inflammatory microenvironment, thus promoting invasive growth of endometriotic lesions.

Cadherins belong to a large family of transmembrane glycoproteins that mediate cell-cell adhesion and may suppress invasion inhibiting the escape of cells from their primary site. In vitro, tumor cells that express E-cadherin are retained by cell-cell adhesions, but when tumor cells do not express E-cadherin are no longer constrained and can invade. Therefore, E-cadherin is considered a central player in the development of cancer metastasis [156–159]. Immunohistochemical studies have reported that epithelial-glandular cells of menstrual effluent, eutopic endometrium, peritoneal fluid, peritoneum, and endometriosis express epithelial cadherin (E-cadherin), suggesting a role of E-cadherin in the maintenance of the endometrial epithelial architecture [151,160]. Endometriosis cells may share molecular mechanisms of invasion and metastasis with carcinoma cells that are related to the level of E-cadherin expression [156,157].

Finally, expression of the transmembrane adhesion molecule and stem cell marker CD44 is dysregulated in endometriosis [161], as exemplified by the correlation of high levels of soluble CD44 in the serum and peritoneal fluid of endometriosis patients with the severity of the disease. Indeed, preclinical data from animal models suggest that interference with CD44 function or with its binding partner, the ECM carbohydrate hyaluronan, may be a worthwhile therapeutic approach [162]. For example, inhibition of CD44 glycosylation was shown to decrease the attachment of endometrial cell lines to peritoneal mesothelial cells [163], and transplantation of endometrium from CD44-deficient mice into wild-type mice and vice versa resulting in a decreased formation of endometriotic lesions in vitro [164], suggesting an important role of CD44 in the adhesion of endometriotic cells to ectopic sites. Finally, pharmacological inhibition of biosynthesis of the CD44 substrate hyaluronan by 4-methylumbelliferone reduced angiogenesis in an in vivo mouse model of endometriosis [165], suggesting that interference with the CD44-hyaluronan axis may represent an approach that synchronously targets multiple molecular mechanisms of endometriosis.

3.6. Extracellular Matrix Remodeling and Matrix Metalloproteinases

The CAM models demonstrate that endometrium is able to adhere and subsequently degrade the ECM, suggesting that endometriotic lesion development requires ECM breakdown. The breakdown and remodeling of the ECM are mainly modulated by matrix metalloproteinases (MMPs) that degrade

ECM components and are reported to be expressed by fragments of endometrium. MMPs are secreted in a latent preform requiring activation to acquire proteolytic activity and are inhibited by specific tissue inhibitors of MMPs (TIMPs). MMPs are structurally related but have different substrate specificity, cellular sources, and inducibility. Based on their substrate specificity, MMPs can be classified into collagenases, gelatinases, stromelysins, membrane-type MMPs, and other MMPs [166].

The activity of MMPs is modulated at the level of gene expression, at the level of latent proenzymes activation, and at the level of the inhibitory activity of TIMPs. Gene expression is modulated by hormones, growth factors, and inflammatory cytokines including IL-6, IL-1, epidermal growth factor, TNF-α, basic fibroblast growth factor (bFGF), and platelet-derived growth factor. Secreted latent proenzymes are activated by the stepwise activation of plasmin, which is considered the most potent activator in vivo, and by the activity of membrane-type MMPs, that are present at the cell surface and intracellularly. TIMPs are expressed by different types of cells and are present in the majority of tissues and body fluids [167–169].

MMPs are involved with highly regulated activity in many reproductive processes, including menstruation, ovulation, and embryo implantation [170,171]. The endometrial expression of MMPs is low during the proliferative phase, declines further during the early secretory phase and increases in the late secretory phase. Although MMPs activity in the endometrium is regulated by different hormones, cytokines, and growth factors, progesterone is a potent repressor both in vitro and in vivo. Progesterone might regulate MMP expression indirectly through the plasminogen activator pathway, increasing the levels of plasminogen activator inhibitor (PAI)-1 and thus reducing the plasmin-mediated activation of latent MMPs [172–174]. Moreover, locally produced retinoic acid and transforming growth factor-β (TGF-β) seem to be mediators of the progesterone suppression enhancing expression of TIMPs. Nevertheless, prematurely decreased progesterone levels not consistent with the peri-menstrual increased expression of MMPs and tissue degradation at focal points rather than throughout the different expression and regulation of MMPs entire endometrium are more likely than progesterone to be the primary modulator of endometrial collagenase activity [175–177].

After the initial attachment, the development of endometriotic lesion requires the invasion of adjacent tissues through the ECM degradation regulated by MMPs activity. This role of MMPs in the pathogenesis of endometriosis was proposed after finding ECM breakdown products in the peritoneal fluid of affected women [174]. Later, studies with artificial induced endometriosis, in mice and in the CAM, reported that endometriotic lesion development could be prevented by inhibiting the activity of MMPs [178,179]. Moreover, different expression and regulation of MMPs were demonstrated in women without and with endometriosis. This included an altered expression of specific MMPs and related TIMPs with an increased MMP/TIMP ratio in women affected by endometriosis as compared to healthy controls [63,166,180–186]. Specifically, in women with endometriosis, as compared to healthy controls, the expression of MMPs was reported enhanced in the secretory phase dominated by progesterone. In vitro studies reported an increased MMP-3 and MMP-7mRNA expression in the eutopic endometrium of women affected by endometriosis in the secretory phase. These results suggest that a contribution to the development of endometriosis comes from a defect in the response to the suppressing action of progesterone, a form of progesterone insensitivity [187].

Furthermore, evidence suggests that MMPs cleave not only ECM components but may also be implicated in the degradation of cytokines and growth factors, regulating tissue organization, angiogenesis, and cell survival. Therefore, MMP activity seems to be able to influence the initial lesion development as well as lesion survival and maintenance [188].

3.7. Angiogenesis

In CAM models, after 72 hours, a complete endometrium with glands and stroma was present in the CAM mesenchyme, and blood vessels were attracted from the CAM inside the endometrium fragment. These studies demonstrated that human endometrium is highly angiogenic and able to attract blood vessels from the surrounding tissue [189]. Angiogenesis is induced when vascular growth factors exceed inhibiting factors, and, although it is reported altered in pathological conditions such as cancer, chronic inflammation, and endometriosis, it is essential in a physiological process such as wound healing, growth, pregnancy and menstrual cycle [190,191]. Therefore, endometrial cells have physiologically angiogenic potential. In the eutopic endometrium during the menstrual cycle, angiogenesis is modulated by many factors, of which VEGF appears to be the most important for its ability to induce proliferation and migration of endothelial cell, vasodilation, and increased vascular permeability [190]. In the proliferative phase, estradiol induces VEGF-A production in endometrium resulting increased in the secretory phase and further increased prior to menstruation when endometrium becomes hypoxic as a result of vasoconstriction [192,193].

Increased endothelial cell proliferation, increased micro-vessel density, and higher levels of VEGF-A and angiopoietin-1 and -2mRNA expression were detected in the eutopic endometrium of patients with endometriosis than in the eutopic endometrium of disease-free women. These factors suggest a dysregulated angiogenic activity in the eutopic endometrium of women affected by endometriosis [64,191,194–196].

Focused studies on the vascularization of endometriotic lesions compared the vascular density and vessel diameter between white, black, and red lesions as well as between deep infiltrating lesions and endometriomas. No differences in the numbers of vessels were reported between different types of lesions, but red lesions have more vessels with a small diameter (<10 µm), whereas black lesions have more vessels with a larger diameter (>20 µm) [197]. The observations of endothelial cell proliferation with the development of blood vessels without smooth muscle in endometriotic lesions suggest that VEGF-A and angiogenesis are of significant value, particularly in early lesions. This was further suggested by studies investigating the soluble VEGF receptor sflt-1 that antagonizes VEGF-A action and was reported able to reduce the number of lesions formed in mice after intraperitoneal injection of endometrium [198]. More support to antiangiogenic therapy as effective in preventing the development of endometriosis has been provided by CAM model studies, in which anti-human VEGF factors administered to the CAM significantly decreased the vascular density of the CAM and prevented endometriosis-like lesion formation after the transplantation of human endometrium [199]. Moreover, after endometriotic lesions had been induced by transplanting human endometrium intraperitoneally, antiangiogenic agents resulted in a significant reduction of the number of endometriotic lesions in treated mice compared to control. The reduction in lesion number was related to a reduction of newly developed vessels, with mature vessels remaining unchanged [200,201]. Although VEGF is the key angiogenetic factor in endometriosis, further factors were reported involved in the angiogenesis of endometriotic lesions, including TGF-α, TGF-β, bFGF, angiopoietin, and hepatocyte growth factor [202–204]. Furthermore, recent results have indicated a role of the stem cell-related notch signaling pathway in sprouting angiogenesis of endometriotic lesions in an in vivo model [205].

3.8. Endometrial Stem Cells

More recently, endometrial stem progenitor cells were proposed as cells that give rise to the origin of endometriotic lesions, both ectopic or transplanted cells [206]. The human endometrium is subject to profound changes in tissue structure and function during the menstrual cycle, and the recovery of epithelial glands and stroma is produced by the endometrial progenitor stem cells within the basal layer, although some studies have suggested the origin may also be from bone marrow [206–208]. Endometrial stem cells demonstrated a high plastic capacity of differentiation by the characterization of several lines of cells with a different expression pattern of cell surface markers, endometrial localization, and clonal efficiency [209]. Recent evidence suggests the monoclonal origin of endometriotic cells within ovarian endometriomas, while peritoneal implants were reported to be polyclonal [210–212]. Moreover, as previously reported, the cells that give rise to endometriotic implants must undergo migration, adhesion, proliferation, and induction of angiogenesis. The endometrial stem cells have demonstrated the ability to activate all these characteristics [213]. As previously reported, it is proposed that physical and biochemical injuries caused by inflammatory cytokines and reactive oxygen species trigger the activation of endometrial stem cells inducing local production of estrogen and tissue injury-repair mechanisms such as cell cycle activation. On that basis, endometrial stem progenitor cells may be involved in the etiopathogenesis of benign and malignant endometrial aberrations such as endometriosis, endometrial hyperplasia, and endometrial cancer [214]. In general, endometrial stem progenitor cells have a long lifespan and trigger epigenetic mechanisms of protection from stress and senescence. They express genes such as Wnt/β-catenin, anti-apoptotic Bcl-2, cell cycle regulatory genes, and enzymes to repair DNA damage [206,209]. For all these characteristics, endometrial stem cells are supposed to be the cells that give rise to endometriotic implants instead of differentiated endometrial tissue fragments [7]. Of interest, endometrial stem progenitor cells can find their potential source from refluxed menstrual endometrium, Müllerian remnants from embryogenesis, as well as an hematogenic origin from the recruitment of circulating stem cell of bone marrow [215]. Notably, several stemness-associated molecular markers have been shown to be upregulated in the eutopic endometrium and ectopic lesions of endometriosis patients, including Msi1, SOX2, notch and numb [82,216,217], supporting the hypothesis of an involvement of stem cells in the pathogenetic process. Preclinical studies demonstrated that the microRNAs miR-145 and miR-200b were suitable tools to alter stemness-related properties of endometriotic cells, opening new therapeutic perspectives [218,219].

4. The Genetics of Endometriosis

The etiopathogenesis of endometriosis is still undefined and debated. To better understand the mechanism leading to the development of endometriosis as a disabling disease instead of spontaneous resolution of peritoneal implants, genetic studies offer an approach of paramount importance [3,220–222]. The evidence for a genetic contribution to the development of endometriosis comes from epidemiological studies that reported familial aggregation of the disease in humans [223–227] and primates [228]. Both hospital- and population-based studies reported higher rates of endometriosis among the relatives of affected women compared to healthy controls [224,225,229]. A study based on siblings, twins and familiars of affected woman reported a higher relative recurrence risk of 2.3 times as compared to the risk in the general population, although it is difficult to perform an accurate estimation because the prevalence in the general population is unknown and there is bias in the surgical diagnosis of endometriosis in siblings [226] and in the daughters of endometriosis patients (personal observation of D.C.M.). A genetic background for endometriosis was further supported by evidence that comes from larger studies in twins and in the population of Iceland [225,226,230–232]. Monozygotic twins show higher concordance for endometriosis than dizygotic twins [230,231], with intra-pair correlation rates of 0.52 versus 0.19 [232]. This data suggest that genetic factors influence about half of the risk for endometriosis development and estimate a heritability of 51% [232]. Further evidence comes from studies in the rhesus macaque animal model, that reported a familial aggregation of spontaneous endometriosis with a significantly higher coefficient of recurrence risk for full siblings (0.75) as compared to maternal (0.26) and paternal (0.18) half-siblings [228].

Although the familial aggregation of confounding risk factors, such as age at menarche, questioned the real role of genetic background in endometriosis risk [233], current evidence supports the genetic contribution to endometriosis development, and genetic approaches can be used to identify genes having a role in endometriosis risk, allowing a better definition of the etiopathogenetic pathways. Moreover, the identification of genetic markers may allow the development of more informative risk predictors as compared to family history, a better understanding of the pathogenesis providing new opportunities for drug discovery, and genetic profiles allow identification of co-morbidity, that may improve diagnosis and treatments.

4.1. Candidate Gene Studies

A general approach to investigate the role of genes in the etiopathogenesis of diseases is the study of specific candidate genes chosen based on the biological mechanisms known as contributors to the disease [234–238]. Nevertheless, for endometriosis, the definition of candidate genes is problematic because of the limited knowledge of etiopathogenetic mechanisms that may involve many genetic pathways and many genes.

Studies have investigated genes involved in sex steroid pathways, detoxification pathways, cytokine signaling pathways, adhesion, and cell cycle regulation molecules and enzymes of the ECM [234,238]. Based on the estrogen-dependent nature of endometriosis, genes from pathways of sex hormones signaling and biosynthesis have been studied. These investigations provided limited evidence supporting the association between either PR or ERα and endometriosis [237], although a further large family-based study failed to demonstrate any association between endometriosis and PR [99]. Similarly, conflicting results were reported for the association between the gene expression of cytochrome P450 and endometriosis [239,240].

Detoxification pathways were investigated based on the supposed role of environmental estrogens in the etiopathogenesis of endometriosis, reporting questionable evidence [73,241]. Glutathione S-transferase enzymes are involved in the detoxification of different toxic compounds and carcinogens. Different studies investigated gene polymorphisms and reported evidence for an increased risk of endometriosis in the presence of specific enzyme variants. Nevertheless, significant heterogeneity between studies and publication bias suggests caution [235]. Similarly, a meta-analysis of studies that investigated the association between polymorphisms in the detoxification enzyme N-acetyltransferase 2 and endometriosis reported no association [236].

In general, many factors have contributed to the failure of candidate gene studies to provide new insights into the pathogenesis of endometriosis. A few of the reported associations have been investigated in an independent sample, as it is suggested before accepting the association with a disease, and the majority of replications failed to confirm previous results [238]. Study power is another cause of concerns both for initial and replication studies [242,243]. In complex diseases such as endometriosis, many genes, as well as environmental factors, may contribute to the etiopathogenesis; therefore, the effect size for the majority of common risk alleles is expected to be low, with odds ratios having a range of 1.1–1.5 [244–246]. On that basis, large sample sizes are required, and most candidate gene studies investigated small samples with inadequate power to detect the small contribution of all genes contributing to the risk of endometriosis [238,247,248]. Moreover, publication bias of significant compared to negative results [242,249], statistical and technical issues, and problems in experimental design provides further concerns [237]. In general, many gene variants with small effects can be considered associated with an increased risk of endometriosis [238].

4.2. Linkage and Association Studies

Linkage studies are performed in families with multiple cases and search for genomic regions shared more frequently than expected between relatives affected by the disease. These regions likely carry gene variants increasing the risk of developing the disease. These studies provided important results in disease related to single-gene mutations with Mendelian segregation [250–252]. Due to the high prevalence of endometriosis, the low recurrence in familiars, and the difficulties in ascertaining the healthy subjects, the best design was to analyze pairs of sisters both affected [252].

A genome analysis of DNA samples from 1176 sister-pair with both laparoscopically confirmed endometriosis and family members from Australian and UK was performed [253]. The study was designed with a power of 80% to detect a region with a recurrence risk to sisters of 1.35 [226]. The analysis identified significant linkage on chromosome 10 and on chromosome 20, although evidence for linkage was confirmed only in chromosome 10 for both Australian and UK families. A separate linkage study was conducted in families with three or more affected women and identified a significant linkage peak on chromosome 7p [254–256]. This suggests that in high-risk families, a locus with high penetrance for endometriosis risk may be located in this region.

Nevertheless, linkage studies are limited by the ability to identify a genomic region of interest but not a specific gene locus. Therefore, association studies are required to identify specific gene variants.

Association studies, with or without family-based designs, compare gene variants frequency in women with endometriosis versus healthy controls. Because most human genome variants are single-base differences, methods to genotype large numbers of single nucleotide polymorphisms (SNPs) are now used for both linkage and association studies. Of interest, common SNPs (with a population frequency > 0.01) that are located close together are not independently inherited (linkage disequilibrium or LD) [257]. Therefore, a SNP can act as a marker for others, allowing the identification of the common variation in a particular region by typing a limited number of SNPs. With this technique, association studies investigated chromosome seven and 10 linkage regions identifying several genes implicated in endometriosis and endometrial cancer such as PTEN, homeobox protein EMX2, and the FGF receptor 2 gene (FGFR2). EMX2 is a transcription factor involved in the development of the reproductive tract and in the cyclicity of eutopic endometrium [258–260]. PTEN regulates proliferation and survival of cells and it is inactivated in the early events of endometrial hyperplasia development and ovarian and endometrial cancer pathogenesis [261]. FGFR2 has been associated with endometrial and breast cancer development [262,263]. Nevertheless, SNP studies, investigating common variants and variants related to endometrial or breast cancer of these three genes, suggested that the linkage signal is not related to these common variants, demonstrating no evidence for any association with the endometriosis [258,264]. However, a role for other unknown variants of these genes in the development of endometriosis cannot be completely excluded. Moreover, the hypothesis that different families may have different mutations of the same gene reduces the probability of identifying these specific variants. It is suggested that the results of linkage studies may be caused by multiple different variants of the same gene; the variant is the same across a single-family but is rare in the general population. Conversely, association studies require that investigated variants are common in the general population [258,264].

4.3. Genome-Wide Association Studies

The complex and multifactorial etiopathogenesis of endometriosis contributes to the failure of candidate gene, association, and linkage studies [245]. Genome-wide association (GWA) provided a new tool to identify genetic variants related to complex human diseases, with the use of genetic markers that include most of the common gene variants (up to 1 million SNPs) and can be screened in a single analysis [257].

Nevertheless, study design, particularly the definition of characteristics, traits of the disease being studied, and the choice of population controls, remains of paramount importance [265]. Moreover, cases and controls need to be well matched for ethnicity to reduce the false-positive rate, and standard, rigorous, and quality control procedures are required to reduce bias. Association results are reported as significant for every SNP that show a significant association as points above a stringent threshold determining the probability of finding a false positive. Once a genetic association is identified, replication provides an important safeguard against false-positive results and gives an independent and better estimate of the effect size [266]. The identified region can be subsequently examined to locate the genes relative to association signals and analyze the variation pattern because SNPs statistically associated with disease are probably not the causal variants, that usually are absent on the gene chip used for SNP detection, but correlate with the common variants genotyped on the chip. The causal variants probably lie near the regions of SNPs statistically associated with disease for the LD [267]. Of note, signals could identify both areas of the genome with genes and intragenic regions identifying regulatory regions of gene expression [244].

Well-powered endometriosis case-control GWA studies identified several genes as possible candidates in the pathogenesis of endometriosis. A Japanese GWA study identified a significant association with LD blocks of chromosome 1 near the cyclin-dependent kinase inhibitor 2B antisense RNA (CDKN2BAS) and the wingless-type MMTV integration site family 4 (WNT4) gene [268]. A smaller Japanese GWA study reported a significant association with LD blocks near IL-1 alpha proprotein. Notably, IL-1α has been shown to be elevated in both the peritoneal fluid and the serum of infertile women with endometriosis compared to healthy controls [269,270]. In a United States

GWA study, SNP-association with endometriosis was reported with LD blocks near nuclear factor erythroid-derived 2-like 3 gene, typically expressed in placenta, and HOXA10 and HOXA11 genes, two candidate genes of the homeobox A transcription factors family. HOXA10 and HOXA11 have key roles in uterine embryogenesis and are expressed at high levels during the luteal phase. Of interest, studies reported that HOXA10 levels were not increased in women affected by endometriosis leading to infertility [271]. A meta-analysis incorporating available data about SNP-association reported different SNPs in the gene of interest between European descents and Japanese, likely reflecting the different genetic backgrounds of investigated populations. Nevertheless, WNT4 was confirmed as a candidate gene for endometriosis, with a signal that overlaps completely with an association signal for ovarian cancer, suggesting some common molecular pathways [220,222,271]. WNT4 is an interesting candidate involved in female reproductive tract embryogenesis, ovarian follicle development, and steroidogenesis. WNT4 was reported to be involved in numerous anomalies of the female genital tract. Moreover, the signaling pathway of WNT genes and WNT/β-catenin were reported to be associated in the control of different types of stem cells and in the resistance to apoptosis by the cell-cell interaction mediated by cadherins [268,272–274].

The International ENDOGENE Consortium, in addition to using SNP–disease associations, applied GWA data to investigate with statistical methods the percentage of disease risk variation attributable to genetic variants, and whether the disease status in an independent sample can be predicted by the disease status in another sample [226,275]. Analyses suggested that in moderate-to-severe endometriosis (Revised American Fertility Society (rAFS) classification stages III-IV) genetic load is higher than in minimal-to-mild disease (rAFS classification stages I-II) with strongest signals of SNP-association. This was subsequently confirmed by prediction analyses with SNP data from moderate-to-severe endometriosis of UK samples that predict moderate-to-severe disease in Australian samples better than data from all endometriosis cases. These results were confirmed by inverted analysis [226,275].

A recent meta-analysis incorporating available data from 11 GWA case-control studies, involving 17,045 endometriosis cases and 191,596 controls, identified five new loci significantly associated with endometriosis risk, that were reported involved in sex steroid hormones pathways. Overall, GWA case-control studies have identified 19 independent SNPs associated with endometriosis risk. Those include SNPs associated with endometriosis identified regions near the gene for ERα, regions upstream of the beta subunit of follicle-stimulating hormone (FSH), and the Growth Regulating Estrogen Receptor Binding 1 (GREB1), previously associated with breast cancer. Other regions identified genes involved in cell migration, adhesion, and proliferation, such as WNT4. Nevertheless, together, these identified SNPs are able to explain only 5.19% of the variance in endometriosis [220,222]. Therefore, the combined effects of all identified genes explain only a small fraction of the estimated 51% heritability of endometriosis [276]. This "missing" heritability may be explained, as reported for other complex diseases, by the small effect size of multiple single variants that contribute to disease risk and do not reach statistical significance. Additionally, SNPs on the current commercial chips may not tag well causal variants. Functional genetic variants that contribute to susceptibility for some common diseases, if rare, limit the performance of GWA studies that are designed to detect common variants and fail to identify low-frequency alleles [277–280].

5. The Epigenetics of Endometriosis

It has been demonstrated that a single lesion of endometriosis is monoclonal [210–212] and, based on gene expression profiling studies, a large number of genes are dysregulated in endometriosis [281–287]. Nevertheless, although the heritability of endometriosis is estimated to be 51% [232], it is difficult to identify specific genes consistently associated with endometriosis and with predictive power in identifying high-risk women [233,234]. During the development of endometriotic lesions from progenitor cells, it was proposed that the aberrations are acquired sequentially and usually without any change in the sequence of DNA (i.e., DNA mutations). Conversely, gene expression dysregulation in the cellular lineage is acquired and maintained by epigenetic processes in a heritable manner. Therefore, sequentially acquired and inherited changes at the level of gene transcription, post-transcriptional modulations, translation, and post-translational modifications are proposed as the common denominator explaining the hormonal, immunological, molecular, histological and cellular aberrations that characterize endometriosis. Furthermore, they may explain the SNPs-association with regulatory regions of gene expression instead of gene loci and the small effect of multiple single-gene variants in GWA studies [244]. At the same time, Bruner-Tran et al. [288] have investigated heritable epigenetic changes in mice in germ cells after exposure to 2,3,7,8-tetrachlorodibenzo-p-dioxin (TCDD) and demonstrated a transgenerational occurrence of several reproductive diseases that have been linked to endometriosis in women, although they could not determine if those changes lead to the development of endometriosis or were a consequence of the inflammatory nature of the disease. However, epigenetic markers occurring within the germline of mice are inheritable and can positively or negatively affect offspring [289,290]. These epigenetic changes potentially include a stable, heritable phenotype caused by chromosomal changes without DNA sequence alterations if they escape epigenetic reprogramming. If so, they are essential in tissue development and cell differentiation [291]. Moreover, epigenetic processes modulate phenomena such as genomic imprinting and X chromosome inactivation, and they are involved in aging and disease development [292–294]. Epigenetic processes involve dynamic changes in the chromatin structure influencing gene expression. Chromatin architecture is modulated by methylation of DNA (hypo- and hypermethylation correspond to gene expression and silencing, respectively), acetylation, ubiquitination, ADP-ribosylation and SUMOylation of histone proteins; and by non-histone proteins DNA-binding [295]. Moreover, epigenetic processes involve the expression of microRNAs (miRNAs). MiRNAs interact with mRNA, inhibiting translation, or inducing mRNA degradation [296–299]. In ectopic endometrial-like cells of endometriosis, the cellular identity and gene expression programs are defined and maintained by epigenetics that may have a key role in the pathogenesis. Of interest, these epigenetic aberrations are dynamic and reversible and may have potential implications for diagnosis, prognosis, and therapy of the disease. In summary, available evidence may suggest a role of epigenetics both in the development of endometriosis lesions and in the heritability of the disease.

5.1. Epigenetics in the Eutopic Endometrium

Epigenetic processes are involved in numerous mechanisms that modulate the gene expression in endometrial development during the menstrual cycle, resulting in coordinated functional and morphological changes [300]. The global methylation level of eutopic endometrium was reported higher in the proliferative phase as compared to the secretory phase of the menstrual cycle. This hypermethylation is consistent with the expression level of DNA methyltransferases 1 (DNMT1) that was reportedly higher in the proliferative and late secretory phase and lower in the mid-secretory phase. A similar expression level was reported for DNMT3A and DNMT3B, for which the gene expression levels were decreased by treatment with estrogen and progestin. Conversely, the expression level of DNMT1 was reported to be unchanged by hormones either due to technical limitations of the used method or because the estrogen and progestin act at the post-transcriptional level, reducing the stability of DNMT1 protein [301].

Similarly, histone modifications by acetylation seem to be involved in endometrial function, with histone acetylation levels reported as globally increased in the early proliferative phase and gradually reduced in the late proliferative phase until ovulation [300]. The histone deacetylase 1 (HDAC1), HDAC3, and two histone acetylases were reported to be constitutively expressed in the endometrium during the menstrual cycle, with HDAC1 having a reduced expression level in the secretory phase [302]. Of note, HDAC inhibitors (HDACIs) were able to determine a differentiation and morphological transformation in endometrium similar to the combined treatment with estrogen and progestin. These results suggest that histone modifications may play a role in the control of decidualization through the regulation of the function of ERs and PGE2-induced 17β-estradiol synthesis [4,303–305].

MiRNAs post-transcriptionally downregulate the expression of genes and seem to be involved in endometrium development during the menstrual cycle, similar to acetylation and methylation [306–308].

MiRNAs were identified in normal endometrium and in eutopic and ectopic endometrium of women affected by endometriosis [101]. An inverse correlation was reported between the expression level of specific miRNAs and the suppression of protein production derived from their target genes, such as aromatase and COX-2 [309]. Moreover, estrogen and progestins were reported able to modify the expression level of miRNAs in endometrial stromal and glandular epithelial cells. Progesterone may oppose estrogen action by fine-tuning gene expression modulating miRNAs, which seems to suppress genes involved in cycle progression and cell proliferation in the secretory-phase [309,310]. This involvement of miRNAs in endometrial cyclicity is consistent with data suggesting that miRNAs seem to have a role in embryo implantation and postnatal uterus development in the mouse [311,312].

5.2. Epigenetics in Endometriosis

Some forms of endometriosis could be considered an epigenetic disorder. A growing body of evidence suggests that epigenetics processes have a key role in the pathogenesis and pathophysiology of endometriosis [313]. Aberrant methylation, acetylation, post-translational modifications, and dysregulation of miRNAs expression were identified in eutopic as well as ectopic endometrium of affected woman and may have great potential as therapeutic targets or as biomarkers for diagnosis and recurrence risk prediction [314].

The first piece of evidence suggesting the role of epigenetic in the etiopathogenesis of endometriosis comes from studies reporting the hypermethylation of the HOXA10 gene promoter in eutopic endometrium of women with endometriosis as compared with healthy controls [315,316]. HOXA10 is a transcription factor belonging to the homeobox gene family and has a role in the development and function of the uterus. Eutopic endometrium expresses HOXA10 during the menstrual cycle with a high expression level in the mid-secretory phase. This high expression, corresponding to increased progesterone levels and to the time of implantation, suggests that HOXA10 may have a key role in establishing the conditions necessary for implantation [316]. Of interest, the hypermethylation of the HOXA10 gene promoter, which means gene silencing, is consistent with studies reporting that HOXA10 levels are reduced in the eutopic endometrium of women affected by endometriosis [271], which may be a cause of the impaired fertility of these women [316]. Animal models further confirmed the key role of HOXA10 gene silencing by promoter hypermethylation both in eutopic and ectopic endometrium [317]. Moreover, animal models suggest that aberrant methylation of the HOXA10 promoter can be induced by in utero exposure to endocrine-disrupting chemicals (EDC) such as diethylstilbestrol, with or without overexpression of DNMTs [318–320].

A growing body of evidence suggests that aberrant expression of interacting homeobox genes and WNT family genes, particularly the WNT/β-catenin pathway, may disrupt organogenesis of the urogenital tract, altering the cell differentiation/migration with ectopic implantation. The WNT/β-catenin signaling pathway is involved in stem cell function and maintenance. These pathways may support the Müllerian remnants hypothesis as well as may be implicated in the survival and implantation of transplanted endometrial stem progenitor cells [7]. Indeed, data suggest that estradiol supports disease progression by upregulating β-catenin, which is degraded when it does not bind E-cadherin. The inhibition of phosphorylation stabilizes β-catenin that reach the nucleus and interacts with transcription factors regulating proliferation and angiogenesis [61].

The epigenetic mechanism of methylation was identified as having a role in progesterone resistance of endometriosis. Studies demonstrated that the promoter of PR-B gene is hypermethylated in endometriosis and adenomyosis with subsequent reduced PR-B expression [321–323]. The relatively permanent nature of hypermethylation of PR-B promoter provides further explanation to the persistent PR-B downregulation and progesterone resistance in endometriosis.

Further evidence confirmed the role of dysregulated methylation in the etiopathogenesis of endometriosis. Genes coding for three DNA methyltransferases, DNMT1, DNMT3A, and DNMT3B, were reported to be overexpressed in endometriosis. The aberrant expression of these enzymes involved in maintenance, as well as de novo methylation, suggests that hypermethylation in endometriosis may be widespread [324–326]. For example, in endometriotic cell lines lacking E-cadherin, whose deregulation was associated with endometriotic cells invasiveness, the gene was hypermethylated, suggesting that methylation of E-cadherin provides invasive properties [327,328]. Notably, E-cadherin expression is also regulated by miR-200b expression, suggesting that this important anti-invasive adhesion molecule is subject to epigenetic regulation [219]. Of interest, both hypoxia and inflammation were reported distinctly able to modulate DNMTs expression and can cause aberrant DNA methylation patterns [4,329].

Endometriosis has both epigenetic mechanisms of hypermethylation as well as hypomethylation. The hypomethylation of specific genes and genes promoters that are hypermethylated in eutopic endometrium explains the altered expression in endometriosis of genes usually silenced in eutopic endometrium. Steroidogenic factor-1 (SF-1) is a transcriptional factor activating multiple genes for the biosynthesis of estrogen. SF-1 is not detected in stromal cells of eutopic endometrium because SF-1 promoter is usually hypermethylated. In endometriotic cells, the SF-1 promoter was reported to be hypomethylated, explaining the aberrant overexpression of SF-1 [330]. Similarly, the ER-β promoter and the aromatase gene were hypomethylated in endometriotic cells, while in eutopic endometrium, they are hypermethylated, providing an explanation as to why these genes are expressed in ectopic but not in normal endometrium. Consistently, the gene coding for 17β-HSD type 2 was reported hypermethylated. Moreover, the promoter of COX-2 was reported to be hypomethylated, explaining the higher expression of COX-2 and subsequent prostaglandin E2 synthesis, which in turn enhances 17β-estradiol production and elevate DNMT3A [4,314,331–333] (Figure 3).

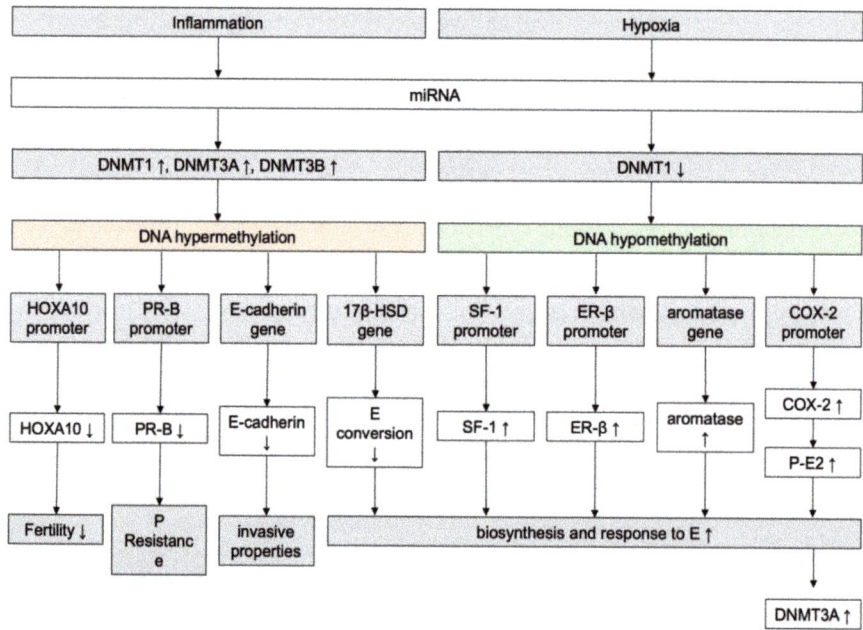

Figure 3. Epigenetic mechanisms of hypermethylation and hypomethylation involved in the etiopathogenesis of endometriosis. Hypoxia and inflammation regulate DNA methylation through microRNAs (miRNA), and genes coding for three DNA methyltransferases (DNMT) were reported overexpressed in endometriosis. microRNAs (miRNA); DNA methyltransferases (DNMT); Homeobox A transcription factor (HOXA10); Progesterone receptor B (PR-B); 17β-hydroxysteroid dehydrogenase (17β-HSD); Steroidogenic factor-1 (SF-1); Estrogen receptor β (ER-β); Cyclo-oxygenase type 2 (COX-2); Prostaglandin E2 (P-E2); Estrogen (E); Progesterone (P).

Regarding the epigenetic regulation by histone acetylation, the balance between the HDACs and histone acetyltransferase activity regulates the gene transcription. Gene expression is promoted by the acetylation of lysine residue by the histone acetyltransferase, whereas is inhibited trough the removal of acetyl group by the HDACs [334]. Endometriotic lesions as well as eutopic endometrium of affected women were reported globally hypoacetylated as compared to the eutopic endometrium of controls, with consequent gene silencing [335]. This observation was consistent with the reported higher expression of HDAC1 and HDAC2 genes and lower levels of SIRT1 in the endometriotic lesions. Moreover, the lost modulation of HDAC expression by estrogen and progesterone was reported in ectopic implants [335–337].

Different genes are known to be involved in the etiopathogenesis of endometriosis by the methylation of their promoters and subsequent downregulation. The same genes and others were reported having the promoter hypoacetylated as well, such as the genes coding ER-α, HOXA10, E-cadherin, and different proapoptotic proteins involved in the cell cycle regulation [335,338].

The global aberrant acetylation is able to explain the altered expression of different genes both for downregulation by hypoacetylation and upregulation by hyperacetylation of the promoter, such as the higher level of SF-1 and hypoxia-inducible factor-1α [335,339].

Interestingly, recent evidence founds not only somatic inactivating mutations of the tumor suppressor ARID1A but also the loss of its expression in endometriotic foci [340]. ARID1A is known to encode the protein BAF250a, which participates in forming SWI/SNF chromatin remodeling complexes. Considering that this gene is frequently mutated in ovarian clear cell and endometrioid carcinomas as well as in uterine endometrioid carcinomas, the epigenetic loss of expression of BAF250a may underlie (at least in part) the potential degeneration of endometriotic tissue toward carcinogenesis. In particular, the loss of expression of the protein encoded by ARID1A (BAF250a) can dysregulate the suppression of cellular proliferation, which is normally modulated through a p53-dependent transcription fashion of several tumor suppressors, including CDKN1A (encoding p21) and SMAD3 [341]. Indeed, published data highlighted that tissue samples from patients who had undergone surgery for endometriosis-associated ovarian cancers or endometriotic ovarian cysts show loss of BAF250a expression in 22% endometrioid cancers, 47% of clear cell cases, 44% of contiguous endometriosis cases, and 8% of benign endometriotic ovarian cysts; in addition, the expression of phosphorylated AKT, γH2AX, BIM, and BAX was higher in endometriosis-associated ovarian cancers and contiguous endometriosis than in benign endometriosis, whereas expression of pATM, pCHK2, and Bcl2 was low [342]. Based on these pieces of evidence, the mutation of ARID1A and/or the loss of expression of BAF250a may appear as a promising strategy for molecular diagnosis of endometriosis-associated ovarian cancer [343].

The epigenetic post-transcriptional mRNA modulation by miRNAs expression has a potential role in the etiopathogenesis of endometriosis [4]. MiRNAs interacting with the correspondent mRNAs downregulate gene expression. Different studies report progressively different expression of many specific miRNAs from eutopic endometrium of healthy women, paired eutopic and ectopic endometrium of women with endometriosis, and ectopic endometrium. Most of these identified miRNAs target genes known to be differentially expressed in eutopic versus ectopic endometrium. Identified miRNA target genes includes those involved in hormone metabolism such as aromatase, PR, ER-α, and ER-β [310]; modulators of the inflammatory response such as COX-2, IL-6, IL-6 receptor, IL-8, and TGF-β; and the induction of apoptosis and angiogenesis such as Bcl-2, cyclin-D, and VEGF [4,136]. The inverse correlation between the expression level of miRNAs and that of target genes supports the hypothesis that altered expression of these specific miRNAs is involved in the pathogenesis of endometriosis [344]. Both upregulated and downregulated expression of specific miRNAs were reported in ectopic endometrium as compared with eutopic endometrium of women with endometriosis [345], as well as in eutopic or ectopic endometrium of women affected by endometriosis as compared with eutopic endometrium of healthy controls [346]. Functional studies in preclinical cell models of endometriosis have confirmed a mechanistic involvement of selected microRNAs in pathogenetically relevant processes, including modulation of cell proliferation by miR-10b and miR-145, of invasive growth by miR-10b, miR-200b, and miR-145, and of stem cell properties, as exemplified by miR-145 and miR-200b [124,218,219]. Of interest, although there is a discrepancy between studies in the identification of miRNAs having altered expression, no miRNAs were "misclassified." These discrepancies can be explained by differences in study design and compared tissues. The comparison between eutopic and ectopic endometrium of affected women may not identify miRNAs associated with endometriosis that are aberrantly expressed in the same direction in both tissues. Finally, it should be noted that the role of miRNAs is more complex than a unidirectional negative regulation of gene expression. Evidence supports that many miRNAs are able to interact with transcription factors forming a network for gene regulation that yield negative as well as positive feedback loops [347]. Moreover, miRNAs have been reported to be both targets and regulators of other epigenetic mechanisms such as methylation and acetylation, and they resulted involved in hypoxia and inflammation signaling pathways [4,344].

5.3. Implications of Epigenetics in Diagnosis, Prognosis, and Therapy

The identification of epigenetic aberrations may provide promising tools for the diagnosis of endometriosis. DNA methylation markers, as well as other epigenetic aberrations that are present in the eutopic endometrium of women with endometriosis and absent in healthy controls, are present in the menstrual blood-derived from eutopic endometrium. The identification of these markers in the menstrual blood could provide high sensitivity and specificity in the identification of endometriosis with a minimally invasive approach [4,294]. These epigenetic markers may also provide prognostic information identifying patients at high risk of recurrence, allowing the tailoring of postoperative therapies and follow-up. For example, hypermethylation of the PR-B promoter identified in surgical tissue samples of endometriotic implants was related to a higher risk of recurrence [321,348].

The therapeutic implications are based on the reversible nature of epigenetic modifications. Therefore, enzymes involved in epigenetic mechanisms could be pharmacological targets. On that basis, HDACIs were investigated in vitro and in animal models as a potential therapy for endometriosis. In vitro, treatment with trichostatin A (TSA), an HDACI, elevated PR-B gene and protein expression, inhibited IL-1β-induced COX-2 expression, and inhibited cellular proliferation with cell cycle arrest in ectopic endometrial stromal cells, but not in eutopic cells [349–351]. In endometrial stromal cells, TSA upregulated Peroxisome proliferator-activated receptor (PPAR)γ expression which inhibits VEGF expression, angiogenesis, and TNF-induced IL-8 production [352–354]. Moreover, TSA attenuated invasion inducing E-cadherin expression [327]. In animal models with induced endometriosis, TSA represses endometriosis, reducing the size of ectopic implants as compared with no-treatment [59,355]. Treatments with other HDACIs and demethylation agents in both in vitro and in vivo studies provided similar promising results [59,323,356].

Data about the use of HDACI in humans derives from the use of Valproic Acid (VPA), an HDACI with known pharmacology. In women with adenomyosis, VPA reduces the amount of menses and dysmenorrhea. This could be explained by the fact that HDACIs suppress the expression of TNF-α-induced tissue factor and VEGF receptor as reported in both in vitro and in vivo studies. Both these pathways are involved in abnormal uterine bleeding and resulted in overexpressed in endometriosis [357–360]. VPA tested on patients was well tolerated, and after two months had reduced pain symptoms, reduced amount of menses, and reduced uterine size [361–363]. This evidence suggests that HDACIs have a potential role as therapy in endometriosis and/or adenomyosis [364].

6. Conclusions

The etiopathogenesis of endometriosis is a multifactorial process that leads to the development of an extremely heterogeneous disease characterized by the variable acquisition and loss of cellular functions. Its origin would appear to be from Müllerian or non-Müllerian stem cells with endometrial differentiation that can potentially originate from stem cells of the endometrial basal layer, present in Müllerian remnants, in the blood originating from bone marrow, or from the peritoneum. These stem cells have the ability of the endometrium to regenerate cyclically by mechanisms of tissue regeneration and angiogenesis in response to hypoxia, which seem to play a key role when they are dysregulated in the development of endometriosis. What determines the presence of such cells in the peritoneal cavity can occur during the development of the embryos as well as during each menstrual cycle, and what leads to the development of endometriosis is a complex process in which play a large number of interconnected factors potentially both inherited and acquired. Genetic studies have confirmed that endometriosis has a genetic nature, but at the same time, this predisposition is complex. It is constituted by the combined action of several genes with limited influence. At the same time, the epigenetic mechanisms underlying endometriosis control many of the processes of acquisition and maintenance of immunologic, immunohistochemical, histological and biological aberrations that characterize both the eutopic and ectopic endometrium in patients affected by endometriosis. However, what triggers such epigenetic alterations is not clear and may be both genetically and epigenetically inherited, or it may be acquired by the particular combination of several factors linked to the persistent presence of menstrual reflux in the peritoneal cavity as well as exogenous factors playing a critical role. Once started, the process is variable and can lead to the development of endometriosis through the progressive acquisition of alterations to the physiological processes of the endometrium, including the altered hormonal physiology, and modulating the interaction between endometriosis and the inflammatory response by subjugating it. However, the heterogeneity of endometriosis and the different contexts in which it develops suggests that a single etiopathogenetic explaining model is not sufficient.

Author Contributions: Conceptualization, A.S.L. and S.G.; methodology, M.F.; data curation, F.G.; writing—original draft preparation, A.S.L. and S.G.; writing—review and editing, M.G., D.C.M., and P.V.; project administration, A.S.L.

Funding: This research received no external funding.

Acknowledgments: None.

Conflicts of Interest: The authors declare no conflict of interest.

Abbreviations

MeSH	Medical Subject Headings
CAM	Chorioallantoic membrane
17β-HSD	17β-hydroxysteroid dehydrogenase
COX-2	Cyclo-oxygenase type 2
TIAR	Tissue injury and repair
TNF	Tumor necrosis factor
IL	Interleukin
VEGF	Vascular endothelial growth factor
Bcl-2	Antiapoptotic protein B cell lymphoma 2
NK cells	Natural Killer cells
sICAM-1	Soluble form of intercellular adhesion molecule-1
LFA-1	Leukocyte function antigen-1
MAPK	Mitogen-activated protein kinase
ECM	Extracellular matrix
HLA-1	Human leukocyte antigen class I
INF	Interferon
TGF-β	Transforming growth factor-β
E-cadherin	Epithelial cadherin
MMPs	Matrix metalloproteinases
TIMPs	Tissue inhibitors of MMPs
bFGF	Basic fibroblast growth factor
PAI	Plasminogen activator inhibitor
PR	Progesterone receptor

ER	Estrogen receptor
SNPs	Single nucleotide polymorphisms
LD	Linkage disequilibrium
FGF	Fibroblast growth factor
FGFR2	FGF receptor 2 gene
GWA	Genome-wide association
CDKN2BAS	Cyclin-dependent kinase inhibitor 2B antisense RNA
MMTV	Mouse mammary tumor virus
WNT4	Wingless-type mouse mammary tumor virus integration site family 4
rAFS	Revised American Fertility Society
FSH	Follicle-stimulating hormone
GREB1	Growth Regulating Estrogen Receptor Binding 1
TCDD	2,3,7,8-tetrachlorodibenzo-p-dioxin
miRNAs	microRNAs
DNMT	DNA methyltransferase
HDAC	Histone deacetylase
HDACIs	Histone deacetylase inhibitors
EDC	Endocrine-disrupting chemicals
SF-1	Steroidogenic factor-1
HOXA10	Homeobox A transcription factor
P-E2	Prostaglandin E2
E	Estrogen
P	Progesterone
TSA	Trichostatin A
PPAR	Peroxisome proliferator-activated receptor
VPA	Valproic acid

References

1. Vercellini, P.; Viganò, P.; Somigliana, E.; Fedele, L. Endometriosis: Pathogenesis and treatment. *Nat. Rev. Endocrinol.* **2014**, *10*, 261–275. [CrossRef] [PubMed]
2. Garai, J.; Molnar, V.; Varga, T.; Koppan, M.; Torok, A.; Bodis, J. Endometriosis: Harmful survival of an ectopic tissue. *Front. Biosci. J. Virtual Libr.* **2006**, *11*, 595–619. [CrossRef] [PubMed]
3. Matalliotakis, M.; Zervou, M.I.; Matalliotaki, C.; Rahmioglu, N.; Koumantakis, G.; Kalogiannidis, I.; Prapas, I.; Zondervan, K.; Spandidos, D.A.; Matalliotakis, I.; et al. The role of gene polymorphisms in endometriosis. *Mol. Med. Rep.* **2017**, *16*, 5881–5886. [CrossRef] [PubMed]
4. Hsiao, K.; Wu, M.; Tsai, S. Epigenetic regulation of the pathological process in endometriosis. *Reprod. Med. Biol.* **2017**, *16*, 314–319. [CrossRef]
5. Clement, P.B. The pathology of endometriosis: A survey of the many faces of a common disease emphasizing diagnostic pitfalls and unusual and newly appreciated aspects. *Adv. Anat. Pathol.* **2007**, *14*, 241–260. [CrossRef]
6. Burney, R.O.; Giudice, L.C. Pathogenesis and pathophysiology of endometriosis. *Fertil. Steril.* **2012**, *98*, 511–519. [CrossRef]
7. Laganà, A.S.; Vitale, S.G.; Salmeri, F.M.; Triolo, O.; Ban Frangež, H.; Vrtačnik-Bokal, E.; Stojanovska, L.; Apostolopoulos, V.; Granese, R.; Sofo, V. Unus pro omnibus, omnes pro uno: A novel, evidence-based, unifying theory for the pathogenesis of endometriosis. *Med. Hypotheses* **2017**, *103*, 10–20. [CrossRef]
8. Laganà, A.S.; La Rosa, V.L.; Rapisarda, A.M.; Valenti, G.; Sapia, F.; Chiofalo, B.; Rossetti, D.; Ban Frangež, H.; Vrtačnik Bokal, E.; Vitale, S.G. Anxiety and depression in patients with endometriosis: Impact and management challenges. *Int. J. Womens Health* **2017**, *9*, 323–330. [CrossRef]
9. Laganà, A.S.; Condemi, I.; Retto, G.; Muscatello, M.R.A.; Bruno, A.; Zoccali, R.A.; Triolo, O.; Cedro, C. Analysis of psychopathological comorbidity behind the common symptoms and signs of endometriosis. *Eur. J. Obstet. Gynecol. Reprod. Biol.* **2015**, *194*, 30–33. [CrossRef]

10. Vitale, S.G.; Petrosino, B.; La Rosa, V.L.; Rapisarda, A.M.C.; Laganà, A.S. A Systematic Review of the Association Between Psychiatric Disturbances and Endometriosis. *J. Obstet. Gynaecol. Can.* **2016**, *38*, 1079–1080. [CrossRef]
11. Laganà, A.S.; La Rosa, V.; Petrosino, B.; Vitale, S.G. Comment on "Risk of developing major depression and anxiety disorders among women with endometriosis: A longitudinal follow-up study". *J. Affect. Disord.* **2017**, *208*, 672–673. [CrossRef] [PubMed]
12. Raffaelli, R.; Garzon, S.; Baggio, S.; Genna, M.; Pomini, P.; Laganà, A.S.; Ghezzi, F.; Franchi, M. Mesenteric vascular and nerve sparing surgery in laparoscopic segmental intestinal resection for deep infiltrating endometriosis. *Eur. J. Obstet. Gynecol. Reprod. Biol.* **2018**, *231*, 214–219. [CrossRef] [PubMed]
13. Baggio, S.; Pomini, P.; Zecchin, A.; Garzon, S.; Bonin, C.; Santi, L.; Festi, A.; Franchi, M.P. Delivery and pregnancy outcome in women with bowel resection for deep endometriosis: A retrospective cohort study. *Gynecol. Surg.* **2015**, *12*, 279–285. [CrossRef]
14. Viganò, P.; Parazzini, F.; Somigliana, E.; Vercellini, P. Endometriosis: Epidemiology and aetiological factors. *Best Pract. Res. Clin. Obstet. Gynaecol.* **2004**, *18*, 177–200. [CrossRef] [PubMed]
15. Buck Louis, G.M.; Hediger, M.L.; Peterson, C.M.; Croughan, M.; Sundaram, R.; Stanford, J.; Chen, Z.; Fujimoto, V.Y.; Varner, M.W.; Trumble, A.; et al. Incidence of endometriosis by study population and diagnostic method: The ENDO study. *Fertil. Steril.* **2011**, *96*, 360–365. [CrossRef] [PubMed]
16. Missmer, S.A.; Cramer, D.W. The epidemiology of endometriosis. *Obstet. Gynecol. Clin. North Am.* **2003**, *30*, 1–19. [CrossRef]
17. Evers, J.L. Endometriosis does not exist; all women have endometriosis. *Hum. Reprod. Oxf. Engl.* **1994**, *9*, 2206–2209. [CrossRef]
18. Evers, J.L. Is adolescent endometriosis a progressive disease that needs to be diagnosed and treated? *Hum. Reprod. Oxf. Engl.* **2013**, *28*, 2023. [CrossRef]
19. Sampson, J.A. Perforating hemorrhage (chocolate) cysts of the ovary: Their importance and especially their relation to pelvic adenomas of endometrial type ("adenomyoma" of the uterus, rectovaginal septum, sigmoid, etc.). *Arch. Surg.* **1921**, *3*, 245–323. [CrossRef]
20. Sampson, J.A. Peritoneal endometriosis due to the menstrual dissemination of endometrial tissue into the peritoneal cavity. *Am. J. Obstet. Gynecol.* **1927**, *14*, 422–469. [CrossRef]
21. Sampson, J.A. The development of the implantation theory for the origin of peritoneal endometriosis. *Am. J. Obstet. Gynecol.* **1940**, *40*, 549–557. [CrossRef]
22. Nisolle, M.; Donnez, J. Peritoneal endometriosis, ovarian endometriosis, and adenomyotic nodules of the rectovaginal septum are three different entities. *Fertil. Steril.* **1997**, *68*, 585–596. [CrossRef]
23. Koninckx, P.R.; Ussia, A.; Adamyan, L.; Wattiez, A.; Donnez, J. Deep endometriosis: Definition, diagnosis, and treatment. *Fertil. Steril.* **2012**, *98*, 564–571. [CrossRef] [PubMed]
24. Koninckx, P.R. Is mild endometriosis a disease?: Is mild endometriosis a condition occurring intermittently in all women? *Hum. Reprod.* **1994**, *9*, 2202–2205. [CrossRef]
25. Donnez, J.; Squifflet, J.; Casanas-Roux, F.; Pirard, C.; Jadoul, P.; Van, A.L. Typical and subtle atypical presentations of endometriosis. *Obstet. Gynecol. Clin. North Am.* **2003**, *30*, 83–93. [CrossRef]
26. Waldeyer, H. "Die epithelialen Eierstockgeschwülste." Ins besonders die Kystome (The epithelial ovarian tumors, especially the cystic tumors). *Arch Gynäkol* **1870**, *1*, 252–316. [CrossRef]
27. van der Linden, P.J. Theories on the pathogenesis of endometriosis. *Hum. Reprod. Oxf. Engl.* **1996**, *11* (Suppl. 3), 53–65. [CrossRef]
28. Miyazaki, K.; Dyson, M.T.; Coon V, J.S.; Furukawa, Y.; Yilmaz, B.D.; Maruyama, T.; Bulun, S.E. Generation of Progesterone-Responsive Endometrial Stromal Fibroblasts from Human Induced Pluripotent Stem Cells: Role of the WNT/CTNNB1 Pathway. *Stem Cell Rep.* **2018**, *11*, 1136–1155. [CrossRef]
29. Lauchlan, S.C. THE SECONDARY MÜLLERIAN SYSTEM. *Obstet. Gynecol. Surv.* **1972**, *27*, 133. [CrossRef]
30. Batt, R.E.; Smith, R.A.; Buck, G.L.; Martin, D.C.; Chapron, C.; Koninckx, P.R.; Yeh, J. Müllerianosis. *Histol. Histopathol.* **2007**, *22*, 1161–1166. [CrossRef]
31. Signorile, P.G.; Baldi, F.; Bussani, R.; D'Armiento, M.; De Falco, M.; Baldi, A. Ectopic endometrium in human foetuses is a common event and sustains the theory of müllerianosis in the pathogenesis of endometriosis, a disease that predisposes to cancer. *J. Exp. Clin. Cancer Res.* **2009**, *28*, 49. [CrossRef] [PubMed]

32. Nawroth, F.; Rahimi, G.; Nawroth, C.; Foth, D.; Ludwig, M.; Schmidt, T. Is there an association between septate uterus and endometriosis? *Hum. Reprod.* **2006**, *21*, 542–544. [CrossRef] [PubMed]
33. Mok-Lin, E.Y.; Wolfberg, A.; Hollinquist, H.; Laufer, M.R. Endometriosis in a Patient with Mayer-Rokitansky-Küster-Hauser Syndrome and Complete Uterine Agenesis: Evidence to Support the Theory of Coelomic Metaplasia. *J. Pediatr. Adolesc. Gynecol.* **2010**, *23*, e35–e37. [CrossRef] [PubMed]
34. Troncon, J.K.; Zani, A.C.T.; Vieira, A.D.D.; Poli-Neto, O.B.; Nogueira, A.A.; Rosa-E-Silva, J.C. Endometriosis in a patient with mayer-rokitansky-küster-hauser syndrome. *Case Rep. Obstet. Gynecol.* **2014**, *2014*, 376231. [CrossRef] [PubMed]
35. Batt, R.E.; Mitwally, M.F.M. Endometriosis from thelarche to midteens: Pathogenesis and prognosis, prevention and pedagogy. *J. Pediatr. Adolesc. Gynecol.* **2003**, *16*, 337–347. [CrossRef] [PubMed]
36. Suginami, H. A reappraisal of the coelomic metaplasia theory by reviewing, endometriosis occurring in unusual sites and instances. *Am. J. Obstet. Gynecol.* **1991**, *165*, 214–218. [CrossRef]
37. Rei, C.; Williams, T.; Feloney, M. Endometriosis in a Man as a Rare Source of Abdominal Pain: A Case Report and Review of the Literature. *Case Rep. Obstet. Gynecol.* **2018**, *2018*, 2083121. [CrossRef]
38. Cullen, T.S. *Adeno-myoma uteri diffusum benignum*; Johns Hopkins Press: Baltimore, Maryland, 1896.
39. Meyer, R. Über eine adenomatöse Wucherung der Serosa in einer Bauchnarbe. *Zeitschr Geburtsh Gynakol* **1903**, *49*, 32–41.
40. Novak, E. Pelvic endometriosis: Spontaneous rupture of endometrial cysts, with a report of three cases. *Am. J. Obstet. Gynecol.* **1931**, *22*, 826–837. [CrossRef]
41. Hu, Z.; Mamillapalli, R.; Taylor, H.S. Increased circulating miR-370-3p regulates steroidogenic factor 1 in endometriosis. *Am. J. Physiol. Endocrinol. Metab.* **2019**, *316*, E373–E382. [CrossRef]
42. Meyer, R. Uber den Stand der Frage der Adenomyositis und Adenomyome im allgeneinen und insbesondere uber Adenomyositis seroepithelialis und Adenomyometritis sarcomatosa. *Zentralbl Gynäkol* **1919**, *36*, 745–750.
43. Munrós, J.; Martínez-Zamora, M.-A.; Tàssies, D.; Reverter, J.C.; Rius, M.; Gracia, M.; Ros, C.; Carmona, F. Total Circulating Microparticle Levels After Laparoscopic Surgical Treatment for Endometrioma: A Pilot, Prospective, Randomized Study Comparing Stripping with CO2 Laser Vaporization. *J. Minim. Invasive Gynecol.* **2019**, *26*, 450–455. [CrossRef] [PubMed]
44. Levander, G.; Normann, P. The Pathogenesis of Endometriosis. *Acta Obstet. Gynecol. Scand.* **1955**, *34*, 366–398. [CrossRef] [PubMed]
45. Merrill, J.A. Endometrial induction of endometriosis across Millipore filters. *Am J Obstet Gynecol* **1966**, *94*, 780–790. [PubMed]
46. Maniglio, P.; Ricciardi, E.; Meli, F.; Vitale, S.G.; Noventa, M.; Vitagliano, A.; Valenti, G.; La Rosa, V.L.; Laganà, A.S.; Caserta, D. Catamenial pneumothorax caused by thoracic endometriosis. *Radiol. Case Rep.* **2018**, *13*, 81–85. [CrossRef] [PubMed]
47. Uğur, M.; Turan, C.; Mungan, T.; Kuşçu, E.; Şenöz, S.; Ağış, H.T.; Gökmen, O. Endometriosis in Association with Müllerian Anomalies. *Gynecol. Obstet. Investig.* **1995**, *40*, 261–264. [CrossRef] [PubMed]
48. Olive, D.L.; Henderson, D.Y. Endometriosis and mullerian anomalies. *Obstet. Gynecol.* **1987**, *69*, 412–415.
49. Javert, C.T. Pathogenesis of endometriosis based on endometrial homeoplasia, direct extension, exfoliation and implantation, lymphatic and hematogenous metastasis. Including five case reports of endometrial tissue in pelvic lymph nodes. *Cancer* **1949**, *2*, 399–410. [CrossRef]
50. Halme, J.; Hammond, M.G.; Hulka, J.F.; Raj, S.G.; Talbert, L.M. Retrograde menstruation in healthy women and in patients with endometriosis. *Obstet. Gynecol.* **1984**, *64*, 151–154.
51. Kruitwagen, R.F.; Poels, L.G.; Willemsen, W.N.; de Ronde, I.J.; Jap, P.H.; Rolland, R. Endometrial epithelial cells in peritoneal fluid during the early follicular phase. *Fertil. Steril.* **1991**, *55*, 297–303. [CrossRef]
52. Koks, C.A.M.; Dunselman, G.A.J.; de Goeij, A.F.P.M.; Arends, J.W.; Evers, J.L.H. Evaluation of a menstrual cup to collect shed endometrium for in vitro studies. *Fertil. Steril.* **1997**, *68*, 560–564. [CrossRef]
53. Vercellini, P.; Aimi, G.; De Giorgi, O.; Maddalena, S.; Carinelli, S.; Crosignani, P.G. Is cystic ovarian endometriosis an asymmetric disease? *Br. J. Obstet. Gynaecol.* **1998**, *105*, 1018–1021. [CrossRef] [PubMed]
54. Vercellini, P.; Abbiati, A.; Vigano, P.; Somigliana, E.D.; Daguati, R.; Meroni, F.; Crosignani, P.G. Asymmetry in distribution of diaphragmatic endometriotic lesions: Evidence in favour of the menstrual reflux theory. *Hum. Reprod.* **2007**, *22*, 2359–2367. [CrossRef] [PubMed]

55. Jenkins, S.; Olive, D.L.; Haney, A.F. Endometriosis: Pathogenetic implications of the anatomic distribution. *Obstet. Gynecol.* **1986**, *67*, 335–338.
56. Martin, D.C. Laparoscopic Appearance of Endometriosis. Available online: https://www.danmartinmd.com/files/lae1988.pdf (accessed on 15 September 2019).
57. Roman, H.; Hennetier, C.; Darwish, B.; Badescu, A.; Csanyi, M.; Aziz, M.; Tuech, J.-J.; Abo, C. Bowel occult microscopic endometriosis in resection margins in deep colorectal endometriosis specimens has no impact on short-term postoperative outcomes. *Fertil. Steril.* **2016**, *105*, 423–429. [CrossRef]
58. Badescu, A.; Roman, H.; Aziz, M.; Puscasiu, L.; Molnar, C.; Huet, E.; Sabourin, J.-C.; Stolnicu, S. Mapping of bowel occult microscopic endometriosis implants surrounding deep endometriosis nodules infiltrating the bowel. *Fertil. Steril.* **2016**, *105*, 430–434. [CrossRef]
59. Bruner-Tran, K.L.; Mokshagundam, S.; Herington, J.L.; Ding, T.; Osteen, K.G. Rodent Models of Experimental Endometriosis: Identifying Mechanisms of Disease and Therapeutic Targets. *Curr. Womens Health Rev.* **2018**, *14*, 173–188. [CrossRef]
60. Laganà, A.S.; Garzon, S.; Franchi, M.; Casarin, J.; Gullo, G.; Ghezzi, F. Translational animal models for endometriosis research: A long and windy road. *Ann. Transl. Med.* **2018**, *6*, 431. [CrossRef]
61. Klemmt, P.A.B.; Starzinski-Powitz, A. Molecular and Cellular Pathogenesis of Endometriosis. *Curr. Womens Health Rev.* **2018**, *14*, 106–116. [CrossRef]
62. Ota, H.; Igarashi, S. Expression of major histocompatibility complex class II antigen in endometriotic tissue in patients with endometriosis and adenomyosis. *Fertil. Steril.* **1993**, *60*, 834–838. [CrossRef]
63. Chung, H.W.; Wen, Y.; Chun, S.H.; Nezhat, C.; Woo, B.H.; Lake Polan, M. Matrix metalloproteinase-9 and tissue inhibitor of metalloproteinase-3 mRNA expression in ectopic and eutopic endometrium in women with endometriosis: A rationale for endometriotic invasiveness. *Fertil. Steril.* **2001**, *75*, 152–159. [CrossRef]
64. Di Carlo, C.; Bonifacio, M.; Tommaselli, G.A.; Bifulco, G.; Guerra, G.; Nappi, C. Metalloproteinases, vascular endothelial growth factor, and angiopoietin 1 and 2 in eutopic and ectopic endometrium. *Fertil. Steril.* **2009**, *91*, 2315–2323. [CrossRef] [PubMed]
65. Redwine, D.B. Was Sampson wrong? *Fertil. Steril.* **2002**, *78*, 686–693. [CrossRef]
66. Suda, K.; Nakaoka, H.; Yoshihara, K.; Ishiguro, T.; Tamura, R.; Mori, Y.; Yamawaki, K.; Adachi, S.; Takahashi, T.; Kase, H.; et al. Clonal Expansion and Diversification of Cancer-Associated Mutations in Endometriosis and Normal Endometrium. *Cell Rep.* **2018**, *24*, 1777–1789. [CrossRef] [PubMed]
67. Leyendecker, G.; Wildt, L.; Mall, G. The pathophysiology of endometriosis and adenomyosis: Tissue injury and repair. *Arch. Gynecol. Obstet.* **2009**, *280*, 529–538. [CrossRef] [PubMed]
68. Young, V.J.; Ahmad, S.F.; Duncan, W.C.; Horne, A.W. The role of TGF-β in the pathophysiology of peritoneal endometriosis. *Hum. Reprod. Update* **2017**, *23*, 548–559. [CrossRef] [PubMed]
69. Maas, J.W.; Groothuis, P.G.; Dunselman, G.A.; de Goeij, A.F.; Struijker-Boudier, H.A.; Evers, J.L. Development of endometriosis-like lesions after transplantation of human endometrial fragments onto the chick embryo chorioallantoic membrane. *Hum. Reprod.* **2001**, *16*, 627–631. [CrossRef]
70. Nap, A.W.; Groothuis, P.G.; Demir, A.Y.; Maas, J.W.; Dunselman, G.A.; de Goeij, A.F.; Evers, J.L. Tissue integrity is essential for ectopic implantation of human endometrium in the chicken chorioallantoic membrane. *Hum. Reprod.* **2003**, *18*, 30–34. [CrossRef]
71. Winterhager, E. Role of Steroid Hormones: Estrogen and Endometriosis. In *Endometriosis: Science and Practice*; John Wiley & Sons, Ltd.: Hoboken, NJ, USA, 2012; pp. 140–144. ISBN 978-1-4443-9851-9.
72. Liang, Y.; Xie, H.; Wu, J.; Liu, D.; Yao, S. Villainous role of estrogen in macrophage-nerve interaction in endometriosis. *Reprod. Biol. Endocrinol.* **2018**, *16*, 122. [CrossRef]
73. Rier, S.E.; Martin, D.C.; Bowman, R.E.; Becker, J.L. Immunoresponsiveness in endometriosis: Implications of estrogenic toxicants. *Environ. Health Perspect.* **1995**, *103*, 151–156.
74. Maruyama, T.; Yoshimura, Y. Molecular and cellular mechanisms for differentiation and regeneration of the uterine endometrium. *Endocr. J.* **2008**, *55*, 795–810. [CrossRef] [PubMed]
75. de Almeida Asencio, F.; Ribeiro, H.A.; Ayrosa Ribeiro, P.; Malzoni, M.; Adamyan, L.; Ussia, A.; Gomel, V.; Martin, D.C.; Koninckx, P.R. Symptomatic endometriosis developing several years after menopause in the absence of increased circulating estrogen concentrations: A systematic review and seven case reports. *Gynecol. Surg.* **2019**, *16*, 3. [CrossRef]

76. Kitawaki, J.; Noguchi, T.; Amatsu, T.; Maeda, K.; Tsukamoto, K.; Yamamoto, T.; Fushiki, S.; Osawa, Y.; Honjo, H. Expression of aromatase cytochrome P450 protein and messenger ribonucleic acid in human endometriotic and adenomyotic tissues but not in normal endometrium. *Biol. Reprod.* **1997**, *57*, 514–519. [CrossRef] [PubMed]
77. Noble, L.S.; Simpson, E.R.; Johns, A.; Bulun, S.E. Aromatase expression in endometriosis. *J. Clin. Endocrinol. Metab.* **1996**, *81*, 174–179. [PubMed]
78. Noble, L.S.; Takayama, K.; Zeitoun, K.M.; Putman, J.M.; Johns, D.A.; Hinshelwood, M.M.; Agarwal, V.R.; Zhao, Y.; Carr, B.R.; Bulun, S.E. Prostaglandin E2 stimulates aromatase expression in endometriosis-derived stromal cells. *J. Clin. Endocrinol. Metab.* **1997**, *82*, 600–606. [CrossRef]
79. Zeitoun, K.; Takayama, K.; Sasano, H.; Suzuki, T.; Moghrabi, N.; Andersson, S.; Johns, A.; Meng, L.; Putman, M.; Carr, B. Deficient 17β-hydroxysteroid dehydrogenase type 2 expression in endometriosis: Failure to metabolize 17β-estradiol. *J. Clin. Endocrinol. Metab.* **1998**, *83*, 4474–4480. [CrossRef]
80. TAKAHAsHI, K.; Nagata, H.; Kitao, M. Clinical usefulness of determination of estradiol level in the menstrual blood for patients with endometriosis. *Nippon Sanka Fujinka Gakkai Zasshi* **1989**, *41*, 1849–1850.
81. Bulun, S.E.; Yang, S.; Fang, Z.; Gurates, B.; Tamura, M.; Zhou, J.; Sebastian, S. Role of aromatase in endometrial disease. *J. Steroid Biochem. Mol. Biol.* **2001**, *79*, 19–25. [CrossRef]
82. Götte, M.; Wolf, M.; Staebler, A.; Buchweitz, O.; Kelsch, R.; Schüring, A.N.; Kiesel, L. Increased expression of the adult stem cell marker Musashi-1 in endometriosis and endometrial carcinoma. *J. Pathol.* **2008**, *215*, 317–329. [CrossRef]
83. Valentijn, A.J.; Palial, K.; Al-Lamee, H.; Tempest, N.; Drury, J.; Von Zglinicki, T.; Saretzki, G.; Murray, P.; Gargett, C.E.; Hapangama, D.K. SSEA-1 isolates human endometrial basal glandular epithelial cells: Phenotypic and functional characterization and implications in the pathogenesis of endometriosis. *Hum. Reprod. Oxf. Engl.* **2013**, *28*, 2695–2708. [CrossRef]
84. Leyendecker, G.; Herbertz, M.; Kunz, G.; Mall, G. Endometriosis results from the dislocation of basal endometrium. *Hum. Reprod.* **2002**, *17*, 2725–2736. [CrossRef] [PubMed]
85. Agic, A.; Djalali, S.; Diedrich, K.; Hornung, D. Apoptosis in endometriosis. *Gynecol. Obstet. Investig.* **2009**, *68*, 217–223. [CrossRef] [PubMed]
86. Zhao, Y.; Gong, P.; Chen, Y.; Nwachukwu, J.C.; Srinivasan, S.; Ko, C.; Bagchi, M.K.; Taylor, R.N.; Korach, K.S.; Nettles, K.W.; et al. Dual suppression of estrogenic and inflammatory activities for targeting of endometriosis. *Sci. Transl. Med.* **2015**, *7*, 271ra9. [CrossRef] [PubMed]
87. Burns, K.A.; Rodriguez, K.F.; Hewitt, S.C.; Janardhan, K.S.; Young, S.L.; Korach, K.S. Role of estrogen receptor signaling required for endometriosis-like lesion establishment in a mouse model. *Endocrinology* **2012**, *153*, 3960–3971. [CrossRef] [PubMed]
88. Han, S.J.; Jung, S.Y.; Wu, S.-P.; Hawkins, S.M.; Park, M.J.; Kyo, S.; Qin, J.; Lydon, J.P.; Tsai, S.Y.; Tsai, M.-J.; et al. Estrogen Receptor β Modulates Apoptosis Complexes and the Inflammasome to Drive the Pathogenesis of Endometriosis. *Cell* **2015**, *163*, 960–974. [CrossRef] [PubMed]
89. Simmen, R.C.M.; Kelley, A.S. Reversal of Fortune: Estrogen Receptor-Beta in Endometriosis. *J. Mol. Endocrinol.* **2016**, *57*, F23–F27. [CrossRef] [PubMed]
90. Hamilton, K.J.; Arao, Y.; Korach, K.S. Estrogen hormone physiology: Reproductive findings from estrogen receptor mutant mice. *Reprod. Biol.* **2014**, *14*, 3–8. [CrossRef]
91. Bulun, S.E.; Monsavais, D.; Pavone, M.E.; Dyson, M.; Xue, Q.; Attar, E.; Tokunaga, H.; Su, E.J. Role of Estrogen Receptor-β in Endometriosis. *Semin. Reprod. Med.* **2012**, *30*, 39–45. [CrossRef]
92. Han, S.J.; Lee, J.E.; Cho, Y.J.; Park, M.J.; O'Malley, B.W. Genomic Function of Estrogen Receptor β in Endometriosis. *Endocrinology* **2019**, *160*, 2495–2516. [CrossRef]
93. McKinnon, B.; Mueller, M.; Montgomery, G. Progesterone Resistance in Endometriosis: An Acquired Property? *Trends Endocrinol. Metab.* **2018**, *29*, 535–548. [CrossRef]
94. Patel, B.G.; Rudnicki, M.; Yu, J.; Shu, Y.; Taylor, R.N. Progesterone resistance in endometriosis: Origins, consequences and interventions. *Acta Obstet. Gynecol. Scand.* **2017**, *96*, 623–632. [CrossRef] [PubMed]
95. Bulun, S.E.; Cheng, Y.-H.; Yin, P.; Imir, G.; Utsunomiya, H.; Attar, E.; Innes, J.; Julie Kim, J. Progesterone resistance in endometriosis: Link to failure to metabolize estradiol. *Mol. Cell. Endocrinol.* **2006**, *248*, 94–103. [CrossRef] [PubMed]

96. Grandi, G.; Mueller, M.D.; Bersinger, N.A.; Facchinetti, F.; McKinnon, B.D. The association between progestins, nuclear receptors expression and inflammation in endometrial stromal cells from women with endometriosis. *Gynecol. Endocrinol. Off. J. Int. Soc. Gynecol. Endocrinol.* **2017**, *33*, 712–715. [CrossRef] [PubMed]
97. Allport, V.C.; Pieber, D.; Slater, D.M.; Newton, R.; White, J.O.; Bennett, P.R. Human labour is associated with nuclear factor-kappaB activity which mediates cyclo-oxygenase-2 expression and is involved with the "functional progesterone withdrawal". *Mol. Hum. Reprod.* **2001**, *7*, 581–586. [CrossRef] [PubMed]
98. Cinar, O.; Seval, Y.; Uz, Y.H.; Cakmak, H.; Ulukus, M.; Kayisli, U.A.; Arici, A. Differential regulation of Akt phosphorylation in endometriosis. *Reprod. Biomed. Online* **2009**, *19*, 864–871. [CrossRef] [PubMed]
99. Treloar, S.A.; Zhao, Z.Z.; Armitage, T.; Duffy, D.L.; Wicks, J.; O'Connor, D.T.; Martin, N.G.; Montgomery, G.W. Association between polymorphisms in the progesterone receptor gene and endometriosis. *Mol. Hum. Reprod.* **2005**, *11*, 641–647. [CrossRef]
100. Ren, Y.; Liu, X.; Ma, D.; Feng, Y.; Zhong, N. Down-regulation of the progesterone receptor by the methylation of progesterone receptor gene in endometrial cancer cells. *Cancer Genet. Cytogenet.* **2007**, *175*, 107–116. [CrossRef]
101. Teague, E.M.C.O.; Print, C.G.; Hull, M.L. The role of microRNAs in endometriosis and associated reproductive conditions. *Hum. Reprod. Update* **2010**, *16*, 142–165. [CrossRef]
102. Rižner, T.L. Diagnostic potential of peritoneal fluid biomarkers of endometriosis. *Expert Rev. Mol. Diagn.* **2015**, *15*, 557–580. [CrossRef]
103. Haney, A.F.; Muscato, J.J.; Weinberg, J.B. Peritoneal fluid cell populations in infertility patients. *Fertil. Steril.* **1981**, *35*, 696–698. [CrossRef]
104. Hill, J.A.; Faris, H.M.; Schiff, I.; Anderson, D.J. Characterization of leukocyte subpopulations in the peritoneal fluid of women with endometriosis. *Fertil. Steril.* **1988**, *50*, 216–222. [CrossRef]
105. Jones, R.K.; Bulmer, J.N.; Searle, R.F. Phenotypic and functional studies of leukocytes in human endometrium and endometriosis. *Hum. Reprod. Update* **1998**, *4*, 702–709. [CrossRef] [PubMed]
106. Darrow, S.L.; Vena, J.E.; Batt, R.E.; Zielezny, M.A.; Michalek, A.M.; Selman, S. Menstrual cycle characteristics and the risk of endometriosis. *Epidemiology* **1993**, 135–142. [CrossRef] [PubMed]
107. Vercellini, P.; De Giorgi, O.; Aimi, G.; Panazza, S.; Uglietti, A.; Crosignani, P.G. Menstrual characteristics in women with and without endometriosis. *Obstet. Gynecol.* **1997**, *90*, 264–268. [CrossRef]
108. Salamanca, A.; Beltrán, E. Subendometrial contractility in menstrual phase visualized by transvaginal sonography in patients with endometriosis. *Fertil. Steril.* **1995**, *64*, 193–195. [CrossRef]
109. Sanfilippo, J.S.; Wakim, N.G.; Schikler, K.N.; Yussman, M.A. Endometriosis in association with uterine anomaly. *Am. J. Obstet. Gynecol.* **1986**, *154*, 39–43. [CrossRef]
110. Oosterlynck, D.J.; Cornillie, F.J.; Waer, M.; Vandeputte, M.; Koninckx, P.R. Women with endometriosis show a defect in natural killer activity resulting in a decreased cytotoxicity to autologous endometrium. *Fertil. Steril.* **1991**, *56*, 45–51. [CrossRef]
111. Laganà, A.S.; Triolo, O.; Salmeri, F.M.; Granese, R.; Palmara, V.I.; Ban Frangež, H.; Vrtčnik Bokal, E.; Sofo, V. Natural Killer T cell subsets in eutopic and ectopic endometrium: A fresh look to a busy corner. *Arch. Gynecol. Obstet.* **2016**, *293*, 941–949. [CrossRef]
112. Semino, C.; Semino, A.; Pietra, G.; Mingari, M.C.; Barocci, S.; Venturini, P.L.; Ragni, N.; Melioli, G. Role of major histocompatibility complex class I expression and natural killer-like T cells in the genetic control of endometriosis*. *Fertil. Steril.* **1995**, *64*, 909–916. [CrossRef]
113. Somigliana, E.; Viganò, P.; Gaffuri, B.; Guarneri, D.; Busacca, M.; Vignali, M. Human endometrial stromal cells as a source of soluble intercellular adhesion molecule (ICAM)-1 molecules. *Hum. Reprod. Oxf. Engl.* **1996**, *11*, 1190–1194. [CrossRef]
114. Viganò, P.; Gaffuri, B.; Somigliana, E.; Busacca, M.; Di Blasio, A.M.; Vignali, M. Expression of intercellular adhesion molecule (ICAM)-1 mRNA and protein is enhanced in endometriosis versus endometrial stromal cells in culture. *Mol. Hum. Reprod.* **1998**, *4*, 1150–1156. [CrossRef] [PubMed]
115. Králíčková, M.; Vetvicka, V. Immunological aspects of endometriosis: A review. *Ann. Transl. Med.* **2015**, *3*, 153. [PubMed]
116. Riccio, L.D.G.C.; Santulli, P.; Marcellin, L.; Abrão, M.S.; Batteux, F.; Chapron, C. Immunology of endometriosis. *Best Pract. Res. Clin. Obstet. Gynaecol.* **2018**, *50*, 39–49. [CrossRef] [PubMed]

117. Santulli, P.; Marcellin, L.; Tosti, C.; Chouzenoux, S.; Cerles, O.; Borghese, B.; Batteux, F.; Chapron, C. MAP kinases and the inflammatory signaling cascade as targets for the treatment of endometriosis? *Expert Opin. Ther. Targets* **2015**, *19*, 1465–1483. [CrossRef]
118. Martínez-Román, S.; Balasch, J.; Creus, M.; Fábregues, F.; Carmona, F.; Vilella, R.; Vanrell, J.A. Transferrin Receptor (CD71) Expression in Peritoneal Macrophages from Fertile and Infertile Women With and Without Endometriosis. *Am. J. Reprod. Immunol.* **1997**, *38*, 413–417. [CrossRef]
119. Raiter-Tenenbaum, A.; Barañao, R.I.; Etchepareborda, J.J.; Meresman, G.F.; Rumi, L.S. Functional and phenotypic alterations in peritoneal macrophages from patients with early and advanced endometriosis. *Arch. Gynecol. Obstet.* **1998**, *261*, 147–157. [CrossRef]
120. Halme, J.; Becker, S.; Wing, R. Accentuated cyclic activation of peritoneal macrophages in patients with endometriosis. *Am. J. Obstet. Gynecol.* **1984**, *148*, 85–90. [CrossRef]
121. McLaren, J.; Prentice, A.; Charnock-Jones, D.S.; Sharkey, A.M.; Smith, S.K. Immunolocalization of the apoptosis regulating proteins Bcl-2 and Bax in human endometrium and isolated peritoneal fluid macrophages in endometriosis. *Hum. Reprod.* **1997**, *12*, 146–152. [CrossRef]
122. Bacci, M.; Capobianco, A.; Monno, A.; Cottone, L.; Di Puppo, F.; Camisa, B.; Mariani, M.; Brignole, C.; Ponzoni, M.; Ferrari, S.; et al. Macrophages Are Alternatively Activated in Patients with Endometriosis and Required for Growth and Vascularization of Lesions in a Mouse Model of Disease. *Am. J. Pathol.* **2009**, *175*, 547–556. [CrossRef]
123. McLaren, J.; Dealtry, G.; Prentice, A.; Charnock-Jones, D.S.; Smith, S.K. Decreased levels of the potent regulator of monocyte/macrophage activation, interleukin-13, in the peritoneal fluid of patients with endometriosis. *Hum. Reprod. Oxf. Engl.* **1997**, *12*, 1307–1310. [CrossRef]
124. Schneider, C.; Kässens, N.; Greve, B.; Hassan, H.; Schüring, A.N.; Starzinski-Powitz, A.; Kiesel, L.; Seidler, D.G.; Götte, M. Targeting of syndecan-1 by micro-ribonucleic acid miR-10b modulates invasiveness of endometriotic cells via dysregulation of the proteolytic milieu and interleukin-6 secretion. *Fertil. Steril.* **2013**, *99*, 871–881. [CrossRef] [PubMed]
125. Götte, M.; Joussen, A.M.; Klein, C.; Andre, P.; Wagner, D.D.; Hinkes, M.T.; Kirchhof, B.; Adamis, A.P.; Bernfield, M. Role of syndecan-1 in leukocyte-endothelial interactions in the ocular vasculature. *Investig. Ophthalmol. Vis. Sci.* **2002**, *43*, 1135–1141. [PubMed]
126. Averbeck, M.; Kuhn, S.; Bühligen, J.; Götte, M.; Simon, J.C.; Polte, T. Syndecan-1 regulates dendritic cell migration in cutaneous hypersensitivity to haptens. *Exp. Dermatol.* **2017**, *26*, 1060–1067. [CrossRef] [PubMed]
127. Pizzo, A.; Salmeri, F.M.; Ardita, F.V.; Sofo, V.; Tripepi, M.; Marsico, S. Behaviour of cytokine levels in serum and peritoneal fluid of women with endometriosis. *Gynecol. Obstet. Investig.* **2002**, *54*, 82–87. [CrossRef]
128. de Barros, I.B.L.; Malvezzi, H.; Gueuvoghlanian-Silva, B.Y.; Piccinato, C.A.; Rizzo, L.V.; Podgaec, S. "What do we know about regulatory T cells and endometriosis? A systematic review". *J. Reprod. Immunol.* **2017**, *120*, 48–55. [CrossRef]
129. Riccio, L.G.C.; Baracat, E.C.; Chapron, C.; Batteux, F.; Abrão, M.S. The role of the B lymphocytes in endometriosis: A systematic review. *J. Reprod. Immunol.* **2017**, *123*, 29–34. [CrossRef]
130. Sattler, M.; Liang, H.; Nettesheim, D.; Meadows, R.P.; Harlan, J.E.; Eberstadt, M.; Yoon, H.S.; Shuker, S.B.; Chang, B.S.; Minn, A.J.; et al. Structure of Bcl-xL-Bak peptide complex: Recognition between regulators of apoptosis. *Science* **1997**, *275*, 983–986. [CrossRef]
131. Tabibzadeh, S.; Zupi, E.; Babaknia, A.; Liu, R.; Marconi, D.; Romanini, C. Site and menstrual cycle-dependent expression of proteins of the tumour necrosis factor (TNF) receptor family, and BCL-2 oncoprotein and phase-specific production of TNF alpha in human endometrium. *Hum. Reprod. Oxf. Engl.* **1995**, *10*, 277–286. [CrossRef]
132. Taniguchi, F.; Kaponis, A.; Izawa, M.; Kiyama, T.; Deura, I.; Ito, M.; Iwabe, T.; Adonakis, G.; Terakawa, N.; Harada, T. Apoptosis and endometriosis. *Front. Biosci. Elite Ed.* **2011**, *3*, 648–662. [CrossRef]
133. Gebel, H.M.; Braun, D.P.; Tambur, A.; Frame, D.; Rana, N.; Dmowski, W.P. Spontaneous apoptosis of endometrial tissue is impaired in women with endometriosis. *Fertil. Steril.* **1998**, *69*, 1042–1047. [CrossRef]
134. Béliard, A.; Noël, A.; Foidart, J.-M. Reduction of apoptosis and proliferation in endometriosis. *Fertil. Steril.* **2004**, *82*, 80–85. [CrossRef] [PubMed]

135. Lac, V.; Verhoef, L.; Aguirre-Hernandez, R.; Nazeran, T.M.; Tessier-Cloutier, B.; Praetorius, T.; Orr, N.L.; Noga, H.; Lum, A.; Khattra, J.; et al. Iatrogenic endometriosis harbors somatic cancer-driver mutations. *Hum. Reprod. Oxf. Engl.* **2019**, *34*, 69–78. [CrossRef] [PubMed]
136. Vetvicka, V.; Laganà, A.S.; Salmeri, F.M.; Triolo, O.; Palmara, V.I.; Vitale, S.G.; Sofo, V.; Králíčková, M. Regulation of apoptotic pathways during endometriosis: From the molecular basis to the future perspectives. *Arch. Gynecol. Obstet.* **2016**, *294*, 897–904. [CrossRef] [PubMed]
137. Sturlese, E.; Salmeri, F.M.; Retto, G.; Pizzo, A.; De Dominici, R.; Ardita, F.V.; Borrielli, I.; Licata, N.; Laganà, A.S.; Sofo, V. Dysregulation of the Fas/FasL system in mononuclear cells recovered from peritoneal fluid of women with endometriosis. *J. Reprod. Immunol.* **2011**, *92*, 74–81. [CrossRef] [PubMed]
138. Rutherford, E.J.; Hill, A.D.K.; Hopkins, A.M. Adhesion in Physiological, Benign and Malignant Proliferative States of the Endometrium: Microenvironment and the Clinical Big Picture. *Cells* **2018**, *7*, e43. [CrossRef] [PubMed]
139. Groothuis, P.G.; Koks, C.A.; de Goeij, A.F.; Dunselman, G.A.; Arends, J.W.; Evers, J.L. Adhesion of human endometrial fragments to peritoneum in vitro. *Fertil. Steril.* **1999**, *71*, 1119–1124. [CrossRef]
140. Koks, C.A.; Groothuis, P.G.; Dunselman, G.A.; de Goeij, A.F.; Evers, J.L. Adhesion of shed menstrual tissue in an in-vitro model using amnion and peritoneum: A light and electron microscopic study. *Hum. Reprod. Oxf. Engl.* **1999**, *14*, 816–822. [CrossRef]
141. Dunselman, G.A.; Groothuis, P.G.; de Goeij, A.F.; Evers, J.L. The Mesothelium, Teflon or Velcro? Mesothelium in endometriosis pathogenesis. *Hum. Reprod. Oxf. Engl.* **2001**, *16*, 605–607. [CrossRef]
142. Canis, M.; Bourdel, N.; Houlle, C.; Gremeau, A.-S.; Botchorishvili, R.; Matsuzaki, S. Trauma and endometriosis. A review. May we explain surgical phenotypes and natural history of the disease? *J. Gynecol. Obstet. Hum. Reprod.* **2017**, *46*, 219–227. [CrossRef]
143. Koks, C.A.; Demir Weusten, A.Y.; Groothuis, P.G.; Dunselman, G.A.; de Goeij, A.F.; Evers, J.L. Menstruum induces changes in mesothelial cell morphology. *Gynecol. Obstet. Investig.* **2000**, *50*, 13–18. [CrossRef]
144. Demir Weusten, A.Y.; Groothuis, P.G.; Dunselman, G.A.; de Goeij, A.F.; Arends, J.W.; Evers, J.L. Morphological changes in mesothelial cells induced by shed menstrual endometrium in vitro are not primarily due to apoptosis or necrosis. *Hum. Reprod. Oxf. Engl.* **2000**, *15*, 1462–1468. [CrossRef] [PubMed]
145. Demir, A.Y.; Groothuis, P.G.; Nap, A.W.; Punyadeera, C.; de Goeij, A.F.P.M.; Evers, J.L.H.; Dunselman, G.A.J. Menstrual effluent induces epithelial-mesenchymal transitions in mesothelial cells. *Hum. Reprod. Oxf. Engl.* **2004**, *19*, 21–29. [CrossRef] [PubMed]
146. Bilyk, O.; Coatham, M.; Jewer, M.; Postovit, L.-M. Epithelial-to-Mesenchymal Transition in the Female Reproductive Tract: From Normal Functioning to Disease Pathology. *Front. Oncol.* **2017**, *5*, 145. [CrossRef] [PubMed]
147. Yang, Y.-M.; Yang, W.-X. Epithelial-to-mesenchymal transition in the development of endometriosis. *Oncotarget* **2017**, *8*, 41679–41689. [CrossRef]
148. Lessey, B.A.; Damjanovich, L.; Coutifaris, C.; Castelbaum, A.; Albelda, S.M.; Buck, C.A. Integrin adhesion molecules in the human endometrium. Correlation with the normal and abnormal menstrual cycle. *J. Clin. Investig.* **1992**, *90*, 188–195. [CrossRef]
149. Lessey, B.A. Endometrial integrins and the establishment of uterine receptivity. *Hum. Reprod.* **1998**, *13*, 247–258. [CrossRef]
150. Tabibzadeh, S. Patterns of expression of integrin molecules in human endometrium throughout the menstrual cycle. *Hum. Reprod.* **1992**, *7*, 876–882. [CrossRef]
151. van der Linden, P.J.Q.; de Goeij, A.F.P.M.; Dunselman, G.A.J.; Erkens, H.W.H.; Evers, J.L.H. Expression of cadherins and integrins in human endometrium throughout the menstrual cycle**Supported in part by a research grant from Organon International B.V., Oss, The Netherlands. *Fertil. Steril.* **1995**, *63*, 1210–1216. [CrossRef]
152. Lessey, B.A.; Castelbaum, A.J.; Sawin, S.W.; Buck, C.A.; Schinnar, R.; Bilker, W.; Strom, B.L. Aberrant integrin expression in the endometrium of women with endometriosis. *J. Clin. Endocrinol. Metab.* **1994**, *79*, 643–649.
153. Lessey, B.A.; Kim, J.J. Endometrial receptivity in the eutopic endometrium of women with endometriosis: It is affected, and let me show you why. *Fertil. Steril.* **2017**, *108*, 19–27. [CrossRef]

154. Germeyer, A.; Klinkert, M.S.; Huppertz, A.-G.; Clausmeyer, S.; Popovici, R.M.; Strowitzki, T.; von Wolff, M. Expression of syndecans, cell-cell interaction regulating heparan sulfate proteoglycans, within the human endometrium and their regulation throughout the menstrual cycle. *Fertil. Steril.* **2007**, *87*, 657–663. [CrossRef] [PubMed]
155. Chelariu-Raicu, A.; Wilke, C.; Brand, M.; Starzinski-Powitz, A.; Kiesel, L.; Schüring, A.N.; Götte, M. Syndecan-4 expression is upregulated in endometriosis and contributes to an invasive phenotype. *Fertil. Steril.* **2016**, *106*, 378–385. [CrossRef] [PubMed]
156. Starzinski-Powitz, A.; Handrow-Metzmacher, H.; Kotzian, S. The putative role of cell adhesion molecules in endometriosis: Can we learn from tumour metastasis? *Mol. Med. Today* **1999**, *5*, 304–309. [CrossRef]
157. Gaetje, R.; Kotzian, S.; Herrmann, G.; Baumann, R.; Starzinski-Powitz, A. Nonmalignant epithelial cells, potentially invasive in human endometriosis, lack the tumor suppressor molecule E-cadherin. *Am. J. Pathol.* **1997**, *150*, 461–467.
158. Guilford, P. E-cadherin downregulation in cancer: Fuel on the fire? *Mol. Med. Today* **1999**, *5*, 172–177. [CrossRef]
159. Wijnhoven, B.P.; Dinjens, W.N.; Pignatelli, M. E-cadherin-catenin cell-cell adhesion complex and human cancer. *Br. J. Surg.* **2000**, *87*, 992–1005. [CrossRef]
160. van der Linden, P.J.; de Goeij, A.F.; Dunselman, G.A.; van der Linden, E.P.; Ramaekers, F.C.; Evers, J.L. Expression of integrins and E-cadherin in cells from menstrual effluent, endometrium, peritoneal fluid, peritoneum, and endometriosis. *Fertil. Steril.* **1994**, *61*, 85–90. [CrossRef]
161. Mashayekhi, F.; Aryaee, H.; Mirzajani, E.; Yasin, A.A.; Fathi, A. Soluble CD44 concentration in the serum and peritoneal fluid samples of patients with different stages of endometriosis. *Arch. Gynecol. Obstet.* **2015**, *292*, 641–645. [CrossRef]
162. Karousou, E.; Misra, S.; Ghatak, S.; Dobra, K.; Götte, M.; Vigetti, D.; Passi, A.; Karamanos, N.K.; Skandalis, S.S. Roles and targeting of the HAS/hyaluronan/CD44 molecular system in cancer. *Matrix Biol. J. Int. Soc. Matrix Biol.* **2017**, *59*, 3–22. [CrossRef]
163. Rodgers, A.K.; Nair, A.; Binkley, P.A.; Tekmal, R.; Schenken, R.S. Inhibition of CD44 N- and O-linked glycosylation decreases endometrial cell lines attachment to peritoneal mesothelial cells. *Fertil. Steril.* **2011**, *95*, 823–825. [CrossRef]
164. Knudtson, J.F.; Tekmal, R.R.; Santos, M.T.; Binkley, P.A.; Krishnegowda, N.; Valente, P.; Schenken, R.S. Impaired Development of Early Endometriotic Lesions in CD44 Knockout Mice. *Reprod. Sci. Thousand Oaks Calif* **2016**, *23*, 87–91. [CrossRef] [PubMed]
165. Olivares, C.N.; Alaniz, L.D.; Menger, M.D.; Barañao, R.I.; Laschke, M.W.; Meresman, G.F. Inhibition of Hyaluronic Acid Synthesis Suppresses Angiogenesis in Developing Endometriotic Lesions. *PloS ONE* **2016**, *11*, e0152302. [CrossRef] [PubMed]
166. Bałkowiec, M.; Maksym, R.B.; Włodarski, P.K. The bimodal role of matrix metalloproteinases and their inhibitors in etiology and pathogenesis of endometriosis. *Mol. Med. Rep.* **2018**, *18*, 3123–3136. [CrossRef] [PubMed]
167. Murphy, G.; Willenbrock, F.; Crabbe, T.; O'Shea, M.; Ward, R.; Atkinson, S.; O'Connell, J.; Docherty, A. Regulation of matrix metalloproteinase activity. *Ann. N. Y. Acad. Sci.* **1994**, *732*, 31–41. [CrossRef]
168. Nagase, H. Activation mechanisms of matrix metalloproteinases. *Biol. Chem.* **1997**, *378*, 151–160.
169. Smigiel, K.S.; Parks, W.C. Matrix Metalloproteinases and Leukocyte Activation. *Prog. Mol. Biol. Transl. Sci.* **2017**, *147*, 167–195.
170. Marbaix, E.; Kokorine, I.; Henriet, P.; Donnez, J.; Courtoy, P.J.; Eeckhout, Y. The expression of interstitial collagenase in human endometrium is controlled by progesterone and by oestradiol and is related to menstruation. *Biochem. J.* **1995**, *305*, 1027–1030. [CrossRef]
171. Hulboy, D.L.; Rudolph, L.A.; Matrisian, L.M. Matrix metalloproteinases as mediators of reproductive function. *Mol. Hum. Reprod.* **1997**, *3*, 27–45. [CrossRef]
172. Rodgers, W.H.; Matrisian, L.M.; Giudice, L.C.; Dsupin, B.; Cannon, P.; Svitek, C.; Gorstein, F.; Osteen, K.G. Patterns of matrix metalloproteinase expression in cycling endometrium imply differential functions and regulation by steroid hormones. *J. Clin. Investig.* **1994**, *94*, 946–953. [CrossRef]

173. Bruner, K.L.; Eisenberg, E.; Gorstein, F.; Osteen, K.G. Progesterone and transforming growth factor-β coordinately regulate suppression of endometrial matrix metalloproteinases in a model of experimental endometriosis. *Steroids* **1999**, *64*, 648–653. [CrossRef]

174. Spuijbroek, M.D.; Dunselman, G.A.; Menheere, P.P.; Evers, J.L. Early endometriosis invades the extracellular matrix. *Fertil. Steril.* **1992**, *58*, 929–933. [CrossRef]

175. Osteen, K.G.; Bruner-Tran, K.L.; Keller, N.R.; Eisenberg, E. Progesterone-Mediated Endometrial Maturation Limits Matrix Metalloproteinase (MMP) Expression in an Inflammatory-like Environment. *Ann. N. Y. Acad. Sci.* **2002**, *955*, 37–47. [CrossRef] [PubMed]

176. Salamonsen, L.A.; Woolley, D.E. Matrix metalloproteinases in normal menstruation. *Hum. Reprod. Oxf. Engl.* **1996**, *11* (Suppl. 2), 124–133. [CrossRef]

177. Salamonsen, L.A.; Zhang, J.; Hampton, A.; Lathbury, L. Regulation of matrix metalloproteinases in human endometrium. *Hum. Reprod. Oxf. Engl.* **2000**, *15* (Suppl. 3), 112–119. [CrossRef]

178. Bruner, K.L.; Matrisian, L.M.; Rodgers, W.H.; Gorstein, F.; Osteen, K.G. Suppression of matrix metalloproteinases inhibits establishment of ectopic lesions by human endometrium in nude mice. *J. Clin. Investig.* **1997**, *99*, 2851–2857. [CrossRef] [PubMed]

179. Nap, A.W.; Dunselman, G.A.J.; de Goeij, A.F.P.M.; Evers, J.L.H.; Groothuis, P.G. Inhibiting MMP activity prevents the development of endometriosis in the chicken chorioallantoic membrane model. *Hum. Reprod.* **2004**, *19*, 2180–2187. [CrossRef] [PubMed]

180. Osteen, K.G.; Bruner, K.L.; Sharpe-Timms, K.L. Steroid and growth factor regulation of matrix metalloproteinase expression and endometriosis. *Semin. Reprod. Endocrinol.* **1996**, *14*, 247–255. [CrossRef] [PubMed]

181. Sillem, M.; Prifti, S.; Neher, M.; Runnebaum, B. Extracellular matrix remodelling in the endometrium and its possible relevance to the pathogenesis of endometriosis. *Hum. Reprod. Update* **1998**, *4*, 730–735. [CrossRef] [PubMed]

182. Sharpe-Timms, K.L.; Keisler, L.W.; McIntush, E.W.; Keisler, D.H. Tissue inhibitor of metalloproteinase-1 concentrations are attenuated in peritoneal fluid and sera of women with endometriosis and restored in sera by gonadotropin-releasing hormone agonist therapy. *Fertil. Steril.* **1998**, *69*, 1128–1134. [CrossRef]

183. Cox, K.E.; Piva, M.; Sharpe-Timms, K.L. Differential regulation of matrix metalloproteinase-3 gene expression in endometriotic lesions compared with endometrium. *Biol. Reprod.* **2001**, *65*, 1297–1303. [CrossRef]

184. Sharpe-Timms, K.L.; Cox, K.E. Paracrine regulation of matrix metalloproteinase expression in endometriosis. *Ann. N. Y. Acad. Sci.* **2002**, *955*, 147–156; discussion 157–158, 396–406. [CrossRef] [PubMed]

185. Pitsos, M.; Kanakas, N. The role of matrix metalloproteinases in the pathogenesis of endometriosis. *Reprod. Sci. Thousand Oaks Calif* **2009**, *16*, 717–726. [CrossRef] [PubMed]

186. Zhou, H.-E.; Nothnick, W.B. The relevancy of the matrix metalloproteinase system to the pathophysiology of endometriosis. *Front. Biosci. J. Virtual Libr.* **2005**, *10*, 569–575. [CrossRef] [PubMed]

187. Osteen, K.G.; Bruner-Tran, K.L.; Eisenberg, E. Reduced progesterone action during endometrial maturation: A potential risk factor for the development of endometriosis. *Fertil. Steril.* **2005**, *83*, 529–537. [CrossRef] [PubMed]

188. Stamenkovic, I. Extracellular matrix remodelling: The role of matrix metalloproteinases. *J. Pathol.* **2003**, *200*, 448–464. [CrossRef] [PubMed]

189. Maas, J.W.; Le Noble, F.A.; Dunselman, G.A.; de Goeij, A.F.; Struyker Boudier, H.A.; Evers, J.L. The chick embryo chorioallantoic membrane as a model to investigate the angiogenic properties of human endometrium. *Gynecol. Obstet. Investig.* **1999**, *48*, 108–112. [CrossRef]

190. Griffioen, A.W.; Molema, G. Angiogenesis: Potentials for pharmacologic intervention in the treatment of cancer, cardiovascular diseases, and chronic inflammation. *Pharmacol. Rev.* **2000**, *52*, 237–268.

191. McLaren, J. Vascular endothelial growth factor and endometriotic angiogenesis. *Hum. Reprod. Update* **2000**, *6*, 45–55. [CrossRef]

192. Charnock-Jones, D.S.; Sharkey, A.M.; Rajput-Williams, J.; Burch, D.; Schofield, J.P.; Fountain, S.A.; Boocock, C.A.; Smith, S.K. Identification and localization of alternately spliced mRNAs for vascular endothelial growth factor in human uterus and estrogen regulation in endometrial carcinoma cell lines. *Biol. Reprod.* **1993**, *48*, 1120–1128. [CrossRef]

193. Smith, S.K. Regulation of angiogenesis in the endometrium. *Trends Endocrinol. Metab. TEM* **2001**, *12*, 147–151. [CrossRef]
194. Donnez, J.; Smoes, P.; Gillerot, S.; Casanas-Roux, F.; Nisolle, M. Vascular endothelial growth factor (VEGF) in endometriosis. *Hum. Reprod. Oxf. Engl.* **1998**, *13*, 1686–1690. [CrossRef] [PubMed]
195. Wingfield, M.; Macpherson, A.; Healy, D.L.; Rogers, P.A. Cell proliferation is increased in the endometrium of women with endometriosis. *Fertil. Steril.* **1995**, *64*, 340–346. [CrossRef]
196. Bourlev, V.; Volkov, N.; Pavlovitch, S.; Lets, N.; Larsson, A.; Olovsson, M. The relationship between microvessel density, proliferative activity and expression of vascular endothelial growth factor-A and its receptors in eutopic endometrium and endometriotic lesions. *Reproduction* **2006**, *132*, 501–509. [CrossRef] [PubMed]
197. Matsuzaki, S.; Canis, M.; Murakami, T.; Dechelotte, P.; Bruhat, M.A.; Okamura, K. Immunohistochemical analysis of the role of angiogenic status in the vasculature of peritoneal endometriosis. *Fertil. Steril.* **2001**, *76*, 712–716. [CrossRef]
198. Hull, M.L.; Charnock-Jones, D.S.; Chan, C.L.K.; Bruner-Tran, K.L.; Osteen, K.G.; Tom, B.D.M.; Fan, T.-P.D.; Smith, S.K. Antiangiogenic agents are effective inhibitors of endometriosis. *J. Clin. Endocrinol. Metab.* **2003**, *88*, 2889–2899. [CrossRef]
199. Nap, A.W.; Dunselman, G.A.J.; Griffioen, A.W.; Mayo, K.H.; Evers, J.L.H.; Groothuis, P.G. Angiostatic agents prevent the development of endometriosis-like lesions in the chicken chorioallantoic membrane. *Fertil. Steril.* **2005**, *83*, 793–795. [CrossRef]
200. Nap, A.W.; Griffioen, A.W.; Dunselman, G.A.J.; Bouma-Ter Steege, J.C.A.; Thijssen, V.L.J.L.; Evers, J.L.H.; Groothuis, P.G. Antiangiogenesis therapy for endometriosis. *J. Clin. Endocrinol. Metab.* **2004**, *89*, 1089–1095. [CrossRef]
201. Van Langendonckt, A.; Donnez, J.; Defrère, S.; Dunselman, G.A.J.; Groothuis, P.G. Antiangiogenic and vascular-disrupting agents in endometriosis: Pitfalls and promises. *Mol. Hum. Reprod.* **2008**, *14*, 259–268. [CrossRef]
202. Becker, C.M.; D'Amato, R.J. Angiogenesis and antiangiogenic therapy in endometriosis. *Microvasc. Res.* **2007**, *74*, 121–130. [CrossRef]
203. May, K.; Becker, C.M. Endometriosis and angiogenesis. *Minerva Ginecol.* **2008**, *60*, 245–254.
204. Taylor, R.N.; Yu, J.; Torres, P.B.; Schickedanz, A.C.; Park, J.K.; Mueller, M.D.; Sidell, N. Mechanistic and Therapeutic Implications of Angiogenesis in Endometriosis. *Reprod. Sci. Thousand Oaks Calif* **2009**, *16*, 140–146. [CrossRef] [PubMed]
205. Körbel, C.; Gerstner, M.D.; Menger, M.D.; Laschke, M.W. Notch signaling controls sprouting angiogenesis of endometriotic lesions. *Angiogenesis* **2018**, *21*, 37–46. [CrossRef] [PubMed]
206. Maruyama, T.; Yoshimura, Y. Stem cell theory for the pathogenesis of endometriosis. *Front. Biosci. Elite Ed.* **2012**, *4*, 2754–2763. [CrossRef] [PubMed]
207. Gargett, C.E.; Masuda, H. Adult stem cells in the endometrium. *Mol. Hum. Reprod.* **2010**, *16*, 818–834. [CrossRef] [PubMed]
208. Taylor, H.S. Endometrial cells derived from donor stem cells in bone marrow transplant recipients. *JAMA* **2004**, *292*, 81–85. [CrossRef] [PubMed]
209. Masuda, H.; Matsuzaki, Y.; Hiratsu, E.; Ono, M.; Nagashima, T.; Kajitani, T.; Arase, T.; Oda, H.; Uchida, H.; Asada, H.; et al. Stem Cell-Like Properties of the Endometrial Side Population: Implication in Endometrial Regeneration. *PLoS ONE* **2010**, *5*, e10387. [CrossRef] [PubMed]
210. Wu, Y.; Basir, Z.; Kajdacsy-Balla, A.; Strawn, E.; Macias, V.; Montgomery, K.; Guo, S.-W. Resolution of clonal origins for endometriotic lesions using laser capture microdissection and the human androgen receptor (HUMARA) assay. *Fertil. Steril.* **2003**, *79*, 710–717. [CrossRef]
211. Nabeshima, H.; Murakami, T.; Yoshinaga, K.; Sato, K.; Terada, Y.; Okamura, K. Analysis of the clonality of ectopic glands in peritoneal endometriosis using laser microdissection. *Fertil. Steril.* **2003**, *80*, 1144–1150. [CrossRef]
212. Mayr, D.; Amann, G.; Siefert, C.; Diebold, J.; Anderegg, B. Does endometriosis really have premalignant potential? A clonal analysis of laser-microdissected tissue. *FASEB J.* **2003**, *17*, 693–695. [CrossRef]
213. Maruyama, T.; Masuda, H.; Ono, M.; Kajitani, T.; Yoshimura, Y. Human uterine stem/progenitor cells: Their possible role in uterine physiology and pathology. *Reprod. Camb. Engl.* **2010**, *140*, 11–22. [CrossRef]

214. Wang, Y.; Sacchetti, A.; van Dijk, M.R.; van der Zee, M.; van der Horst, P.H.; Joosten, R.; Burger, C.W.; Grootegoed, J.A.; Blok, L.J.; Fodde, R. Identification of Quiescent, Stem-Like Cells in the Distal Female Reproductive Tract. *PLOS ONE* **2012**, *7*, e40691. [CrossRef] [PubMed]
215. Laganà, A.S.; Salmeri, F.M.; Vitale, S.G.; Triolo, O.; Götte, M. Stem Cell Trafficking During Endometriosis: May Epigenetics Play a Pivotal Role? *Reprod. Sci. Thousand Oaks Calif* **2018**, *25*, 978–979. [CrossRef] [PubMed]
216. Schüring, A.N.; Dahlhues, B.; Korte, A.; Kiesel, L.; Titze, U.; Heitkötter, B.; Ruckert, C.; Götte, M. The endometrial stem cell markers notch-1 and numb are associated with endometriosis. *Reprod. Biomed. Online* **2018**, *36*, 294–301. [CrossRef] [PubMed]
217. Götte, M.; Wolf, M.; Staebler, A.; Buchweitz, O.; Kiesel, L.; Schüring, A.N. Aberrant expression of the pluripotency marker SOX-2 in endometriosis. *Fertil. Steril.* **2011**, *95*, 338–341. [CrossRef] [PubMed]
218. Adammek, M.; Greve, B.; Kässens, N.; Schneider, C.; Brüggemann, K.; Schüring, A.N.; Starzinski-Powitz, A.; Kiesel, L.; Götte, M. MicroRNA miR-145 inhibits proliferation, invasiveness, and stem cell phenotype of an in vitro endometriosis model by targeting multiple cytoskeletal elements and pluripotency factors. *Fertil. Steril.* **2013**, *99*, 1346–1355. [CrossRef]
219. Eggers, J.C.; Martino, V.; Reinbold, R.; Schäfer, S.D.; Kiesel, L.; Starzinski-Powitz, A.; Schüring, A.N.; Kemper, B.; Greve, B.; Götte, M. microRNA miR-200b affects proliferation, invasiveness and stemness of endometriotic cells by targeting ZEB1, ZEB2 and KLF4. *Reprod. Biomed. Online* **2016**, *32*, 434–445. [CrossRef]
220. Sapkota, Y.; Steinthorsdottir, V.; Morris, A.P.; Fassbender, A.; Rahmioglu, N.; De Vivo, I.; Buring, J.E.; Zhang, F.; Edwards, T.L.; Jones, S.; et al. Meta-analysis identifies five novel loci associated with endometriosis highlighting key genes involved in hormone metabolism. *Nat. Commun.* **2017**, *8*, 15539. [CrossRef]
221. Bouaziz, J.; Mashiach, R.; Cohen, S.; Kedem, A.; Baron, A.; Zajicek, M.; Feldman, I.; Seidman, D.; Soriano, D. How Artificial Intelligence Can Improve Our Understanding of the Genes Associated with Endometriosis: Natural Language Processing of the PubMed Database. *BioMed Res. Int.* **2018**, *2018*, 6217812. [CrossRef]
222. Gajbhiye, R.; Fung, J.N.; Montgomery, G.W. Complex genetics of female fertility. *NPJ Genomic Med.* **2018**, *3*, 29. [CrossRef]
223. Kennedy, S. The genetics of endometriosis. *J. Reprod. Med.* **1998**, *43*, 263–268.
224. Simpson, J.L.; Bischoff, F.Z. Heritability and molecular genetic studies of endometriosis. *Ann. N. Y. Acad. Sci.* **2002**, *955*, 239–251; discussion 293–295, 396–406. [CrossRef] [PubMed]
225. Stefansson, H.; Geirsson, R.T.; Steinthorsdottir, V.; Jonsson, H.; Manolescu, A.; Kong, A.; Ingadottir, G.; Gulcher, J.; Stefansson, K. Genetic factors contribute to the risk of developing endometriosis. *Hum. Reprod. Oxf. Engl.* **2002**, *17*, 555–559. [CrossRef] [PubMed]
226. Treloar, S.; Hadfield, R.; Montgomery, G.; Lambert, A.; Wicks, J.; Barlow, D.H.; O'Connor, D.T.; Kennedy, S.; International Endogene Study Group. The International Endogene Study: A collection of families for genetic research in endometriosis. *Fertil. Steril.* **2002**, *78*, 679–685. [CrossRef]
227. Zondervan, K.T.; Cardon, L.R.; Kennedy, S.H. The genetic basis of endometriosis. *Curr. Opin. Obstet. Gynecol.* **2001**, *13*, 309–314. [CrossRef]
228. Zondervan, K.T.; Weeks, D.E.; Colman, R.; Cardon, L.R.; Hadfield, R.; Schleffler, J.; Trainor, A.G.; Coe, C.L.; Kemnitz, J.W.; Kennedy, S.H. Familial aggregation of endometriosis in a large pedigree of rhesus macaques. *Hum. Reprod. Oxf. Engl.* **2004**, *19*, 448–455. [CrossRef]
229. Kennedy, S.; Mardon, H.; Barlow, D. Familial endometriosis. *J. Assist. Reprod. Genet.* **1995**, *12*, 32–34. [CrossRef]
230. Hadfield, R.M.; Mardon, H.J.; Barlow, D.H.; Kennedy, S.H. Endometriosis in monozygotic twins. *Fertil. Steril.* **1997**, *68*, 941–942. [CrossRef]
231. Moen, M.H. Endometriosis in monozygotic twins. *Acta Obstet. Gynecol. Scand.* **1994**, *73*, 59–62. [CrossRef]
232. Treloar, S.A.; O'Connor, D.T.; O'Connor, V.M.; Martin, N.G. Genetic influences on endometriosis in an Australian twin sample. *Fertil. Steril.* **1999**, *71*, 701–710. [CrossRef]
233. Di, W.; Guo, S.-W. The search for genetic variants predisposing women to endometriosis. *Curr. Opin. Obstet. Gynecol.* **2007**, *19*, 395–401. [CrossRef]
234. Falconer, H.; D'Hooghe, T.; Fried, G. Endometriosis and genetic polymorphisms. *Obstet. Gynecol. Surv.* **2007**, *62*, 616–628. [CrossRef] [PubMed]
235. Guo, S.-W. Glutathione S-transferases M1/T1 gene polymorphisms and endometriosis: A meta-analysis of genetic association studies. *Mol. Hum. Reprod.* **2005**, *11*, 729–743. [CrossRef] [PubMed]

236. Guo, S.-W. The association of endometriosis risk and genetic polymorphisms involving dioxin detoxification enzymes: A systematic review. *Eur. J. Obstet. Gynecol. Reprod. Biol.* **2006**, *124*, 134–143. [CrossRef] [PubMed]
237. Guo, S.-W. Association of endometriosis risk and genetic polymorphisms involving sex steroid biosynthesis and their receptors: A meta-analysis. *Gynecol. Obstet. Investig.* **2006**, *61*, 90–105. [CrossRef] [PubMed]
238. Montgomery, G.W.; Nyholt, D.R.; Zhao, Z.Z.; Treloar, S.A.; Painter, J.N.; Missmer, S.A.; Kennedy, S.H.; Zondervan, K.T. The search for genes contributing to endometriosis risk. *Hum. Reprod. Update* **2008**, *14*, 447–457. [CrossRef] [PubMed]
239. Çayan, F.; Ayaz, L.; Aban, M.; Dilek, S.; Gümüş, L.T. Role of CYP2C19 polymorphisms in patients with endometriosis. *Gynecol. Endocrinol.* **2009**, *25*, 530–535. [CrossRef] [PubMed]
240. Bozdag, G.; Alp, A.; Saribas, Z.; Tuncer, S.; Aksu, T.; Gurgan, T. CYP17 and CYP2C19 gene polymorphisms in patients with endometriosis. *Reprod. Biomed. Online* **2010**, *20*, 286–290. [CrossRef]
241. Guo, S.-W.; Simsa, P.; Kyama, C.M.; Mihályi, A.; Fülöp, V.; Othman, E.-E.R.; D'Hooghe, T.M. Reassessing the evidence for the link between dioxin and endometriosis: From molecular biology to clinical epidemiology. *MHR Basic Sci. Reprod. Med.* **2009**, *15*, 609–624. [CrossRef]
242. Ioannidis, J.P.A.; Ntzani, E.E.; Trikalinos, T.A.; Contopoulos-Ioannidis, D.G. Replication validity of genetic association studies. *Nat. Genet.* **2001**, *29*, 306–309. [CrossRef]
243. Lohmueller, K.E.; Pearce, C.L.; Pike, M.; Lander, E.S.; Hirschhorn, J.N. Meta-analysis of genetic association studies supports a contribution of common variants to susceptibility to common disease. *Nat. Genet.* **2003**, *33*, 177–182. [CrossRef]
244. Hindorff, L.A.; Sethupathy, P.; Junkins, H.A.; Ramos, E.M.; Mehta, J.P.; Collins, F.S.; Manolio, T.A. Potential etiologic and functional implications of genome-wide association loci for human diseases and traits. *Proc. Natl. Acad. Sci.* **2009**, *106*, 9362–9367. [CrossRef] [PubMed]
245. McCarthy, M.I.; Abecasis, G.R.; Cardon, L.R.; Goldstein, D.B.; Little, J.; Ioannidis, J.P.A.; Hirschhorn, J.N. Genome-wide association studies for complex traits: Consensus, uncertainty and challenges. *Nat. Rev. Genet.* **2008**, *9*, 356–369. [CrossRef] [PubMed]
246. Visscher, P.M.; Montgomery, G.W. Genome-wide association studies and human disease: From trickle to flood. *JAMA* **2009**, *302*, 2028–2029. [CrossRef] [PubMed]
247. Zondervan, K.; Cardon, L.; Desrosiers, R.; Hyde, D.; Kemnitz, J.; Mansfield, K.; Roberts, J.; Scheffler, J.; Weeks, D.E.; Kennedy, S. The Genetic Epidemiology of Spontaneous Endometriosis in the Rhesus Monkey. *Ann. N. Y. Acad. Sci.* **2002**, *955*, 233–238. [CrossRef]
248. Zondervan, K.T.; Cardon, L.R. The complex interplay among factors that influence allelic association. *Nat. Rev. Genet.* **2004**, *5*, 89–100. [CrossRef]
249. Hirschhorn, J.N.; Lohmueller, K.; Byrne, E.; Hirschhorn, K. A comprehensive review of genetic association studies. *Genet. Med.* **2002**, *4*, 45–61. [CrossRef]
250. Kruglyak, L.; Lander, E.S. Complete multipoint sib-pair analysis of qualitative and quantitative traits. *Am. J. Hum. Genet.* **1995**, *57*, 439–454.
251. Lander, E.; Kruglyak, L. Genetic dissection of complex traits: Guidelines for interpreting and reporting linkage results. *Nat. Genet.* **1995**, *11*, 241. [CrossRef]
252. Risch, N. Linkage strategies for genetically complex traits. II. The power of affected relative pairs. *Am. J. Hum. Genet.* **1990**, *46*, 229–241.
253. Treloar, S.A.; Wicks, J.; Nyholt, D.R.; Montgomery, G.W.; Bahlo, M.; Smith, V.; Dawson, G.; Mackay, I.J.; Weeks, D.E.; Bennett, S.T.; et al. Genomewide Linkage Study in 1,176 Affected Sister Pair Families Identifies a Significant Susceptibility Locus for Endometriosis on Chromosome 10q26. *Am. J. Hum. Genet.* **2005**, *77*, 365–376. [CrossRef]
254. Miki, Y.; Swensen, J.; Shattuck-Eidens, D.; Futreal, P.A.; Harshman, K.; Tavtigian, S.; Liu, Q.; Cochran, C.; Bennett, L.M.; Ding, W.; et al. A strong candidate for the breast and ovarian cancer susceptibility gene BRCA1. *Science* **1994**, *266*, 66–71. [CrossRef] [PubMed]
255. Wooster, R.; Bignell, G.; Lancaster, J.; Swift, S.; Seal, S.; Mangion, J.; Collins, N.; Gregory, S.; Gumbs, C.; Micklem, G.; et al. Identification of the breast cancer susceptibility gene BRCA2. *Nature* **1995**, *378*, 789. [CrossRef] [PubMed]
256. Zondervan, K.T.; Treloar, S.A.; Lin, J.; Weeks, D.E.; Nyholt, D.R.; Mangion, J.; MacKay, I.J.; Cardon, L.R.; Martin, N.G.; Kennedy, S.H.; et al. Significant evidence of one or more susceptibility loci for endometriosis

with near-Mendelian inheritance on chromosome 7p13–15. *Hum. Reprod.* **2007**, *22*, 717–728. [CrossRef] [PubMed]
257. The International HapMap Consortium A second generation human haplotype map of over 3.1 million SNPs. *Nature* **2007**, *449*, 851–861. [CrossRef]
258. Treloar, S.A.; Zhao, Z.Z.; Le, L.; Zondervan, K.T.; Martin, N.G.; Kennedy, S.; Nyholt, D.R.; Montgomery, G.W. Variants in EMX2 and PTEN do not contribute to risk of endometriosis. *MHR Basic Sci. Reprod. Med.* **2007**, *13*, 587–594. [CrossRef] [PubMed]
259. Daftary, G.S.; Taylor, H.S. EMX2 Gene Expression in the Female Reproductive Tract and Aberrant Expression in the Endometrium of Patients with Endometriosis. *J. Clin. Endocrinol. Metab.* **2004**, *89*, 2390–2396. [CrossRef] [PubMed]
260. Troy, P.J.; Daftary, G.S.; Bagot, C.N.; Taylor, H.S. Transcriptional Repression of Peri-Implantation EMX2 Expression in Mammalian Reproduction by HOXA10. *Mol. Cell. Biol.* **2003**, *23*, 1–13. [CrossRef]
261. Maxwell, G.L.; Risinger, J.I.; Gumbs, C.; Shaw, H.; Bentley, R.C.; Barrett, J.C.; Berchuck, A.; Futreal, P.A. Mutation of the PTEN Tumor Suppressor Gene in Endometrial Hyperplasias. *Cancer Res.* **1998**, *58*, 2500–2503.
262. Easton, D.F.; Pooley, K.A.; Dunning, A.M.; Pharoah, P.D.P.; Thompson, D.; Ballinger, D.G.; Struewing, J.P.; Morrison, J.; Field, H.; Luben, R.; et al. Genome-wide association study identifies novel breast cancer susceptibility loci. *Nature* **2007**, *447*, 1087–1093. [CrossRef]
263. Pollock, P.M.; Gartside, M.G.; Dejeza, L.C.; Powell, M.A.; Mallon, M.A.; Cancer Genome Project; Davies, H.; Mohammadi, M.; Futreal, P.A.; Stratton, M.R.; et al. Frequent activating FGFR2 mutations in endometrial carcinomas parallel germline mutations associated with craniosynostosis and skeletal dysplasia syndromes. *Oncogene* **2007**, *26*, 7158–7162. [CrossRef]
264. Zhao, Z.Z.; Pollock, P.M.; Thomas, S.; Treloar, S.A.; Nyholt, D.R.; Montgomery, G.W. Common variation in the fibroblast growth factor receptor 2 gene is not associated with endometriosis risk. *Hum. Reprod.* **2008**, *23*, 1661–1668. [CrossRef] [PubMed]
265. Zondervan, K.T.; Cardon, L.R. Designing candidate gene and genome-wide case–control association studies. *Nat. Protoc.* **2007**, *2*, 2492–2501. [CrossRef] [PubMed]
266. Zöllner, S.; Pritchard, J.K. Overcoming the Winner's Curse: Estimating Penetrance Parameters from Case-Control Data. *Am. J. Hum. Genet.* **2007**, *80*, 605–615. [CrossRef] [PubMed]
267. Sabeti, P.C.; Varilly, P.; Fry, B.; Lohmueller, J.; Hostetter, E.; Cotsapas, C.; Xie, X.; Byrne, E.H.; McCarroll, S.A.; Gaudet, R.; et al. Genome-wide detection and characterization of positive selection in human populations. *Nature* **2007**, *449*, 913–918. [CrossRef]
268. Uno, S.; Zembutsu, H.; Hirasawa, A.; Takahashi, A.; Kubo, M.; Akahane, T.; Aoki, D.; Kamatani, N.; Hirata, K.; Nakamura, Y. A genome-wide association study identifies genetic variants in the *CDKN2BAS* locus associated with endometriosis in Japanese. *Nat. Genet.* **2010**, *42*, 707–710. [CrossRef]
269. Kondera-Anasz, Z.; Sikora, J.; Mielczarek-Palacz, A.; Jońca, M. Concentrations of interleukin (IL)-1α, IL-1 soluble receptor type II (IL-1 sRII) and IL-1 receptor antagonist (IL-1 Ra) in the peritoneal fluid and serum of infertile women with endometriosis. *Eur. J. Obstet. Gynecol. Reprod. Biol.* **2005**, *123*, 198–203. [CrossRef]
270. Adachi, S.; Tajima, A.; Quan, J.; Haino, K.; Yoshihara, K.; Masuzaki, H.; Katabuchi, H.; Ikuma, K.; Suginami, H.; Nishida, N.; et al. Meta-analysis of genome-wide association scans for genetic susceptibility to endometriosis in Japanese population. *J. Hum. Genet.* **2010**, *55*, 816–821. [CrossRef]
271. Zanatta, A.; Rocha, A.M.; Carvalho, F.M.; Pereira, R.M.A.; Taylor, H.S.; Motta, E.L.A.; Baracat, E.C.; Serafini, P.C. The role of the Hoxa10/HOXA10 gene in the etiology of endometriosis and its related infertility: A review. *J. Assist. Reprod. Genet.* **2010**, *27*, 701–710. [CrossRef]
272. Naillat, F.; Prunskaite-Hyyryläinen, R.; Pietilä, I.; Sormunen, R.; Jokela, T.; Shan, J.; Vainio, S.J. Wnt4/5a signalling coordinates cell adhesion and entry into meiosis during presumptive ovarian follicle development. *Hum. Mol. Genet.* **2010**, *19*, 1539–1550. [CrossRef]
273. Boyer, A.; Lapointe, É.; Zheng, X.; Cowan, R.G.; Li, H.; Quirk, S.M.; DeMayo, F.J.; Richards, J.S.; Boerboom, D. WNT4 is required for normal ovarian follicle development and female fertility. *FASEB J.* **2010**, *24*, 3010–3025. [CrossRef]
274. MacDonald, B.T.; Tamai, K.; He, X. Wnt/β-Catenin Signaling: Components, Mechanisms, and Diseases. *Dev. Cell* **2009**, *17*, 9–26. [CrossRef] [PubMed]

275. Yang, J.; Benyamin, B.; McEvoy, B.P.; Gordon, S.; Henders, A.K.; Nyholt, D.R.; Madden, P.A.; Heath, A.C.; Martin, N.G.; Montgomery, G.W.; et al. Common SNPs explain a large proportion of the heritability for human height. *Nat. Genet.* **2010**, *42*, 565–569. [CrossRef] [PubMed]
276. Painter, J.N.; Anderson, C.A.; Nyholt, D.R.; Macgregor, S.; Lin, J.; Lee, S.H.; Lambert, A.; Zhao, Z.Z.; Roseman, F.; Guo, Q.; et al. Genome-wide association study identifies a locus at 7p15.2 associated with endometriosis. *Nat. Genet.* **2011**, *43*, 51–54. [CrossRef] [PubMed]
277. Bodmer, W.; Bonilla, C. Common and rare variants in multifactorial susceptibility to common diseases. *Nat. Genet.* **2008**, *40*, 695–701. [CrossRef]
278. Gorlov, I.P.; Gorlova, O.Y.; Sunyaev, S.R.; Spitz, M.R.; Amos, C.I. Shifting Paradigm of Association Studies: Value of Rare Single-Nucleotide Polymorphisms. *Am. J. Hum. Genet.* **2008**, *82*, 100–112. [CrossRef]
279. Curtin, K.; Iles, M.M.; Camp, N.J. Identifying Rarer Genetic Variants for Common Complex Diseases: Diseased Versus Neutral Discovery Panels. *Ann. Hum. Genet.* **2009**, *73*, 54–60. [CrossRef]
280. Iles, M.M. What Can Genome-Wide Association Studies Tell Us about the Genetics of Common Disease? *PLOS Genet.* **2008**, *4*, e33. [CrossRef]
281. Mettler, L.; Salmassi, A.; Schollmeyer, T.; Schmutzler, A.G.; Püngel, F.; Jonat, W. Comparison of c-DNA microarray analysis of gene expression between eutopic endometrium and ectopic endometrium (endometriosis). *J. Assist. Reprod. Genet.* **2007**, *24*, 249–258. [CrossRef]
282. Eyster, K.M.; Klinkova, O.; Kennedy, V.; Hansen, K.A. Whole genome deoxyribonucleic acid microarray analysis of gene expression in ectopic versus eutopic endometrium. *Fertil. Steril.* **2007**, *88*, 1505–1533. [CrossRef]
283. Flores, I.; Rivera, E.; Ruiz, L.A.; Santiago, O.I.; Vernon, M.W.; Appleyard, C.B. Molecular profiling of experimental endometriosis identified gene expression patterns in common with human disease. *Fertil. Steril.* **2007**, *87*, 1180–1199. [CrossRef]
284. Hull, M.L.; Escareno, C.R.; Godsland, J.M.; Doig, J.R.; Johnson, C.M.; Phillips, S.C.; Smith, S.K.; Tavaré, S.; Print, C.G.; Charnock-Jones, D.S. Endometrial-Peritoneal Interactions during Endometriotic Lesion Establishment. *Am. J. Pathol.* **2008**, *173*, 700–715. [CrossRef] [PubMed]
285. Zafrakas, M.; Tarlatzis, B.C.; Streichert, T.; Pournaropoulos, F.; Wölfle, U.; Smeets, S.J.; Wittek, B.; Grimbizis, G.; Brakenhoff, R.H.; Pantel, K.; et al. Genome-wide microarray gene expression, array-CGH analysis, and telomerase activity in advanced ovarian endometriosis: A high degree of differentiation rather than malignant potential. *Int. J. Mol. Med.* **2008**, *21*, 335–344. [CrossRef] [PubMed]
286. Pelch, K.E.; Schroder, A.L.; Kimball, P.A.; Sharpe-Timms, K.L.; Davis, J.W.; Nagel, S.C. Aberrant gene expression profile in a mouse model of endometriosis mirrors that observed in women. *Fertil. Steril.* **2010**, *93*, 1615–1627. [CrossRef] [PubMed]
287. Umezawa, M.; Tanaka, N.; Tainaka, H.; Takeda, K.; Ihara, T.; Sugamata, M. Microarray analysis provides insight into the early steps of pathophysiology of mouse endometriosis model induced by autotransplantation of endometrium. *Life Sci.* **2009**, *84*, 832–837. [CrossRef] [PubMed]
288. Bruner-Tran, K.L.; Gnecco, J.; Ding, T.; Glore, D.R.; Pensabene, V.; Osteen, K.G. Exposure to the environmental endocrine disruptor TCDD and human reproductive dysfunction: Translating lessons from murine models. *Reprod. Toxicol. Elmsford N* **2017**, *68*, 59–71. [CrossRef] [PubMed]
289. Morgan, H.D.; Santos, F.; Green, K.; Dean, W.; Reik, W. Epigenetic reprogramming in mammals. *Hum. Mol. Genet.* **2005**, *14*, R47–R58. [CrossRef]
290. Gabory, A.; Attig, L.; Junien, C. Epigenetic mechanisms involved in developmental nutritional programming. *World J. Diabetes* **2011**, *2*, 164–175. [CrossRef]
291. Berger, S.L.; Kouzarides, T.; Shiekhattar, R.; Shilatifard, A. An operational definition of epigenetics. *Genes Dev.* **2009**, *23*, 781–783. [CrossRef]
292. Robertson, K.D. DNA methylation and human disease. *Nat. Rev. Genet.* **2005**, *6*, 597–610. [CrossRef]
293. Robertson, K.D.; Wolffe, A.P. DNA methylation in health and disease. *Nat. Rev. Genet.* **2000**, *1*, 11–19. [CrossRef]
294. Rodenhiser, D.; Mann, M. Epigenetics and human disease: Translating basic biology into clinical applications. *CMAJ Can. Med. Assoc. J. J. Assoc. Medicale Can.* **2006**, *174*, 341–348. [CrossRef] [PubMed]
295. Li, E. Chromatin modification and epigenetic reprogramming in mammalian development. *Nat. Rev. Genet.* **2002**, *3*, 662–673. [CrossRef] [PubMed]

296. Ritchie, W. microRNA Target Prediction. *Methods Mol. Biol. Clifton NJ* **2017**, *1513*, 193–200.
297. Sun, K.; Lai, E.C. Adult-specific functions of animal microRNAs. *Nat. Rev. Genet.* **2013**, *14*, 535–548. [CrossRef]
298. Kurokawa, R.; Rosenfeld, M.G.; Glass, C.K. Transcriptional regulation through noncoding RNAs and epigenetic modifications. *RNA Biol.* **2009**, *6*, 233–236. [CrossRef]
299. Saare, M.; Rekker, K.; Laisk-Podar, T.; Rahmioglu, N.; Zondervan, K.; Salumets, A.; Götte, M.; Peters, M. Challenges in endometriosis miRNA studies - From tissue heterogeneity to disease specific miRNAs. *Biochim. Biophys. Acta Mol. Basis Dis.* **2017**, *1863*, 2282–2292. [CrossRef]
300. Munro, S.K.; Farquhar, C.M.; Mitchell, M.D.; Ponnampalam, A.P. Epigenetic regulation of endometrium during the menstrual cycle. *Mol. Hum. Reprod.* **2010**, *16*, 297–310. [CrossRef]
301. Yamagata, Y.; Asada, H.; Tamura, I.; Lee, L.; Maekawa, R.; Taniguchi, K.; Taketani, T.; Matsuoka, A.; Tamura, H.; Sugino, N. DNA methyltransferase expression in the human endometrium: Down-regulation by progesterone and estrogen. *Hum. Reprod. Oxf. Engl.* **2009**, *24*, 1126–1132. [CrossRef]
302. Krusche, C.A.; Vloet, A.J.; Classen-Linke, I.; von Rango, U.; Beier, H.M.; Alfer, J. Class I histone deacetylase expression in the human cyclic endometrium and endometrial adenocarcinomas. *Hum. Reprod. Oxf. Engl.* **2007**, *22*, 2956–2966. [CrossRef]
303. Sakai, N.; Maruyama, T.; Sakurai, R.; Masuda, H.; Yamamoto, Y.; Shimizu, A.; Kishi, I.; Asada, H.; Yamagoe, S.; Yoshimura, Y. Involvement of histone acetylation in ovarian steroid-induced decidualization of human endometrial stromal cells. *J. Biol. Chem.* **2003**, *278*, 16675–16682. [CrossRef]
304. Uchida, H.; Maruyama, T.; Ohta, K.; Ono, M.; Arase, T.; Kagami, M.; Oda, H.; Kajitani, T.; Asada, H.; Yoshimura, Y. Histone deacetylase inhibitor-induced glycodelin enhances the initial step of implantation. *Hum. Reprod. Oxf. Engl.* **2007**, *22*, 2615–2622. [CrossRef] [PubMed]
305. Uchida, H.; Maruyama, T.; Nagashima, T.; Ono, M.; Masuda, H.; Arase, T.; Sugiura, I.; Onouchi, M.; Kajitani, T.; Asada, H.; et al. Human endometrial cytodifferentiation by histone deacetylase inhibitors. *Hum. Cell* **2006**, *19*, 38–42. [CrossRef] [PubMed]
306. Galliano, D.; Pellicer, A. MicroRNA and implantation. *Fertil. Steril.* **2014**, *101*, 1531–1544. [CrossRef] [PubMed]
307. Hull, M.L.; Nisenblat, V. Tissue and circulating microRNA influence reproductive function in endometrial disease. *Reprod. Biomed. Online* **2013**, *27*, 515–529. [CrossRef]
308. Pan, Q.; Chegini, N. MicroRNA signature and regulatory functions in the endometrium during normal and disease states. *Semin. Reprod. Med.* **2008**, *26*, 479–493. [CrossRef]
309. Kuokkanen, S.; Chen, B.; Ojalvo, L.; Benard, L.; Santoro, N.; Pollard, J.W. Genomic profiling of microRNAs and messenger RNAs reveals hormonal regulation in microRNA expression in human endometrium. *Biol. Reprod.* **2010**, *82*, 791–801. [CrossRef]
310. Lessey, B.A. Fine tuning of endometrial function by estrogen and progesterone through microRNAs. *Biol. Reprod.* **2010**, *82*, 653–655. [CrossRef]
311. Pastorelli, L.M.; Wells, S.; Fray, M.; Smith, A.; Hough, T.; Harfe, B.D.; McManus, M.T.; Smith, L.; Woolf, A.S.; Cheeseman, M.; et al. Genetic analyses reveal a requirement for Dicer1 in the mouse urogenital tract. *Mamm. Genome Off. J. Int. Mamm. Genome Soc.* **2009**, *20*, 140–151. [CrossRef]
312. Hong, X.; Luense, L.J.; McGinnis, L.K.; Nothnick, W.B.; Christenson, L.K. Dicer1 is essential for female fertility and normal development of the female reproductive system. *Endocrinology* **2008**, *149*, 6207–6212. [CrossRef]
313. Koninckx, P.R.; Ussia, A.; Adamyan, L.; Wattiez, A.; Gomel, V.; Martin, D.C. Pathogenesis of endometriosis: The genetic/epigenetic theory. *Fertil. Steril.* **2019**, *111*, 327–340. [CrossRef]
314. Yamagata, Y.; Nishino, K.; Takaki, E.; Sato, S.; Maekawa, R.; Nakai, A.; Sugino, N. Genome-wide DNA methylation profiling in cultured eutopic and ectopic endometrial stromal cells. *PloS ONE* **2014**, *9*, e83612. [CrossRef] [PubMed]
315. Signorile, P.G.; Severino, A.; Santoro, M.; Spyrou, M.; Viceconte, R.; Baldi, A. Methylation analysis of HOXA10 regulatory elements in patients with endometriosis. *BMC Res. Notes* **2018**, *11*. [CrossRef] [PubMed]
316. Wu, Y.; Halverson, G.; Basir, Z.; Strawn, E.; Yan, P.; Guo, S.-W. Aberrant methylation at HOXA10 may be responsible for its aberrant expression in the endometrium of patients with endometriosis. *Am. J. Obstet. Gynecol.* **2005**, *193*, 371–380. [CrossRef] [PubMed]

317. Lee, B.; Du, H.; Taylor, H.S. Experimental Murine Endometriosis Induces DNA Methylation and Altered Gene Expression in Eutopic Endometrium. *Biol. Reprod.* **2009**, *80*, 79–85. [CrossRef]
318. Bromer, J.G.; Wu, J.; Zhou, Y.; Taylor, H.S. Hypermethylation of Homeobox A10 by in Utero Diethylstilbestrol Exposure: An Epigenetic Mechanism for Altered Developmental Programming. *Endocrinology* **2009**, *150*, 3376–3382. [CrossRef]
319. Bromer, J.G.; Zhou, Y.; Taylor, M.B.; Doherty, L.; Taylor, H.S. Bisphenol-A exposure in utero leads to epigenetic alterations in the developmental programming of uterine estrogen response. *FASEB J.* **2010**, *24*, 2273–2280. [CrossRef]
320. Kulp, J.L.; Mamillapalli, R.; Taylor, H.S. Aberrant HOXA10 Methylation in Patients With Common Gynecologic Disorders. *Reprod. Sci.* **2016**, *23*, 455–463. [CrossRef]
321. Wu, Y.; Strawn, E.; Basir, Z.; Halverson, G.; Guo, S.-W. Promoter hypermethylation of progesterone receptor isoform B (PR-B) in endometriosis. *Epigenetics* **2006**, *1*, 106–111. [CrossRef]
322. Attia, G.R.; Zeitoun, K.; Edwards, D.; Johns, A.; Carr, B.R.; Bulun, S.E. Progesterone receptor isoform A but not B is expressed in endometriosis. *J. Clin. Endocrinol. Metab.* **2000**, *85*, 2897–2902. [CrossRef]
323. Nie, J.; Liu, X.; Guo, S.W. Promoter hypermethylation of progesterone receptor isoform B (PR-B) in adenomyosis and its rectification by a histone deacetylase inhibitor and a demethylation agent. *Reprod. Sci. Thousand Oaks Calif* **2010**, *17*, 995–1005.
324. Wu, Y.; Strawn, E.; Basir, Z.; Halverson, G.; Guo, S.-W. Aberrant expression of deoxyribonucleic acid methyltransferases DNMT1, DNMT3A, and DNMT3B in women with endometriosis. *Fertil. Steril.* **2007**, *87*, 24–32. [CrossRef] [PubMed]
325. Dyson, M.T.; Kakinuma, T.; Pavone, M.E.; Monsivais, D.; Navarro, A.; Malpani, S.S.; Ono, M.; Bulun, S.E. Aberrant expression and localization of deoxyribonucleic acid methyltransferase 3B in endometriotic stromal cells. *Fertil. Steril.* **2015**, *104*, 953–963. [CrossRef] [PubMed]
326. Aznaurova, Y.B.; Zhumataev, M.B.; Roberts, T.K.; Aliper, A.M.; Zhavoronkov, A.A. Molecular aspects of development and regulation of endometriosis. *Reprod. Biol. Endocrinol. RBE* **2014**, *12*, 50. [CrossRef] [PubMed]
327. Wu, Y.; Starzinski-Powitz, A.; Guo, S.-W. Trichostatin A, a histone deacetylase inhibitor, attenuates invasiveness and reactivates E-cadherin expression in immortalized endometriotic cells. *Reprod. Sci. Thousand Oaks Calif* **2007**, *14*, 374–382. [CrossRef]
328. KOUKOURA, O.; SIFAKIS, S.; SPANDIDOS, D.A. DNA methylation in endometriosis (Review). *Mol. Med. Rep.* **2016**, *13*, 2939–2948. [CrossRef]
329. Arosh, J.A.; Lee, J.; Starzinski-Powitz, A.; Banu, S.K. Selective inhibition of prostaglandin E2 receptors EP2 and EP4 modulates DNA methylation and histone modification machinery proteins in human endometriotic cells. *Mol. Cell. Endocrinol.* **2015**, *409*, 51–58. [CrossRef]
330. Xue, Q.; Lin, Z.; Yin, P.; Milad, M.P.; Cheng, Y.-H.; Confino, E.; Reierstad, S.; Bulun, S.E. Transcriptional activation of steroidogenic factor-1 by hypomethylation of the 5' CpG island in endometriosis. *J. Clin. Endocrinol. Metab.* **2007**, *92*, 3261–3267. [CrossRef]
331. Xue, Q.; Lin, Z.; Cheng, Y.-H.; Huang, C.-C.; Marsh, E.; Yin, P.; Milad, M.P.; Confino, E.; Reierstad, S.; Innes, J.; et al. Promoter methylation regulates estrogen receptor 2 in human endometrium and endometriosis. *Biol. Reprod.* **2007**, *77*, 681–687. [CrossRef]
332. Izawa, M.; Taniguchi, F.; Uegaki, T.; Takai, E.; Iwabe, T.; Terakawa, N.; Harada, T. Demethylation of a nonpromoter cytosine-phosphate-guanine island in the aromatase gene may cause the aberrant up-regulation in endometriotic tissues. *Fertil. Steril.* **2011**, *95*, 33–39. [CrossRef]
333. Wang, D.; Chen, Q.; Zhang, C.; Ren, F.; Li, T. DNA hypomethylation of the COX-2 gene promoter is associated with up-regulation of its mRNA expression in eutopic endometrium of endometriosis. *Eur. J. Med. Res.* **2012**, *17*, 12. [CrossRef]
334. Nasu, K.; Kawano, Y.; Kai, K.; Aoyagi, Y.; Abe, W.; Okamoto, M.; Narahara, H. Aberrant histone modification in endometriosis. *Front. Biosci. Landmark Ed.* **2014**, *19*, 1202–1214. [CrossRef] [PubMed]
335. Monteiro, J.B.; Colón-Díaz, M.; García, M.; Gutierrez, S.; Colón, M.; Seto, E.; Laboy, J.; Flores, I. Endometriosis Is Characterized by a Distinct Pattern of Histone 3 and Histone 4 Lysine Modifications. *Reprod. Sci.* **2014**, *21*, 305–318. [CrossRef] [PubMed]

336. Xiaomeng, X.; Ming, Z.; Jiezhi, M.; Xiaoling, F. Aberrant histone acetylation and methylation levels in woman with endometriosis. *Arch. Gynecol. Obstet.* **2013**, *287*, 487–494. [CrossRef]
337. Samartzis, E.P.; Noske, A.; Samartzis, N.; Fink, D.; Imesch, P. The Expression of Histone Deacetylase 1, But Not Other Class I Histone Deacetylases, Is Significantly Increased in Endometriosis. *Reprod. Sci.* **2013**, *20*, 1416–1422. [CrossRef] [PubMed]
338. Kawano, Y.; Nasu, K.; Li, H.; Tsuno, A.; Abe, W.; Takai, N.; Narahara, H. Application of the histone deacetylase inhibitors for the treatment of endometriosis: Histone modifications as pathogenesis and novel therapeutic target. *Hum. Reprod. Oxf. Engl.* **2011**, *26*, 2486–2498. [CrossRef]
339. Imesch, P.; Samartzis, E.P.; Schneider, M.; Fink, D.; Fedier, A. Inhibition of transcription, expression, and secretion of the vascular epithelial growth factor in human epithelial endometriotic cells by romidepsin. *Fertil. Steril.* **2011**, *95*, 1579–1583. [CrossRef] [PubMed]
340. Ayhan, A.; Mao, T.-L.; Seckin, T.; Wu, C.-H.; Guan, B.; Ogawa, H.; Futagami, M.; Mizukami, H.; Yokoyama, Y.; Kurman, R.J.; et al. Loss of ARID1A expression is an early molecular event in tumor progression from ovarian endometriotic cyst to clear cell and endometrioid carcinoma. *Int. J. Gynecol. Cancer Off. J. Int. Gynecol. Cancer Soc.* **2012**, *22*, 1310–1315. [CrossRef]
341. Lowery, W.J.; Schildkraut, J.M.; Akushevich, L.; Bentley, R.; Marks, J.R.; Huntsman, D.; Berchuck, A. Loss of ARID1A-associated Protein Expression Is a Frequent Event in Clear Cell and Endometrioid Ovarian Cancers. *Int. J. Gynecol. Cancer* **2012**, *22*, 9–14. [CrossRef]
342. Chene, G.; Ouellet, V.; Rahimi, K.; Barres, V.; Provencher, D.; Mes-Masson, A.M. The ARID1A pathway in ovarian clear cell and endometrioid carcinoma, contiguous endometriosis, and benign endometriosis. *Int. J. Gynaecol. Obstet. Off. Organ Int. Fed. Gynaecol. Obstet.* **2015**, *130*, 27–30. [CrossRef]
343. Er, T.-K.; Su, Y.-F.; Wu, C.-C.; Chen, C.-C.; Wang, J.; Hsieh, T.-H.; Herreros-Villanueva, M.; Chen, W.-T.; Chen, Y.-T.; Liu, T.-C.; et al. Targeted next-generation sequencing for molecular diagnosis of endometriosis-associated ovarian cancer. *J. Mol. Med. Berl. Ger.* **2016**, *94*, 835–847. [CrossRef]
344. Nothnick, W.B. MicroRNAs and Endometriosis: Distinguishing Drivers from Passengers in Disease Pathogenesis. *Semin. Reprod. Med.* **2017**, *35*, 173–180. [CrossRef] [PubMed]
345. Filigheddu, N.; Gregnanin, I.; Porporato, P.E.; Surico, D.; Perego, B.; Galli, L.; Patrignani, C.; Graziani, A.; Surico, N. Differential Expression of MicroRNAs between Eutopic and Ectopic Endometrium in Ovarian Endometriosis. *J. Biomed. Biotechnol.* **2010**, *2010*. [CrossRef] [PubMed]
346. Burney, R.O.; Hamilton, A.E.; Aghajanova, L.; Vo, K.C.; Nezhat, C.N.; Lessey, B.A.; Giudice, L.C. MicroRNA expression profiling of eutopic secretory endometrium in women with versus without endometriosis. *Mol. Hum. Reprod.* **2009**, *15*, 625–631. [CrossRef] [PubMed]
347. Vasudevan, S.; Tong, Y.; Steitz, J.A. Switching from repression to activation: MicroRNAs can up-regulate translation. *Science* **2007**, *318*, 1931–1934. [CrossRef] [PubMed]
348. Han, A.R.; Lee, T.H.; Kim, S.; Lee, H.Y. Risk factors and biomarkers for the recurrence of ovarian endometrioma: About the immunoreactivity of progesterone receptor isoform B and nuclear factor kappa B. *Gynecol. Endocrinol. Off. J. Int. Soc. Gynecol. Endocrinol.* **2017**, *33*, 70–74. [CrossRef] [PubMed]
349. Wu, Y.; Guo, S.-W. Inhibition of Proliferation of Endometrial Stromal Cells by Trichostatin A, RU486, CDB-2914, N-Acetylcysteine, and ICI 182780. *Gynecol. Obstet. Investig.* **2006**, *62*, 193–205. [CrossRef] [PubMed]
350. Wu, Y.; Guo, S.-W. Histone deacetylase inhibitors trichostatin A and valproic acid induce cell cycle arrest and p21 expression in immortalized human endometrial stromal cells. *Eur. J. Obstet. Gynecol. Reprod. Biol.* **2008**, *137*, 198–203. [CrossRef]
351. Wu, Y.; Guo, S.-W. Suppression of IL-1β-induced COX-2 expression by trichostatin A (TSA) in human endometrial stromal cells. *Eur. J. Obstet. Gynecol. Reprod. Biol.* **2007**, *135*, 88–93. [CrossRef]
352. Wu, Y.; Guo, S.-W. Peroxisome proliferator-activated receptor-gamma and retinoid X receptor agonists synergistically suppress proliferation of immortalized endometrial stromal cells. *Fertil. Steril.* **2009**, *91*, 2142–2147. [CrossRef]
353. Peeters, L.L.H.; Vigne, J.-L.; Tee, M.K.; Zhao, D.; Waite, L.L.; Taylor, R.N. PPARgamma represses VEGF expression in human endometrial cells: Implications for uterine angiogenesis. *Angiogenesis* **2006**, *8*, 373–379. [CrossRef]

354. Ohama, Y.; Harada, T.; Iwabe, T.; Taniguchi, F.; Takenaka, Y.; Terakawa, N. Peroxisome proliferator-activated receptor-γ ligand reduced tumor necrosis factor-α-induced interleukin-8 production and growth in endometriotic stromal cells. *Fertil. Steril.* **2008**, *89*, 311–317. [CrossRef]
355. Lu, Y.; Nie, J.; Liu, X.; Zheng, Y.; Guo, S.-W. Trichostatin A, a histone deacetylase inhibitor, reduces lesion growth and hyperalgesia in experimentally induced endometriosis in mice. *Hum. Reprod. Oxf. Engl.* **2010**, *25*, 1014–1025. [CrossRef] [PubMed]
356. Imesch, P.; Fink, D.; Fedier, A. Romidepsin reduces histone deacetylase activity, induces acetylation of histones, inhibits proliferation, and activates apoptosis in immortalized epithelial endometriotic cells. *Fertil. Steril.* **2010**, *94*, 2838–2842. [CrossRef] [PubMed]
357. Wang, J.; Mahmud, S.A.; Bitterman, P.B.; Huo, Y.; Slungaard, A. Histone Deacetylase Inhibitors Suppress TF-κB-dependent Agonist-driven Tissue Factor Expression in Endothelial Cells and Monocytes. *J. Biol. Chem.* **2007**, *282*, 28408–28418. [CrossRef] [PubMed]
358. Dong, X.-F.; Song, Q.; Li, L.-Z.; Zhao, C.-L.; Wang, L.-Q. Histone deacetylase inhibitor valproic acid inhibits proliferation and induces apoptosis in KM3 cells via downregulating VEGF receptor. *Neuro Endocrinol. Lett.* **2007**, *28*, 775–780.
359. Deroanne, C.F.; Bonjean, K.; Servotte, S.; Devy, L.; Colige, A.; Clausse, N.; Blacher, S.; Verdin, E.; Foidart, J.-M.; Nusgens, B.V.; et al. Histone deacetylases inhibitors as anti-angiogenic agents altering vascular endothelial growth factor signaling. *Oncogene* **2002**, *21*, 427–436. [CrossRef]
360. Lockwood, C.J.; Krikun, G.; Hickey, M.; Huang, S.J.; Schatz, F. Decidualized Human Endometrial Stromal Cells Mediate Hemostasis, Angiogenesis, and Abnormal Uterine Bleeding. *Reprod. Sci. Thousand Oaks Calif* **2009**, *16*, 162–170. [CrossRef]
361. Liu, X.; Guo, S.-W. A pilot study on the off-label use of valproic acid to treat adenomyosis. *Fertil. Steril.* **2008**, *89*, 246–250. [CrossRef]
362. Liu, X.; Yuan, L.; Guo, S.W. Valproic acid as a therapy for adenomyosis: A comparative case series. *Reprod. Sci. Thousand Oaks Calif* **2010**, *17*, 904–912.
363. Liu, M.; Liu, X.; Zhang, Y.; Guo, S.-W. Valproic acid and progestin inhibit lesion growth and reduce hyperalgesia in experimentally induced endometriosis in rats. *Reprod. Sci. Thousand Oaks Calif* **2012**, *19*, 360–373.
364. Barra, F.; Ferrero, S. Epigenetic Drugs in the Treatment of Endometriosis. *Reprod. Sci. Thousand Oaks Calif* **2018**, 1933719118765987. [CrossRef] [PubMed]

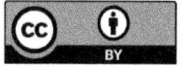

© 2019 by the authors. Licensee MDPI, Basel, Switzerland. This article is an open access article distributed under the terms and conditions of the Creative Commons Attribution (CC BY) license (http://creativecommons.org/licenses/by/4.0/).

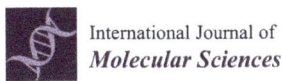

Review

Biomarkers for the Noninvasive Diagnosis of Endometriosis: State of the Art and Future Perspectives

Costin Vlad Anastasiu [1], Marius Alexandru Moga [1], Andrea Elena Neculau [2,*], Andreea Bălan [1,*], Ioan Scârneciu [1], Roxana Maria Dragomir [1], Ana-Maria Dull [3] and Liana-Maria Chicea [4]

1. Department of Medical and Surgical Specialties, Faculty of Medicine, Transilvania University of Brasov, 500019 Brasov, Romania; canastasiu@gmail.com (C.V.A.); moga.og@gmail.com (M.A.M.); urologie_scarneciu@yahoo.com (I.S.); roxana.gidinceanu@unitbv.ro (R.M.D.)
2. Department of Fundamental, Prophylactic and Clinical Sciences, Faculty of Medicine, University Transilvania Brasov, 500019 Brasov, Romania
3. Regina Maria Hospital, 500091 Brasov, Romania; dullana2005@yahoo.com
4. "Victor Papilian" Medical School, University "Lucian Blaga" of Sibiu, 550024 Sibiu, Romania; liana.chicea@gmail.com
* Correspondence: andrea.neculau@unitbv.ro (A.E.N.); dr.andreeabalan@gmail.com (A.B.); Tel.: +40-268-41-30-00 (A.E.N.); +40-268-412-185 (A.B.)

Received: 19 December 2019; Accepted: 2 March 2020; Published: 4 March 2020

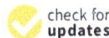

Abstract: Background: Early and accurate diagnosis of endometriosis is crucial for the management of this benign, yet debilitating pathology. Despite the advances of modern medicine, there is no common ground regarding the pathophysiology of this disease as it continues to affect the quality of life of millions of women of reproductive age. The lack of specific symptoms often determines a belated diagnosis. The gold standard remains invasive, surgery followed by a histopathological exam. A biomarker or a panel of biomarkers is easy to measure, usually noninvasive, and could benefit the clinician in both diagnosing and monitoring the treatment response. Several studies have advanced the idea of biomarkers for endometriosis, thereby circumventing unnecessary invasive techniques. Our paper aims at harmonizing the results of these studies in the search of promising perspectives on early diagnosis. Methods: We selected the papers from Google Academic, PubMed, and CrossRef and reviewed recent articles from the literature, aiming to evaluate the effectiveness of various putative serum and urinary biomarkers for endometriosis. Results: The majority of studies focused on a panel of biomarkers, rather than a single biomarker and were unable to identify a single biomolecule or a panel of biomarkers with sufficient specificity and sensitivity in endometriosis. Conclusion: Noninvasive biomarkers, proteomics, genomics, and miRNA microarray may aid the diagnosis, but further research on larger datasets along with a better understanding of the pathophysiologic mechanisms are needed.

Keywords: biomarker; angiogenesis; cytokines; urinary biomarkers; endometriosis

1. Introduction

Endometriosis is considered a debilitating gynecological pathology with a high prevalence among young women [1]. The incidence of the disease varies between 6–10% [2]. Various sources indicate a constant increase in the number of cases, reaching almost 15% worldwide [3]. Endometriosis is characterized by the migration of endometrial-like cells in ectopic places outside the uterus. The clinical manifestations thereof consist of chronic pelvic pain, dysmenorrhea, and infertility, the latter being reported in 30–50% of cases, while 20–25% of patients remain asymptomatic [4].

Given the nonspecific symptoms of this disease that can usually mimic those associated with pelvic inflammatory disease or other conditions associated with chronic pelvic pain, the gold standard for a definitive diagnosis consists of surgical procedures, followed by histopathological exams [5]. Under these circumstances, a considerable diagnostic delay is explicable [6,7], leading to 8–12 years of belated appropriate treatment [8]. As of yet, reliable laboratory biomarkers for this gynecological pathology remain elusive. The increased incidence of this pathology in women with early menarche compels the development of novel noninvasive diagnostic biomarkers for faster diagnosis, appropriate treatment, and for triaging potential patients for surgery [9,10]. A biomarker is a biological molecule that can be "objectively measured and evaluated as an indicator of normal biological processes, pathogenic processes, or pharmacological responses to a therapeutic intervention" [11]. Therefore, a biomarker or a panel of biomarkers found in the biological fluids of the affected women could be an expedient diagnostic tool for endometriosis as well as an objective assessment of the effectiveness of the treatment [12].

The pathophysiology of this disease is not thoroughly understood. Sampson's theory of retrograde menstruation is still viewed as the principal etiopathogenic factor of endometriosis. However, approximately 90% of non-affected women undergo retrograde menstruation [13]. Novel pieces of evidence support the hypothesis that endometriosis development is caused by the occurrence of primitive endometrial cells outside the uterus, during organogenesis. Following puberty, these cells differentiate into functional endometriotic implants [14]. Other authors suggested that the principal source of extrapelvic endometriosis is represented by bone marrow-derived stem cells, which are able to migrate through the peripheral circulation and induce endometriosis in remote sites [15].

According to the "embryonic theory" or epigenetic theory, during organogenesis, the genes of the Homeobox and Wingless family are essential for the differentiation of the anatomical structures of the urogenital tract. Any dysregulation of these genes through the Wnt/b-catenin signaling pathway will lead to various anomalies and may cause aberrant placement of the stem cells. The abnormal placement of these cells, associated with immune alterations and the pro-inflammatory peritoneal environment, will determine the progression towards endometriosis [14]. An ectopic endometrium displays a distinctive epigenetic expression profile, which involves homeobox A (HOXA) clusters and Wnt signaling pathway genes [16]. Furthermore, miRNAs dysregulations were found to modulate the proliferation and invasiveness of ectopic endometrial cells. Eggers et al. [17] pointed out that dysregulation of miR-200b family affects the differentiation of ectopic cells by regulating epithelial-to-mesenchymal transition. Moreover, epigenetics plays an important indirect role in the recruitment and differentiation of bone marrow-derived stem cells by modulating the relationship between the inflammatory microenvironment and steroid action. This interaction represents the trigger for the recruitment of bone marrow-derived stem cells, and it is highly influenced by the epigenetic expression profile [16].

Endometriosis is considered an inflammatory disease, due to increased levels of activated macrophages and cytokines such as interleukins (IL-6, IL-8, IIL-1β), tumor necrosis factor-alpha (TNF-α), and macrophage migration inhibitory factor (MIF), in the peritoneal fluid of affected women [2]. Furthermore, several inflammatory biomarkers registered increased levels in the serum of endometriotic women: C-reactive protein (CRP), IL-4, TNF-α, monocyte chemoattractant protein-1 (MCP-1), IL-6, IL-8, and regulated on activation, normal T cell expressed and secreted (RANTES) [13].

Recently, a wide range of papers revealed the importance and effectiveness of various putative biomarkers from the biological fluids of affected patients. Despite considerable research on this topic, noninvasive biomarkers of endometriosis have eluded the transition from bench to bedside. Some of the limitations of biomarker studies consist of reduced datasets, methodological flaws (the variability of biomarkers under physiological conditions such as menstrual phases), the lack of reproducibility across multiple studies, and, last but not least, high costs of the complex assays.

This paper aims to synthesize the expanding body of knowledge regarding the putative noninvasive biomarkers (Figure 1) of endometriosis. Furthermore, it presents the opportunities offered by the newest technologies such as proteomics, genomics, and miRNA microarray, which may represent the future perspective of diagnosis.

2. Material and Methods

This study is a synthesis of noninvasive biomarkers of endometriosis, based on literature review, highlighting their possible use for early and precise diagnosis while emphasizing the newest perspectives and opportunities in the diagnostic field.

Our research included all the publications in Google Scholar, PubMed and Cross Ref related to noninvasive biomarkers for endometriosis, during the period January 2000 to December 2019, using the following Medical Subject Headings (MeSH) keywords: biomarker, angiogenesis, cytokine, urinary biomarkers, and endometriosis. Two authors independently identified and selected relevant articles based on the following inclusion criteria: full-text articles, written in English, human-based studies, biomarkers retrieved from serum, plasma, or urine. All the studies included patients and controls that have either tested positive or negative for endometriosis. The exclusion criteria were, as follows: studies on animals or involving cell cultures, biomarkers retrieved from any invasive procedure (endometriotic tissue, endometriomas content or peritoneal fluid), papers written in other languages than English, duplicate papers, abstracts and papers that only compared biomarker levels between affected women with different stages of endometriosis, without the inclusion of healthy controls. A total number of 55 studies met our criteria.

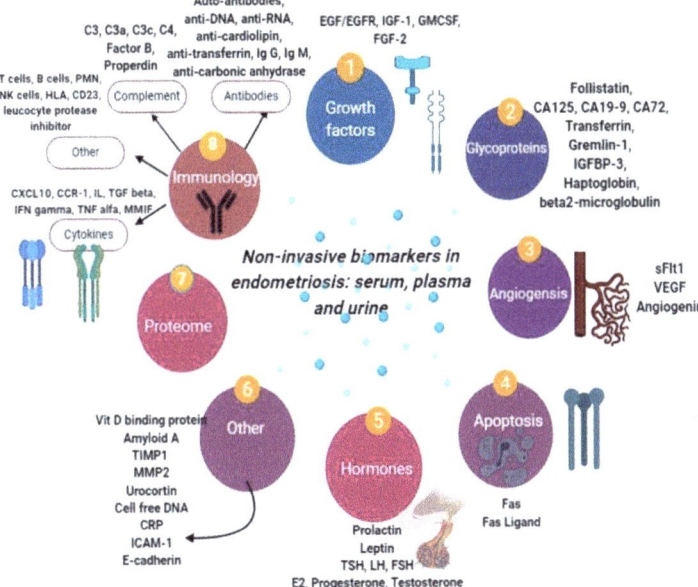

Figure 1. Putative noninvasive biomarkers for endometriosis [12].

3. Endometriosis—An Inflammatory Disease

A thorough understanding of the pathogenic and molecular mechanisms of endometriosis represents the springboard in finding various molecules that could serve as noninvasive biomarkers for early diagnosis.

Endometriosis is characterized by chronic abdominal pain, infertility, dysmenorrhea, and sometimes anxiety, related to the degree of the pelvic pain [18,19]. This pathology is the result of interactions between various hormonal, immunological, and genetic factors, and it is characterized by an increased expression of inflammatory factors and angiogenesis [20].

The central role in endometriosis belongs to local inflammation, which triggers the development of the disease and induces pain and infertility [21]. In support of this statement, a wide range of studies reported that the peritoneal fluid of endometriotic patients contained high levels of macrophages and immune cells, which secrete cytokines, angiogenic factors, and growth factors [22]. A further factor influencing the expression of these cytokines and of other cell adhesion molecules is represented by oxidative stress, thought to be an associated compound of endometriosis-related inflammation [23].

Normally, the peritoneal fluid contains 85% macrophages, as well as mast cells, lymphocytes, and mesothelial cells [24]. During menstruation and in endometriosis, this percentage is increased, and macrophages are more able to release prostaglandins (PG), cytokines, complement components, hydrolytic enzymes, and growth factors, which are central contributors to the endometriosis pathogenesis [25], and thus, possible biomarkers for the early diagnosis of this pathology. Since elevated values of PGs have been discovered in the peritoneal fluid of affected women, it is considered that PGs can trigger the progression of the disease by their inhibitory action through macrophage function, and their capacity to increase cellular proliferation and angiogenesis rate [25].

The inflammatory environment of this disease points out an increased production of estrogens, which in turn will raise the production of PGs through the activation of both NF-kB and cyclooxygenase-2 (COX-2) [26]. A paper by Banu et al. highlighted the influence of COX-2 and prostaglandin E2 (PGE2) on the migration and invasion of endometrial cells. Furthermore, the inhibition of COX-2 was able to decrease the invasion of epithelial and stromal cells in endometriosis [27].

COX-2 usually presents high values in ectopic endometrioid implants. Some studies found increased COX-2 expression and increased COX-2-derived PGE2 production in ectopic implants [27]. PGE2 and other proinflammatory cytokines induce increased values of COX-2 in normal and ectopic endometrial cells [28]. In ectopic endometriotic stromal cells, proinflammatory cytokines, such as interleukine-1β (IL-1β), are able to increase mRNA stability and to upregulate COX-2 promoter activity. This positive regulation of COX-2 is achieved via mitogen-activated protein kinase (MAPK)-dependent signaling pathways, which facilitate the binding of COX-2 promoter to the cAMP-responding element site. The subsequent dysregulation of MAPK signaling pathways increases inflammation, thereby recruiting immune cells and amplifying the inflammatory response [29].

Human endometrial cells have been shown to express NF-kappa B subunits [30,31], which are activated during normal menstruation [32]. In vitro, the activation of NF-kappa B in endometriotic stromal cells has proven a positive modulation of the proinflammatory cytokines, interleukins (IL-8, IL-6), RANTES, TNF-alpha, macrophage migration inhibitory factor (MIF), MCP-1, intercellular adhesion molecule (ICAM)-1, and granulocyte-macrophage colony-stimulating factor (GM-CSF) [33]. Alternatively, in vivo, the integrative activation of NF-kappa B subunits has been highlighted in ectopic areas of endometrial tissue [34]. The researcher's common point of view is that in endometriosis, NF-kappa B activated macrophages release IL-1, 6, 8, COX-2, TNF-alpha, and vascular endothelial growth factor (VEGF); thus, perpetuating the inflammatory pathway [21].

Several studies also suggested the contribution of oxidative stress in endometriosis-associated inflammation. Increased production of reactive oxygen species (ROS) inside the peritoneal environment may promote the inflammatory process through the positive regulation of several proinflammatory genes [35]. Zeller et al. [36] reported increased production of ROS into the peritoneal fluid of affected women. Portz and collab. [37] suggested that injecting antioxidant enzymes into the peritoneal cavity of endometriotic subjects could prevent the formation of intraperitoneal adhesions. However, other researchers, which directly measured the production of ROS in the peritoneal cavity of the affected patients did not find any obvious oxidant or antioxidant imbalance [38,39]

4. Immunological Aspects of Endometriosis

Immune dysfunction characterized by hyperactive peritoneal macrophages with altered phagocytic ability represents another key-point in endometriosis development and progression. The phagocytic ability of macrophages is mediated by matrix metalloproteinases (MMP), enzymes capable of destroying the structure of the extracellular matrix, and by the expression of several macrophage surface receptors, that can promote the dissolution of cellular debris [40]. Lagana et al. [41] suggested that macrophages are classified into M1 macrophages, and M2 macrophages, which display anti-inflammatory and pro-fibrotic activities. Moreover, these molecules are able to induce immunotolerance. In their study, Lagana and coworkers collected tissues from the ovarian endometriomas of women at different stages of endometriosis and measured M1 and M2 macrophage levels. They observed that the number of both M1 and M2 macrophages was significantly higher in the endometriosis group compared to controls. Furthermore, a progressive decrease of M1 macrophages and an increase of M2 macrophages from stage I to stage IV endometriosis was also noted [41].

Tie-2-expressing macrophages is a subset of macrophages that have been proved to promote tumor growth and angiogenesis. Using a murine model, these molecules were observed surrounding recently developed endometriotic blood vessels [42]. Should this hypothesis be proven accurate, it would infer the progression from endometriosis to ovarian cancer, thus explaining the increased risk of ovarian cancer in women affected by endometriosis [43].

Natural Killer cells (NK) activity is usually significantly decreased in endometriosis patients. This immunosuppressive effect, which consists of the reduction of T cell-mediated cytotoxicity, is not related to steroid hormone levels or to the day of the menstrual period. Wu et al. [44] explained this low activity of NK cells through highly increased levels of killer cell inhibitory receptors (KIRs) on NK cells of women with stage III-IV endometriosis. Recently, a new subset of T cells was identified, Invariant Natural Killer T cells (iNKT). They combine both classically innate and adaptive immunologic characteristics. These molecules are able to secrete both Th1 and Th2 cytokine patterns, and their actions in the eutopic and ectopic endometrium are subject to further research [45].

The contribution of IL-10 to endometriosis has also been suggested. Elevated levels of this cytokine-induced a decreased activity of cytotoxic T lymphocytes and CD+ helper cells into the peritoneal fluid of affected patients [46]. Furthermore, M1 to M2 macrophage polarization is promoted by the increased expression of IL-10 [47].

Several studies were conducted on transgenic mice in order to asses the levels of mucin 1 (MUC1) and Foxp3+ CD4 lymphocytes (Tregs). Under normal conditions, MUC1 is present on eutopic endometrial glands but is overexpressed in ectopic lesions. Preclinical investigations have revealed that upon disease development, endometriotic mice displayed high titers of anti-MUC1 antibodies and increased levels of Tregs [48]. These findings suggest that Treg lymphocytes could represent a promising venue for additional research.

Further immunological factors involved in the development of endometriosis are represented by T helper cells (Th), IL-17A and IL-4, as showed by Osuga et al. [49]. They observed increased levels of Th2 and Th17 cells in endometriotic tissues. IL-4 stimulates the proliferation of endometriotic stromal cells and IL-17A induces neutrophil migration in endometriotic tissues. Moreover, IL-17A, combined with TNFα, enhances the secretion of IL-8 and CCL-20, suggesting the cooperation of inflammation and Th17 immune response. Given the body of scientific proof, these molecules could be the focus of further reasearch for endometriosis treatment as well as potentially viable biomarkers for the disease development.

Since endometriosis is now considered an immune dysregulation with profound changes in the activities of various cells involved in immune reactions, further studies might offer novel therapeutic targets as well as biomarkers for early detection of endometriosis.

5. Angiogenesis in Endometriosis

Endometriosis is a polygenic and multifactorial disease, and increased angiogenesis and proteolysis may trigger its development and progression [50]. Studies have shown an essential involvement of several angiogenesis-related factors in endometriosis, such as the Delta-like 4 (Dll4)-Notch signal pathways, angiopoietin, vascular endothelial growth factor (VEGF), and vascular endothelial growth factor receptor (VEGFR) [51].

Vascular endothelial growth factor (VEGF), and vascular endothelial growth factor receptor (VEGFR) are the most well-known molecules involved in the angiogenesis process. They are able to regulate the proliferation, migration, and permeability of the cells. A study by Ahn et al. [52] pointed out that IL-17A is emerging as a potent angiogenic factor, and it can upregulate VEGF and IL-8. This mechanism promotes intraperitoneal angiogenesis in order to maintain the ectopic foci and to facilitate the development of new ones. Furthermore, plasmatic concentrations of IL-17A displayed a significant decrease following surgical removal of ectopic endometrial tissue.

The expression of VEGF microRNA (mRNA) is more increased in hypoxic areas. The growth of endometriotic cells creates hypoxia, enhancing the production of several molecules with pro-angiogenic potentials, such as TNF-α, VEGF, IL-8, bFGF, and TGF-β. All these factors trigger vessel hyperpermeability, release plasmatic proteins, induce the formation of fibrin, endothelial cells proliferation, and promote angiogenesis and fibrinolysis [53].

Several studies reported that interleukins also display a pro-angiogenic effect. Interleukins with a Glutamic Acid-Leucine-Arginine-amino-terminal site, such as IL-8, increase the angiogenesis rate, while those lacking this sequence, such as IL-4, impede this process [54]. Volpert et al. [55] highlighted that in vivo, IL-4 inhibits the vessel's neoformation induced by bFGF, while in vitro, it impedes the transmigration of endothelial cells towards bFGF. Another interleukin involved in endometriosis-related angiogenesis is IL-1α, which promotes this process through the augmented expression of various angiogenic factors such as VEGF, IL-8, and bFGF, according to the results published by Torisu and collab [56].

Donnez et al. [57] highlighted that red and white endometriosis foci exhibit different degrees of expression of pro-angiogenic factors. Consequently, they have shown that red endometriosis lesions display a more pronounced vascularization and a higher cell proliferative activity.

Figure 2 is a schematic representation of the mechanism of development and progression of endometriosis, illustrating the inflammatory and angiogenetic pathways.

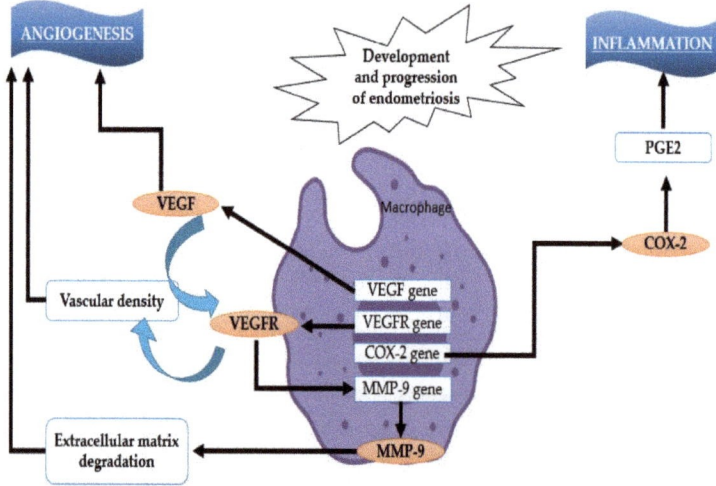

Figure 2. Angiogenesis process—In endometriosis, the central role in pathophysiological mechanisms is attributed to macrophages. These cells increase the intranuclear expression of vascular endothelial growth factor (VEGF) and cyclooxygenase 2 (COX-2) genes, leading to increased angiogenesis and an inflammatory environment [58].

6. Studies of New Noninvasive Biomarkers in Endometriosis

A noninvasive biomolecule for endometriosis diagnosis could be extracted and quantified from serum, plasma, or urine and would be beneficial for patients with chronic pelvic pain, infertility, and dysmenorrhea, in the context of a regular ultrasound.

Blood and urine make for excellent sources of biomarkers due to their reproducibility, ease of access, and measurement [59]. Promising potential endometriosis biomarkers that underwent testing were: glycoproteins, growth factors, miRNAs, lncRNAs, as well as proteins related to the angiogenesis process or immunology [12]. Despite extensive research, neither a single biomarker nor a panel of biomolecules has been considered sufficiently specific and sensitive to be used as a diagnostic test for endometriosis [12].

6.1. Serum/Plasma Biomarkers of Endometriosis

6.1.1. Glycoproteins

Although lacking both specificity and sensitivity for this pathology, the most representative glycoprotein used as a biomarker for endometriosis is CA-125 [60]. However, the simultaneous measurement of CA-125 with other molecules and their combination showed different sensitivities and specificities for endometriosis. For example, Mihalyi et al. combined CA-125 with IL-8 and TNF-α during the secretory phase of the menstrual cycle and observed that this combination gives a sensitivity of 89.7% and specificity of 71.1% for endometriosis [61]. Furthermore, the combination of CA-125, chemokine receptor (CCR) type1, mRNA, and MCP1 proved to be efficient as a biomarker panel, with a sensitivity of 92.2% and specificity of 81.6%, according to Agic et al. [62]. Vodolazkaia combined four biomarkers, namely: VEGF, CA-125, Annexin V, and glycodelin resulting in a sensitivity and a specificity of 74–94% and 55–75%, respectively [63].

Another tumor marker, CA-19-9, was investigated as a possible biomarker for endometriosis diagnosis. Elevated values of this glycoprotein were detected in endometriotic women in comparison to healthy patients, but the sensitivity of this molecule was significantly lower when compared to CA-125 [12]. It is worthwhile mentioning that CA-19-9 has shown a positive correlation with the severity of the disease [64].

Glycodelin is a glycoprotein that promotes cell proliferation and neovascularization. Serum levels of this molecule have been found higher in endometriotic women when compared to non-affected patients. Mosbah et al. conducted a study that included women 21–48 years old with endometriosis and measured the levels of intercellular adhesion molecule 2 (ICAM-2), IL-6, and glycodelin A in their serum samples. Their results showed that IL-6 and glycodelin A displayed higher serum as well as peritoneal fluid levels in affected subjects compared to controls, with a sensitivity and specificity of 91.7% and 75.0% for serum glycodelin A, 93.8% and 80.0% for serum IL-6, 58.3%, and 60.0%, respectively for ICAM-1 [65]. Kocbek et al. [66] also identified significantly increased concentrations of glycodelin-A in the serum of cases compared to controls. Furthermore, combinations that included leptin/glycodelin-A ratio and ficolin 2/glycodelin-A ratio displayed a sensitivity and specificity of 72.5% to 84.2% and 78.4% to 91.2%, respectively.

Prentice Crapper [67] analyzed eight putative serum biomarkers for endometriosis, and they observed a significant elevation of only two of these molecules. Its results indicated that glycodelin has a sensitivity and specificity of 81.6% and 69.6%, respectively, for disease diagnosis. Zinc alpha 2-glycoprotein also registered increased values in affected women, with a sensitivity of 46% and a specificity of 100%. The combination of these two markers showed a greater specificity and sensitivity for the detection of this gynecological disorder (65% and 90%, respectively).

Follistatin is an inhibitor of activin, produced by the endometrium. It is increased in endometriosis, and thus, it could be used as a noninvasive biomarker for endometriosis diagnosis. Reis et al. simultaneously evaluated the levels of serum activin A and follistatin in healthy and affected subjects (with ovarian endometrioma, peritoneal endometriosis, and deep infiltrating endometriosis). Their study concluded that follistatin and activin A are not significantly modified in peritoneal or deep infiltrating endometriosis, but their serum concentrations in ovarian endometrioma were slightly higher [68].

Intercellular adhesion molecule-1 (ICAM-1) is a glycoprotein that seems to be involved in the development and promotion of endometriosis. It plays an essential role in the promotion of the inflammatory and immunological reactions, and recent studies associated the polymorphism of the ICAM-1 gene with the severity of this gynecological disorder. Vigano et al. [69] analyzed two polymorphic sites of the ICAM-1 gene, known as G/R241 and E/K469, using a cohort of 188 women with confirmed endometriosis and 175 controls. They observed that the frequency of the R241 allele was slightly higher in the endometriosis cohort than in the control group, while the frequency of the second allele was approximately the same in both groups. In conclusion, genetic polymorphism in the ICAM-1 gene domain G/R241 offers a promising perspective in the field of noninvasive biomarkers. Furthermore, concomitantly with the development of genomics, this glycoprotein could prove conducive in diagnosing endometriosis, as well as in predicting the degree of severity of this pathology.

6.1.2. Inflammatory Cytokines and Immunological Molecules

In the last decades, immunological molecules and inflammatory cytokines have been extensively studied for their potential as noninvasive biomarkers for endometriosis, with the most representative being IL-1, IL-6, IL-8, interferon-γ (IFN-γ), MCP-1, and TNF-α. Othman et al. tested three serum cytokines, both separately and in various combinations. They collected blood samples and measured cytokines levels with the Bio-Plex Protein Array System. The final results concluded that Il-6, MCP-1, and IFN-γ were significantly increased in the serum of affected women, in comparison with non-affected subjects. No difference has been found between serum concentration levels of tumor necrosis factor-alpha (TNF-α), or granulocyte macrophage colony-stimulating factor (GM-CSF). IL-2, IL-8 and, IL-15 were undetectable both in endometriosis and healthy group [70]. Borrelli et al. determined increased levels of IL-8, MCP-1, and RANTES in the peripheral blood of affected patients vs. controls, in 46.1%, 50%, and 75%, of the assessed cases, suggesting their potential use as noninvasive biomarkers for endometriosis [71].

Interleukin 6 is a proinflammatory cytokine that has shown increased serum levels in affected women. A study of Martinez et al. [72] pointed out that patients with Stage I-II endometriosis had increased levels of IL-6, with a sensitivity of approximately 75% and a specificity of 83.3%. In 2010, Socolov et al. [73] included 24 cases of endometriosis and 24 controls in a study and investigated their serum levels of IL-6, IL-8, IL-1, CA-125, and TNF. Their results indicated that IL-6 was above the cut-off threshold of 2 pg/mL in 71% of the cases and 87% of controls, with a sensitivity and specificity of 71% and 12%, respectively. They concluded that the difference between the two groups was not statistically significant.

Interleukin-8 is a chemokine derived from monocyte/macrophage that has also been considered for the noninvasive diagnosis of endometriosis. While some studies found no differences between cases and controls in terms of IL-8 levels [74]. Pizzo et al. [75] pointed out that this interleukin has increased levels in affected women with Stage I–II endometriosis and even higher levels in endometriomas [76].

Tumor necrosis factor alpha (TNF-α) is a proinflammatory cytokine with pro-angiogenic potential. Its role as a biomarker for endometriosis is controversial; while several studies proved increased serum levels of TNF-α in women with endometriosis [77–79], others showed no difference between affected patients and healthy controls [70,80]. Cho et al. [79] concluded that TNF-α increases only in the serum of endometriotic women, while urinary levels remain unchanged. The severity of endometriosis has also been associated with elevated serum TNF-α levels [75]. A recent study conducted by Steff et al. [81] revealed that the level of soluble TNF receptor in affected patients registered a significant increase during the follicular phase of the menstrual cycle.

Choi et al. [82] collected serum samples from 50 patients with endometriosis and 35 healthy individuals and used enzyme-linked immunosorbent assay (ELISA) in order to measure the levels of IL-32, 6, 10, 1β, TNF-α, and CA-125. Only IL-32 displayed significantly higher levels in patients compared to controls. When IL-32 was associated with CA-125, the specificity and sensitivity of this combination reached 60% and 82.9%, respectively, thereby suggesting IL-32 as a potential biomarker for endometriosis diagnosis.

Several studies have also assessed Natural killer (NK) cells as potentially viable biomarkers. Kikuchi et al. [83] reported declining levels in the subset of NK cells (CD57 + CD16) in endometriosis, followed by significantly elevated levels of these cells one month following surgery.

Copeptin is a molecule that has augmented values in inflammatory conditions. Tuten et al. [84] determined the serum levels of copeptin, CA-125, C-reactive protein, CA-15-3, and CA-19-9 in a study on 50 women laparoscopically diagnosed with endometriosis and 36 controls. Their results indicated that the level of copeptin was significantly higher in affected women in comparison to controls. Furthermore, these levels were positively correlated with the stage of the disease. However, there is no consensus indicating that cytokines are suitable for early-stage detection of endometriosis, or discriminating patients with endometriosis from patients with other pelvic pathologies.

6.1.3. Oxidative Stress Markers

Despite being still inconclusive, the pathophysiology of endometriosis seems to be based on several theories, including the imbalance between reactive oxygen species (ROS) and antioxidants [85]. This causes an inflammatory response in the peritoneal cavity and ROS to modulate the proliferation of the endometriotic cells [86].

Malondialdehyde (MDA) is a lipid peroxidase which can be considered an oxidative stress marker. A study conducted by Nasiri et al. [87] concluded that, in the serum of endometriotic patients, there are higher values of MDA in comparison with healthy individuals. Furthermore, women with endometriosis have higher levels of lipid hydroperoxides [88], vitamin E [89], and catalase [90], without any conclusive explanation yet.

Superoxide dismutase (SOD) is an enzyme involved in oxidative stress. It registered diminished activity in the plasma of affected patients, supporting the theory of a decreased antioxidant capacity in endometriosis [91]. Andrisani and coworkers [92] studied the activity of carbonic anhydrase in endometriotic women, in comparison to healthy controls. They observed increased enzymatic activity in response to oxidative stress, along with a cytosolic decrease of glutathione content in affected patients.

The major limitations of all the above-mentioned research papers consist of interlaboratory variations. As such, in order to compare the results across different studies, an all-encompassing methodology is needed.

6.1.4. Growth Factors and Peptides

Our research revealed a scarce number of studies conducted on growth factors and peptides, with a large body of uncertainty and controversy regarding their possible use as biomarkers.

Insulin-like growth factor-1 (IGF-1) has been increased in stages III–IV of endometriosis, but not in stages I–II [93]. However, Steff et al. [94] revealed no statistically significant difference between patients and controls in terms of IGF-1. IGFBP3 is a protein that ensures the transport of IGF-1 and is involved in endometrial cell growth. There are two studies that have proven no difference between serum levels of IGFBP3 in healthy women compared to endometriotic patients [93,95].

Nesfatin-1 was initially described as a hypothalamic neuropeptide, with the ability to lower the intake of food [96]. Sengul et al. [97] investigated the level of serum nesfatin-1 in women with endometriosis, before and after the adjustment for body mass index (BMI). At the end of the study, their results indicated that serum nesfatin-1 levels were significantly decreased in the group of subjects, compared to healthy controls, with unchanged results following BMI adjustment.

Urocortin is a neuropeptide that can be found in both endometrium and ovary, and several research papers highlighted the similarity of serum urocortin levels in endometriotic subjects and healthy controls [98,99]. A further study indicated that serum levels of urocortin were significantly increased in women with ovarian endometriosis in comparison to women with other benign ovarian cysts with a sensitivity of 88% and specificity of 90% [100].

Leptin is a helical cytokine that regulates the process of steroidogenesis as well as the decidual transformation of the endometrium. Chmaj-Wierzchowska et al. [99] revealed that the serum level of this molecule was slightly lower in women with ovarian endometriomas compared to control. However, these differences were not statistically significant.

6.1.5. Angiogenesis Molecules

While some studies suggested that VEGF-A levels following laparoscopic excision of endometriosis foci are reduced [101,102], Szubert et al. [103] concluded that following danazol treatment, plasmatic VEGF concentrations were significantly increased, therefore implying that this molecule could not be associated with the disease.

Pigment epithelium-derived factor (PEDF) is an inhibitor of angiogenesis with neurotrophic and anti-inflammatory properties, and modified values of this molecule have been found in endometriotic patients. Chen et al. [104] analyzed the serum levels of PEDF in 43 women with laparoscopically confirmed endometriosis and 28 controls, using the enzyme-linked immunosorbent assay. The results of their study indicated that PEDF was significantly decreased (16.3 ± 6.6 ng/mL) in cases compared to controls (24.5 ± 7.3 ng/mL) and was correlated with the severity of the symptoms.

While elevated values of serum fibroblast growth factor-2 (FGF-2), and angiogenin have also been recorded in the quest for viable biomarkers, soluble endothelial growth factor (EGF) and platelet-derived growth factor (PDGF) revealed no sizable differences between cases and controls; therefore, being sidelined as potential candidates [12].

6.1.6. Autoantibodies

In the last years, several authors focused on the role of circulating antibodies that could be involved in the pathogenesis of endometriosis. The close interrelation of the endometrium with the immune system justifies and partly explains the mechanism of development, as well as the progression of endometriosis.

Anti-endometrial antibodies and total immunoglobulin have also been considered as noninvasive biomarkers for endometriosis. The antibodies with the highest potential as biomarkers for this pelvic pathology were antibodies against α2-HS glycoprotein, malondialdehyde-modified low-density lipoprotein, laminin-I, lipid peroxide, modified rabbit serum albumin, cardiolipin, and specific antibodies against carbonic anhydrase and transferrin [12]. Ozhan et al. [105] researched serum syntaxin-5, anti-endometrial antibody, and other molecules as noninvasive biomarkers. They concluded that the blood serum levels of syntaxin-5 were significantly increased in the endometriosis group, compared to the control group. Furthermore, serum levels of syntaxin-5 in stage I and II endometriosis were found to have different levels compared to controls.

Gajbhiye et al. [106] included 40 endometriosis patients in their study and noted higher serum levels of autoantibodies compared to tropomodulin 3 (TMOD3), tropomyosin 3 (TPM3), and stomatin-like protein 2 (SLP2) in contrast to control's serum samples. Elevated values were associated with both minimal to mild and moderate to severe disease. Additionally, in women with endometriomas, autoantibodies against IGF-2 mRNA-binding protein 1 (IMP1) were identified by Yi et al. to be significantly elevated compared to healthy controls [107].

Anti-α-enolase antibodies in endometriotic subjects were significantly elevated compared to non-affected subjects. The sensitivity and specificity of serum Anti-α-enolase antibodies were comparable to CA125 values, and the combination of these molecules revealed potentially high diagnostic utility [108].

Anti-laminin-1 antibodies were associated with recurrent miscarriage, and increased levels were described in infertile women, as well as in patients with endometriosis. However, this biomarker has not yet passed a diagnostic threshold in current medical practice [109,110].

Two studies conducted by Mathur et al. [111] and Odukoya et al. [112] identified a potential correlation between IgG and endometriosis. IgG antibodies were identified in 56% of affected women and 5% of healthy controls. Another investigation highlighted the presence of IgG in 33% of cases, and of IgM in 27% of them [113].

Given the results of these studies, some autoantibodies could be considered as noninvasive biomarkers for the diagnosis of endometriosis, but further research is necessary.

6.1.7. Proteomics, Metabolomics, and Genomics: The Novel Perspectives of Noninvasive Biomarkers

Proteomics is a new and challenging perspective in the field of noninvasive biomarkers for early detection of endometriosis, which includes all the protein "fingerprints" used for endometriosis diagnosis. Despite promising results, these technologies need better standardization and are cost and time-intensive [12].

Long et al. [113] collected serum samples from several affected women and compared them to controls, in order to detect different protein fingerprints of this disease, by using MALDI-TOF–MS. Their results indicated that 13 protein peaks were over-expressed, and five protein peaks were down-regulated in the affected group compared to healthy subjects.

A further study analyzed distinct patterns of serum proteins in 90 endometriotic women, using SELDI-TOF MS. Following surgical intervention, 51 out of 90 patients were diagnosed with endometriosis, while 39 were unaffected. The researchers concluded that a unique combination of proteins, with molecular weights ranging between 2000 and 20,000 Da made a difference between affected women and controls. The sensitivity of this technique was 81.3%, with a specificity of 60.3% [114]. According to Zheng et al. [115], a proteomic fingerprint model including three peptide peaks showed a sensitivity and specificity of 91.4% and 95%, respectively, for the detection of endometriosis, when compared to controls. In an independent cohort, this combination of peptides revealed a sensitivity of 89.3% and a specificity of 90%.

Wang and collab. [116] illustrated a panel of five protein peaks with a specificity of 90% and a sensitivity of 91.7% for endometriosis, and Jing et al. [117] highlighted two protein peaks with specificity and sensitivity of 97% and 87%, respectively.

Given the inflammatory nature of the disease, inflammation-related proteins have also been investigated for their utility as noninvasive biomarkers. Plasma levels of AXIN1 and ST1A1 were analyzed using ELISA in both affected subjects and healthy controls. AXIN1 and ST1A1 had higher values in endometriosis when compared to healthy controls, regardless of the anatomical location of the lesions [118]. AXIN1 is a promising protein that should be further investigated as a biomarker for endometriosis diagnosis.

Signorile and coworkers [119] used 2D gel analysis in order to describe the potential of two proteins (serum albumin and complement C3 precursor) as diagnostic markers for endometriosis. Their technique was easily reproducible, and their results indicated a sensitivity/specificity for albumin and the complement C3 of 83.3%/83.3% and 58.1%/100%, respectively. In conclusion, this study confirmed the statistical significance of the differential expression for these two proteins in endometriotic women with respect to unaffected individuals. The same authors conducted, in the year 2014, a study comprising 120 women with endometriosis and 20 healthy controls, in order to highlight their serum levels of Zn-alpha2-glycoprotein. After performing ELISA, they observed that the serum levels of this protein were significantly increased in the endometriosis group than in healthy women [120]. In the issue of this observation, the analysis of Zn-alpha2-glycoprotein levels in the serum could become an innovative noninvasive diagnostic test for endometriosis.

Additionally, several studies regarding the metabolome of endometriotic patients have been conducted. Dutta et al. [121] included 22 endometriotic patients and 23 healthy women. They revealed elevated values of Lactate, 3-Hydroxybutyrate, Alanine, Glycerophosphatidylcholine, Valine, Leucine, Threonine, 2-Hydroxybutyrate, Lysine, and Succinic acid in the serum samples of affected women. Furthermore, lower values of glucose, L-Isoleucine, and L-Arginine were discovered in the endometriosis group.

Another study, conducted by Vouk et al. [122] analyzed plasma samples from 40 women with ovarian endometriosis and 52 controls, who underwent laparoscopy. The researchers used electrospray ionization tandem mass spectrometry for more than 140 targeted analytes, including sphingolipids, glycerophospholipids, and acylcarnitines. The results concluded that a model containing hydroxysphingomyelin C16:1 and the ratio between phosphatidylcholine PCaa C36:2 to ether-phospholipid PCae C34:2, had a sensitivity and specificity of 90% and 84.3%, respectively.

In order to establish if the metabolomic profile of affected patients could serve as a noninvasive biomarker for the diagnosis of this pathology, further thorough research is needed.

Genomics may prove an untapped biomarker source with a promising perspective in early diagnosis of endometriosis. Gene-based technologies include cDNA microarray techniques and cDNA hybridization. Recent studies suggested higher plasma concentrations of circulating cell-free cDNA in women with endometriosis [123], in comparison to healthy individuals.

The mitochondrial genome represents another unexplored and potentially promising biomarker pool [108]. Creed et al. [124], highlighted two Mitochondrial DNA (mtDNA) deletions (1.2 and 3.7 kb) which could serve as noninvasive biomarkers.

6.1.8. miRNAs

MicroRNAs (miRNA) are non-coding RNAs with approximately 21–25 nucleotides and represent major modulators of gene expression in a wide range of pathologies, including endometriosis [125]. miRNA profiling is usually achieved by microarray, followed by qRT-PCR validation. Due to their high stability in the biological fluids and tissue specificity, miRNAs might prove desirable molecules for the diagnosis of endometriosis and other pathologies [126], giving a whole new dimension to the noninvasive diagnosis of endometriosis [127].

Despite several studies on miRNA in endometriosis, the results are still equivocal, with no single miRNA or panel of biomarkers showing enough specificity and sensitivity for this pathology, but with promising results.

MiR-200 is a miRNAs family consisting of three members: miR-200a, miR-200b, and miR-141, which have been thoroughly studied for their dysregulations associated with endometriosis. A study performed by Ohlsson et al. [127] revealed a sensitivity of 84.4% and a specificity of 66.7% in endometriotic patients.

Although not highly specific, miR-20 can be potentially used as a biomarker in early diagnosis of endometriosis. Furthermore, it has been proven that miR-20a targets TGF-β and Il-8, and its down-regulation leads to increased concentrations of these pro-inflammatory molecules [128].

MiR-199a revealed a specificity and sensitivity of 78.33% and 76%, respectively, for endometriosis, according to the results of Wang and collab. [129]. Furthermore, this molecule targets CLIC4 and VCL, inducing a high infiltration proclivity of endometrial cells [129]. Kozomara et al. [130] quantified miR-145 in the peripheral blood of endometriotic patients and compared the values with those from healthy controls. They observed that miR-145 is up-regulated in advanced stages of endometriosis, but in early stages, its down-regulated values are not suitable for diagnosis.

Wang and collab [129] analyzed various miRNAs in 765 serum samples from both cases and healthy controls. Their results showed that miR-199a and miR-122 were up-regulated in affected women in comparison to controls, while miR-9, mi-R-141, mi-R-145, miR-542-3p registered decreased values in endometriosis.

miRNA-200 family is one of the most studied groups of miRNAs molecules, and Rekker et al. [131] concluded that miR-200a-3p and miR-141-3p are more sensitive and specific for endometriosis and that these members of miR-200 family are down-regulated in endometriosis, in comparison with the control group.

As previously mentioned, the results regarding the role of miRNAs as a diagnostic tool in endometriosis are controversial and still equivocal. While several studies support the considerable potential of miRNAs as biomarkers for early stages diagnosis, others revealed a modest specificity of these molecules. Nisenblat et al. [132] determined 49 miRNAs, differentially expressed in endometriotic women. A panel formed by miR-155, miR574-3p, and miR139-3p revealed a sensitivity of 83% and a specificity of only 51%.

Vanhie et al. [133] considered 42 miRNAs, out of which only one panel, namely: hsa-miR-125b-5p, hsa-miR-28-5p and hsa-miR-29a-3p revealed a moderate sensitivity and modest specificity of 78% and 37%, respectively.

In Table 1, we summarized the previous studies illustrating the sensitivity and specificity of different dysregulated miRNAs in endometriosis.

Table 1. Studies reporting the sensitivity and specificity of dysregulated miRNAs in endometriosis.

Author, Reference	Dysregulated miRNA	Specificity	Sensitivity
Ohlsson et al., 2009 [127]	miR-200a, miR-200b, and miR-141	66,7%	84,4%
	miR-22	90%	90%
Jia et al., 2013 [134]	miR-17-5p	80%	60%
	miR-20a	90%	60%
	miR-145	96%	70%
Wang et al., 2013 [129]	miR-122	76%	80%
	miR-199a	76%	78,3%
	miR-141-5p	96%	71,7%
Suryavanshi et al., 2013 [135]	miR-195, miR-16, miR-191	60%	88%
	miR-200a-3p	70.8%	71.9%
Rekker et al., 2015 [131]	miR-200b-3p	90.6%	70.8%
	miR-141-3p	70.8%	71.9%
Cosar et al., 2016 [136]	miR-125b	96%	100%
Nisenblat et al., 2019 [132]	miR-155, miR574-3p and miR139-3p	51%	83%
Vanhie et al., 2019 [133]	hsa-miR-125b-5p, hsa-miR-28-5p and hsa-miR-29a-3p	37%	78%

Long non-coding RNAs (lncRNAs) represent a class of molecules with a length of more than 200 nucleotides. They lack the ability of protein-coding [137]. Wang W. et al. [138] applied genome-wide profiling in order to investigate serum lncRNAs differentially expressed in endometriosis women in comparison to healthy controls. They concluded that these molecules presented significant deregulated expressions. Using the PCR quantification method, the authors revealed that 16 lncRNAs were clearly able to distinguish endometriosis from healthy patients—the levels of NR_038452 and ENST00000393610 lncRNA molecules were significantly higher in the serum of affected women, while ENST00000529000, ENST00000482343, ENST00000544649, NR_038395, NR_033688, and ENST00000465368 were decreased in endometriosis. Furthermore, they highlighted an optimal panel of lncRNAs (NR_038395, NR_038452, ENST00000482343, ENST00000544649, and ENST00000393610) able to differentiate between affected and healthy patients. This study concluded that the lncRNAs panel with the highest potential for early detection of endometriosis contains five molecules, namely: NR_038395, NR_038452, ENST00000482343, ENST00000544649, and ENST00000393610.

TC0101441 is a lncRNA molecule with high potential as a biomarker for endometriosis diagnosis, severity, and recurrence prediction. A recent study [139] analyzed the expression of TC0101441 in the serum of affected women versus healthy controls. The authors observed increased TC0101441 levels in the exosomes derived from the serum of endometriotic patients, and a positive and statistically significant correlation between these levels and infertility, chronic pelvic pain, and recurrence of the disease.

6.2. Urinary Biomarkers in Endometriosis

Given its ease of access and fluid composition, urine is one of the most widely used biological samples. As such, the increased accuracy of a urinary test could ideally establish the diagnosis of endometriosis without the need for undergoing invasive surgical interventions. Similar to serum, urinary biomarkers have been measured by a wide range of protein detection methods and have been reported both alone and in combinations [7].

Several urinary peptides and proteins were analyzed for their potential as biomarkers, but further studies are required, with larger sample sizes, in a more diverse population [140]. Creatinine-corrected soluble fms-like tyrosine kinase (sFlt-1) is one of these promising urinary biomarkers for endometriosis.

Cho et al. [79] described increased urinary sFlt-1 levels in endometriotic patients. Furthermore, serum sFlt-1 and urinary sFlt-1 levels, corrected for creatinine, were increased in women with endometriosis stage I and II.

Cytokeratin-19 (CK19) is another molecule that could be used in the detection of endometriosis. Kuessel et al. [141] measured urinary levels of CK19 by ELISA on a cohort of 76 women. The study concluded that there was no significant correlation between urinary levels of CK19 and endometriosis. Tokushige et al. [142] used an immunoblot technique to prove that CK19 is expressed only in the urine of women with confirmed endometriosis while absent in the urine of healthy women.

Matrix metalloproteinases (MMP) have been proven to be involved in the pathophysiology of endometriosis, and thus, several authors studied their level in affected women. A panel composed of MMP-2, MMP-9, and MMP-9/neutrophil gelatinase-associated lipocalin was found to increase in 33 subjects with confirmed endometriosis when compared to controls [143].

Using MALDI-TOF MS (matrix-assisted laser desorption/ionization mass spectrometry (MALDI MS) and time-of-flight analyzer (TOF)), differential peptide profiles have been described in the urine of endometriotic women, compared to healthy subjects. Tokushige and colleagues [144], revealed a 12-fold higher expression of five proteins in affected women by combining MALDI-TOF with two-dimensional polyacrylamide gel electrophoresis and El-Kasti et al. [145] highlighted a 3280.9 Da periovulatory peptide that differentiates women with all stages of endometriosis from healthy subjects (sensitivity 82% and specificity 88%).

Cho et al. [146] used western blot and ELISA to investigate urinary proteins of patients with endometriosis. They concluded that 22 protein spots were differentially expressed in the urine of endometriotic women, and one of them was urinary vitamin D-binding protein (VDBP). The conclusion was that urinary VDBP corrected for creatinine (VDBP-Cr) was significantly elevated in patients with endometriosis. The sensitivity of this biomarker was 58%, and the specificity, 76%. When combined with serum CA-125 levels, the authors observed that the positive predictive value was not significantly increased compared to CA-125 alone.

Potlog-Nahari et al. [147] included 40 affected women, with histologically confirmed endometriosis, and 22 healthy controls. They measured the urinary level of VEGF corrected for creatinine. The results of this study revealed no significant difference between urinary levels of VEGF in women with and without endometriosis. Furthermore, these values have not significantly varied between groups according to the phase of the menstrual cycle, hence the unlikeliness that urinary VEGF could serve as a biomarker for endometriosis. No other authors investigated this molecule with respect to endometriosis.

Chen and coworkers [148] were the first to identify histone 4 as a potential urinary biomarker in endometriosis. The authors observed an elevated level of histone 4 in the urine of endometriotic women with a sensitivity and specificity of 70% and 80%, respectively. Considering this research as a key stone, further studies could be conducted in order to validate and strengthen the hypothesis of Chen et al.

In Table 2, we summarize the studies illustrating the main noninvasive biomarkers assessed for endometriosis.

Table 2. Studies assessing the main noninvasive biomarkers for endometriosis.

Author, Reference	Source	Investigated Biomarkers
Agic et al, 2008 [62]	Serum	CA-125, CCR-1, miRNA, MCP-1
Borrelli et al., 2014 [71]	Serum	IL-8, MCP-1, RANTES
Chen et al., 2012 [104]	Serum	Serum pigment epithelium-derived factor
Chen et al., 2019 [148]	Urine	Histone 4
Chmaj-Wierzchowska et al., 2015 [99]	Serum	Urocortin, ghrelin, leptin
Cho et al., 2007 [79]	Serum, Urine	TNF-α, urinary sFlt-1

Table 2. Cont.

Author, Reference	Source	Investigated Biomarkers
Cho et al., 2012 [146]	Urine	Vitamin D-binding protein
Choi et al., 2019 [82]	Serum	IL-32, IL-6, IL-10, IL-1β, TNF-α, CA-125
Cosar et al., 2016 [136]	Serum	miR-125b
Creed et al., 2019 [124]	Serum	mtDNA
Darai et al., 2003 [77]	Serum	IL-6, IL-8, TNF-α
Dutta et al., 2012 [91]	Serum	Lactate, 3-Hydroxybutyrate, Alanine, Glycerophosphatidylcholine, Valine, Leucine, Threonine, 2-Hydroxybutyrate, Lysine, Succinic acid
Gajbhiye et al., 2012 [106]	Serum	Autoantibodies against tropomodulin 3 (TMOD3), tropomyosin 3 (TPM3), stomatin-like protein 2 (SLP2)
Gmyrek et al., 2005 [149]	Serum	MCP-1
Gungor et al., 2009 [150]	Serum	Leptin
Huang et al., 2004 [151]	Serum	MMP2
Jia et al., 2013 [134]	Serum	miR-22, miR-17-5p, miR-20a
Jing et al., 2008 [117]	Plasma	Proteomics-mass spectrometry
Kocbek et al., 2015 [66]	Serum	Glycodelin-A
Kuessel et al., 2014 [141]	Urine	CK19
Liu et al., 2007 [139]	Plasma	Proteomics – mass spectrometry
Malin et al., 2019 [118]	Serum	AXIN1
Martinez et al., 2007 [70]	Serum	IL-6
May et al., 2010 [12]	Serum	FGF-2, angiogenin
Mihalyi et al., 2010 [61]	Serum	CA-125, IL-8, TNF-α
Morin et al., 2005 [152]	Peripheral blood	Macrophage migration inhibitory factor
Mosbah et al., 2016 [65]	Serum	ICAM-1, glycodelin
Nabeta et al., 2009 [108]	Serum	Anti-α-enolase antibodies
Nasiri et al., 2017 [87]	Serum	Malondialdehyde (MDA)
Nisenblat et al., 2019 [132]	Serum	miR-155, miR574-3p, and miR139-3p
Ohata et al., 2008 [76]	Seum	IL-8
Ohlsson et al., 2009 [127]	Serum	miR-200a, miR-200b, and miR-141
Othman et al., 2008 [70]	Serum	Il-6, MCP-1, IFN-γ, IL-2, IL-8, IL-15
Ozhan et al., 2014 [105]	Serum	Syntaxin-5, anti-endometrial antibody
Philippoussis et al., 2004 [95]	Serum	IGFBP3, EGF
Pizzo et al., 2002 [75]	Serum	IL-8
Potlog-Nahar.i, 2004 [147]	Urine	VEGF
Qui et al., 2019 [139]	Serum	lncRNA
Reis et al., 2012 [68]	Serum	Activin A, follistatin
Rekker et al., 2015 [125]	Serum	miR-200a-3p, miR-200b-3p, miR-141-3p
Seeber et al., 2008 [80]	Serum	TNF-α
Sengul et al., 2014 [97]	Serum	Nesfatin-1
Socolov et al., 2010 [73]	Serum	IL-6, IL-8, IL-1, CA-125, TNF
Steff et al., 2004 [94]	Serum	IGF-1, IGFBP3
Suryavanshi et al., 2013 [135]	Serum	miR-195, miR-16, miR-191
Tokmak et al., 2011 [98]	Serum	Urocortin
Tokushige et al., 2011 [144]	Urine	CK19
Becker et al., 2010 [143]	Urine	MMP-2, MMP-9
Tuten et al., 2014 [64]	Serum	Copeptin, CA-125, C-reactive protein, CA-15-3, CA-19-9
Vanhie et al., 2019 [133]	Serum	hsa-miR-125b-5p, hsa-miR-28-5p and hsa-miR-29a-3p
Vigano et al., 2003 [69]	Serum	ICAM-1
Vodolazkaia et al., 2012 [63]	Serum	VEGF, CA-125, Annexin V, glycodelin
Wang et al., 2013 [129]	Serum	miR-145, miR-122, miR-199a, miR-141-5p
Wang et al., 2016 [138]	Serum	lncRNA
Xavier et al., 2006 [78]	Serum	TNF-α, VEGF

7. Conclusions

Despite its benign character, endometriosis remains a debilitating disease that interferes with the quality of life of millions of women. The main symptoms: pelvic pain, infertility, and severe dysmenorrhea are nonspecific, and thus, invariably lead to a long-term delay in establishing the appropriate diagnosis. An invasive procedure, surgery, followed by a histopathological exam, represents the gold standard for diagnosis. As such, literature review proved to be a saga of noninvasive biomarkers, with researchers focusing their efforts into developing noninvasive putative biomarkers for this pathology in hope for promising perspectives on early diagnosis.

Various lines of evidence support the potential role of many biomolecules or panels of biomolecules, but, as of yet, none of them have the test proof sensitivity and specificity. Therefore, they can only complement the diagnosis of this pathology, in conjunction with imaging techniques or laparoscopic surgery.

Inflammatory cytokines proved to be the most non-suitable candidates for noninvasive diagnosis of endometriosis, despite the ability of several panels of cytokines to discriminate between affected and non-affected patients. Similarly, no single miRNA or lncRNA was considered as a sole noninvasive biomarker. According to various authors, a panel of miRNAs or lncRNAs could be more conducive indicators of this gynecological pathology.

The latest technologies consisting of proteomics, metabolomics, and genomics that investigate a complete panel of molecules or a profile of genes could evolve into the gold standard diagnostic tool and thus eliminate invasive laparoscopies.

Furthermore, increased knowledge of the pathophysiologic mechanisms of endometriosis is crucial for a more expedient and accurate diagnosis, improving the overall health-related quality of life.

Author Contributions: C.V.A., M.A.M., I.S.: conceptualization, formal analysis, investigation, A.B., A.E.N., A.-M.D.: writing original draft, editing, drawing figures. R.M.D., L.-M.C.: methodology, supervision, validation. All authors read and approved the final manuscript.

Funding: The authors received no financial support for the research, authorship, and/or publication of this article.

Conflicts of Interest: The authors declare no conflict of interest.

Abbreviations

BMI	Body mass index
C3	Complement
CK 19	Cytokeratin 19
COX-2	Cyclooxygenase 2
CRP	C-reactive protein
DNA	Deoxiribonucleic acid
EGF	Endothelial growth factor
EGFR	Endothelial growth factor receptor
ELISA	Enzyme-linked immunosorbent assay
FGF	Fibroblast growth factor
GM-CSF	Granulocyte macrophage colony-stimulating factor
HOXA	Homebox A
ICAM	Intercellular adhesion molecule
IFN	Interferon
IGF	Insulin-like growth factor
Il	Interleukin
iNKT	Invariant natural killer T cells
lncRNA	Long non-coding ribonucleic acid
MCP-1	Monocyte chemoattractant protein 1
MIF	Macrophage inhibitory factor
MMP	Matrix metalloproteinase
miRNA	Micro ribonucleic acid

mtDNA	Mitochondrial DNA
NK	Natural killer
NF-KB	Nuclear factor-kappa beta
PDGF	Platelet-derived growth factor
PG	Prostaglandins
PGE2	Prostaglandin E2
PK-1	Prokinetitsin 1
RANTES	Regulated on Activation, Normal T Cell Expressed and Secreted
ROS	Reactive oxygen species
SOD	Superoxide dismutase
sFlt1	Soluble fms-like tyrosine kinase
TNF	Tumor-necrosis factor
TSP-1	Thrombospondin 1
VDBP	Urinary vitamin D binding protein
VEGF	Vascular endothelial growth factor
VEGFR	Vascular endothelial growth factor receptor
Wnt/b-catenin	Wingless-type mouse mammary tumor virus integration site family

References

1. Bratila, E.; Comandasu, D.-E.; Coreleuca, C.; Cirstoiu, M.; Bohiltea, R.; Mehedintu, C.; Vladareanu, S.; Berceanu, C. Gatrointestinal Symptoms in Endometriosis Correlated With the Disease Stage. 2016. Available online: https://www.researchgate.net/publication/312552546_Gastrointestinal_symptoms_in_endometriosis_correlated_with_the_disease_stage (accessed on 27 October 2019).
2. Giudice, L.C.; Kao, L.C. Endometriosis. *Lancet* **2004**, *364*, 1789–1799. [CrossRef]
3. Moga, M.A.; Balan, A.; Dimienescu, O.G.; Burtea, V.; Dragomir, R.M.; Anastasiu, V.C. Circulating miRNAs as biomarkers for endometriosis and endometriosis-related ovarian cancer—An overview. *J. Clin. Med.* **2019**, *8*, 735. [CrossRef]
4. Bulletti, C.; Coccia, M.E.; Battistoni, S.; Borini, A. Endometriosis and infertility. *J. Assist. Reprod. Genet.* **2010**, *27*, 441–447. [CrossRef]
5. Argawal, S.K.; Chapron, C.; Giudice, L.C.; Laufer, M.R.; Lyland, N.; Missmer, S.A.; Singh, S.S.; Taylor, H.S. Clinical diagnosis of endometriosis: A call to action. *Am. J. Obstet. Gynecol.* **2019**, *220*, 354.e1–354.e12. [CrossRef]
6. Nnoaham, K.E.; Hummelshoj, L.; Webster, P.; D'Hooghe, T.; de Cicco Nardone, F.; de Cicco Nardone, C.; de Cicco Nardone, C.; Jerkinson, C.; Kennedy, S.H.; Zondervan, K.T.; et al. Impact of endometriosis on quality of life and work productivity: A multicenter study across ten countries. *Fertil. Steril.* **2011**, *96*, 366–373. [CrossRef]
7. Fassbender, A.; Burney, R.O.; D'Hooghe, T.; Giudice, L. Update on biomarkers for the detection of endometriosis. *BioMed Res. Int.* **2015**, *2015*, 130854. [CrossRef]
8. Hadfield, R.; Mardon, H.; Barlow, D.; Kennedy, S. Delay in the diagnosis of endometriosis: A survey of women from the USA and the UK. *Hum. Reprod.* **1996**, *11*, 878–880. [CrossRef]
9. Ahn, S.H.; Singh, V.; Tayade, C. Biomarkers in endometriosis: Challenges and opportunities. *Fertil. Steril.* **2017**, *107*, 523–532. [CrossRef] [PubMed]
10. Irungu, S.; Mavrelos, D.; Worthington, J.; Blyuss, O.; Saridogan, E.; Timms, J.F. Discovery of non-invasive biomarkers for the diagnosis of endometriosis. *Clin. Proteom.* **2019**, *16*, 14. [CrossRef] [PubMed]
11. Biomarkers Definitions Working Group. Biomarkers and surrogate endpoints: Preferred definitions and conceptual framework. *Clin. Pharmacol. Ther.* **2001**, *69*, 89–95. [CrossRef] [PubMed]
12. May, K.E.; Conduit-Hulbert, S.A.; Villar, J.; Kirtley, S.; Kennedy, S.H.; Becker, C.M. Peripheral biomarkers of endometriosis: A systematic review. *Hum. Reprod. Update* **2010**, *16*, 651–674. [CrossRef] [PubMed]
13. Halme, J.; Hammond, M.G.; Hulka, J.F.; Raj, S.G.; Talbert, L.M. Retrograde menstruation in healthy women and in patients with endometriosis. *Obstet. Gynecol.* **1984**, *64*, 151–154. [PubMed]
14. Lagana, A.S.; Vitale, S.G.; Salmeri, F.M.; Triolo, O.; Ban Frangez, H.; Vrtacnik-Bokal, E.; Stojanovska, L.; Apostolopoulos, V.; Granese, R.; Sofo, V. Unus pro omnibus, omnes pro uno: A novel, evidence-based, unifying theory for the pathogenesis of endometriosis. *Med. Hypotheses* **2017**, *103*, 10–20. [CrossRef] [PubMed]

15. Pluchino, N.; Taylor, H.S. Endometriosis and stem cell trafficking. *Reprod. Sci.* **2016**, *23*, 1616–1619. [CrossRef] [PubMed]
16. Lagana, A.S.; Salmeri, F.M.; Vitale, S.G.; Triolo, O.; Gotte, M. Stem cell trafficking during endometriosis: May epigenetics play a pivotal role? *Reprod. Sci.* **2017**, *25*, 978–979. [CrossRef]
17. Eggers, J.C.; Martino, V.; Reinbold, R.; Schafer, S.D.; Kiesel, L.; Starzinski-Powitz, A.; Schuring, A.N.; Kemper, B.; Greve, B.; Gotte, M. microRNA miR-200b affects proliferation, invasiveness and stemness of endometriotic cells by targeting ZEB1, ZEB2 and KLF4. *Reprod. Biomed. Online* **2016**, *32*, 434–445. [CrossRef]
18. Marki, G.; Bokor, A.; Rigo, J.; Rigo, A. Physical pain and emotion regulation as the main predictive factors of health-related quality of life in women living with endometriosis. *Hum. Reprod.* **2017**, *32*, 1432–1438. [CrossRef]
19. Lagana, A.S.; La Rosa, V.L.; Rapisarda, A.M.C. Anxiety and depression in patients with endometriosis: Impact and management challenges. *Int. J. Women Health.* **2017**, *9*, 323–330. [CrossRef]
20. Zheng, W.; Cao, L.; Zheng, X.; Yuanyuan, M.; Liang, X. Anti-Angiogenic Alternative and complementary medicines for the treatment of endometriosis: A review of potential molecular mechanisms. *Evid. Based Complement. Alternat. Med.* **2018**, *2018*, 4128984. [CrossRef]
21. Lousse, J.C.; Van Langendonckt, A.; Defrere, S.; Gonzalez Ramos, R.; Colette, S. Peritoneal endometriosis is an inflammatory disease. *Frontiers Biosci.* **2012**, *E4*, 23–40. [CrossRef]
22. Gazvani, R.; Templeton, A. Peritoneal environment, cytokines and angiogenesis in the pathophysiology of endometriosis. *Reprod.* **2002**, *123*, 217–226. [CrossRef] [PubMed]
23. Van Langendonckt, A.; Casanas-Roux, F.; Donnez, J. Oxidative stress and peritoneal endometriosis. *Fertil. Steril.* **2002**, *77*, 861–870. [CrossRef]
24. Oral, E.; Olive, D.L.; Arici, A. The peritoneal environment in endometriosis. *Hum. Reprod. Update* **1996**, 385–398. [CrossRef] [PubMed]
25. Wu, M.H.; Shoji, Y.; Chuang, P.; Tsai, S. Endometriosis: Disease pathophysiology and the role of prostaglandins. *Expert Rev Mol Med.* **2007**, *9*, 1–20. [CrossRef] [PubMed]
26. Sugino, N.; Karube-Harada, A.; Taketani, T.; Sakata, A.; Nakamura, Y. Withdrawal of ovarian steroids stimulates prostaglandin F2-alpha production through nuclear factor-kappaB activation via oxygen radicals in human endometrial stromal cells: Potential relevance to menstruation. *J. Reprod. Dev.* **2004**, *50*, 215–225. [CrossRef]
27. Banu, S.K.; Lee, J.; Speights, V.O.; Starzinski-Powitz, A.; Arosh, J.A. Cyclooxygenase-2 regulates survival, migration, and invasion of human endometriotic cells through multiple mechanisms. *Endocrinol* **2008**, *149*, 1180–1189. [CrossRef]
28. Wu, M.H.; Wang, C.A.; Lin, C.C.; Chen, L.-C.; Chang, W.-C.; Tsai, S.-J. Distinct regulation of cyclooxygenase-2 by interleukin-1 beta in normal and endometriotic stromal cells. *J. Clin. Endocrinol. Metab.* **2005**, *90*, 286–295. [CrossRef]
29. Lagana, A.S.; Garzon, S.; Gotte, M.; Vigano, P.; Franchi, M.; Ghezzi, F.; Martin, D.C. The pathogenesis of endometriosis: Molecular and cell biology insights. *Int. J. Mol. Sci.* **2019**, *20*, 5615. [CrossRef]
30. Laird, S.M.; Tuckerman, E.M.; Cork, B.A.; Li, T.C. Expression of nuclear factor kappa B in human endometrium; role in the control of interleukin 6 and leukaemia inhibitory factor production. *Mol. Hum. Reprod.* **2000**, *6*, 34–40. [CrossRef]
31. Page, M.; Tuckerman, E.M.; Li, T.C.; Laird, S.M. Expression of nuclear factor kappa-B components in human endometrium. *J. Reprod. Immunol.* **2002**, *54*, 1–13. [CrossRef]
32. King, A.E.; Critchley, H.; Kelly, R.W. The NF-kappaB pathway in human endometrium and first trimester decidua. *Mol. Hum. Reprod.* **2001**, *7*, 175–183. [CrossRef] [PubMed]
33. González Ramos, R.; Van Langendonckt, A.; Defrère, S.; Lousse, J.C.; Colette, S.; Devoto, L.; Donnez, J. Involvement of the nuclear factor-kappaB (NF-kappa B) pathway in the pathogenesis of endometriosis. *Fertil Steril* **2010**, *94*, 1985–1994. [CrossRef] [PubMed]
34. Lousse, J.C.; Van Langendonckt, A.; González Ramos, R.; Defrère, S.; Renkin, E.; Donnez, J. Increased activation of nuclear factor-kappa B (NF-kappa B) in isolated peritoneal macrophages of patients with endometriosis. *Fertil. Steril.* **2008**, *90*, 217–220. [CrossRef] [PubMed]
35. Agarwal, A.; Gupta, S.; Sikka, S. The role of oxidative stress in endometriosis. *Curr. Opin. Obstet. Gynecol.* **2006**, *18*, 325–332. [CrossRef] [PubMed]

36. Zeller, J.M.; Henig, I.; Radwanska, E.; Dmowski, W.P. Enhancement of human monocyte and peritoneal macrophage chemiluminescence activities in women with endometriosis. *Am. J. Reprod. Immunol. Microbiol.* **1987**, *13*, 78–82. [CrossRef]
37. Portz, D.M.; Elkins, T.E.; White, R.; Warren, J.; Adadevoh, S.; Randolph, J. Oxygen free radicals and pelvic adhesion formation: Blocking oxygen free radical toxicity to prevent adhesion formation in an endometriosis model. *Int. J. Fertil.* **1991**, *36*, 39–42. [CrossRef]
38. Wang, Y.; Sharma, R.K.; Falcone, T.; Goldberg, J.; Agarwal, A. Importance of reactive oxygen species in the peritoneal fluid of women with endometriosis or idiopathic infertility. *Fertil. Steril.* **1997**, *68*, 826–830. [CrossRef]
39. Polak, G.; Koziol-Montewka, M.; Gogacz, M.; Blaszkowska, I.; Kotarski, J. Total antioxidant status of the peritoneal fluid in infertile women. *Eur. J. Obstet. Gynecol. Reprod. Biol.* **2001**, *94*, 261–263. [CrossRef]
40. Wu, M.H.; Hsiao, K.Y.; Tsai, S.J. Endometriosis and possible inflammation markers. *Gynecol. Minim. Invasive Ther.* **2015**, *4*, 61–67. [CrossRef]
41. Lagana, A.S.; Salmeri, F.M.; Ban Frangez, H.; Ghezzi, F.; Vrtacnik-Bokal, E.; Granese, R. Evaluation of M1 and M2 macrophages in ovarian endometriomas from women affected by endometriosis at different stages of the disease. *Gynecol. Endocrinol.* **2019**, *30*, 1–4. [CrossRef]
42. Capobianco, A.; Monno, A.; Cottone, L.; Venneri, M.A.; Biziato, D.; Di Puppo, F.; Ferrari, S.; De Palma, M.; Manfredi, A.A.; Rovere-Querini, P. Proangiogenic Tie2(+) macrophages infiltrate human and murine endometriotic lesions and dictate their growth in a mouse model of the disease. *Am. J. Pathol.* **2011**, *179*, 2651–2659. [CrossRef] [PubMed]
43. Lagana, A.S.; Ghezzi, F.; Vetvicka, V. Endometriosis and risk of ovarian cancer: What do we know? *Arch. Gynecol. Obstet.* **2019**, *301*, 1–10. [CrossRef]
44. Wu, M.Y.; Yang, J.H.; Chao, K.H.; Hwang, J.L.; Yang, Y.S.; Ho, H.N. Increase in the expression of killer cell inhibitory receptors on peritoneal natural killer cells in women with endometriosis. *Fertil. Steril.* **2000**, *74*, 1187–1191. [CrossRef]
45. Lagana, A.S.; Triolo, O.; Salmeri, F.M.; Granese, R.; Palmara, V.I.; Ban Frangez, H.; Vrtcnik Bokal, E.; Sofo, V. Natural Killer T cell subsets in eutopic and ectopic endometrium: A fresh look to a busy corner. *Arch. Gynecol. Obstet.* **2016**, *293*, 941–949. [CrossRef] [PubMed]
46. Ho, H.N.; Wu, M.Y.; Chao, K.H.; Der Chen, C.; Chen, S.U.; Yang, Y.S. Peritoneal interleukin-10 increases with decrease in activated CD4+ T lymphocytes in women with endometriosis. *Hum. Reprod.* **1997**, *12*, 2528–2533. [CrossRef] [PubMed]
47. Nie, M.-F.; Xie, Q.; Wu, Y.-H.; He, H.; Zou, L.-J.; She, X.-L.; Wu, X.-Q. Serum and Ectopic Endometrium from Women with Endometriosis Modulate Macrophage M1/M2 Polarization via the Smad2/Smad3 Pathway. *J. Immun. Res.* **2018**, *2018*, 14. [CrossRef] [PubMed]
48. Kralickova, M.; Vetvicka, V. Immunological aspects of endometriosis: Review. *Ann. Transl. Med.* **2015**, *3*, 153. [CrossRef]
49. Osuga, Y.; Hirota, Y.; Hirata, T.; Takamura, M.; Urata, Y.; Harada, M.; Izumi, G.; Fujii, T.; Koga, K. Th2 Cells and Th17 cells in the development of endometriosis—Possible roles of interleukin-4 and interleukin-17A. *J. Endometr. Pelvic Pain Dis.* **2016**, *8*, 136–140. [CrossRef]
50. Asante, A.; Taylor, R.N. Endometriosis: The role of neuroangiogenesis. *Ann. Rev. Physiol.* **2011**, *73*, 163–182. [CrossRef]
51. Hanahan, D.; Folkman, J. Patterns and emerging mechanisms of the angiogenic switch during tumorigenesis. *Cell* **1996**, *86*, 353–364. [CrossRef]
52. Ahn, S.H.; Edwards, A.K.; Singh, S.S.; Young, S.L.; Lessey, B.A.; Tayade, C. Il-17A contributes to the pathogenesis of endometriosis bu triggering proinflammatory cytokines and angiogenic growth factors. *J. Immunol.* **2015**, *195*, 2591–2600. [CrossRef] [PubMed]
53. Gupta, M.K.; Qin, R.Y. Mechanism and its regulation of tumor-induced angiogenesis. *World J. Gastroenterol.* **2003**, *9*, 1144–1155. [CrossRef] [PubMed]
54. Strieter, R.M.; Polverini, P.J.; Kunkel, S.L.; Arenberg, D.A.; Burdick, M.D.; Kasper, J.; Dzuiba, J.; Van Damme, J.; Walz, A.; Marriott, D.; et al. The functional role of the ELR motif in CXC chemokine-mediated angiogenesis. *J. Biol. Chem.* **1995**, *270*, 27348–27357. [CrossRef] [PubMed]
55. Volpert, O.V.; Fong, T.; Koch, A.E.; Peterson, J.D.; Waltenbaugh, C.; Tepper, R.I.; Bouck, N.P. Inhibition of angiogenesis by interleukin 4. *J. Exp. Med.* **1998**, *188*, 1039–1046. [CrossRef]

56. Torisu, H.; Ono, M.; Kiryu, H.; Furue, M.; Ohmoto, Y.; Nakayama, J.; Nishioka, Y.; Sone, S.; Kuwano, M. Macrophage infiltration correlates with tumor stage and angiogenesis in human malignant melanoma: Possible involvement of TNFalpha and IL-1alpha. *Int. J. Cancer* **2000**, *85*, 182–188. [CrossRef]
57. Donnez, J.; Smoes, P.; Gillerot, S.; Casanas-Roux, F.; Nisolle, M. Vascular endothelial growth factor (VEGF) in endometriosis. *Hum. Reprod.* **1998**, *3*, 1686–1690. [CrossRef]
58. Machado, D.E.; Rodrigues-Baptista, K.C.; Perini, J.A. Soares de Moura, R. Euterpe oleracea extract (Açaí) is a promising novel pharmacological therapeutic treatment for experimental endometriosis. *PLoS ONE* **2016**, *11*, e0166059. [CrossRef]
59. Thambisetty, M.; Lovestone, S. Blood-based biomarkers of Alzheimers disease: Challenging but feasible. *Biomark. Med.* **2010**, *4*, 65–79. [CrossRef]
60. Mol, B.W.J.; Bayram, N.; Lijmer, J.G.; Wiegerinck, M.A.H.M.; Bongers, M.Y.; Van der Veen, F.; Bossuyt, P. The performance of CA-125 measurement in the detection of endometriosis: A meta-analysis. *Fertil. Steril.* **1998**, *70*, 1101–1108. [CrossRef]
61. Mihalyi, A.; Gevaert, O.; Kyama, C.M.; Simsa, P.; Pochet, N.; De Smet, F.; De Moor, B.; Meuleman, C.; Billen, J.; Blanckaert, N.; et al. Non-invasive diagnosis of endometriosis based on a combined analysis of six plasma biomarkers. *Hum. Reprod.* **2010**, *25*, 654–664. [CrossRef]
62. Agic, A.; Djalali, S.; Wolfler, M.M.; Halis, G.; Diedrich, K.; Hornung, D. Combination of CCR1 mRNA, MCP1, and CA125 measurements in peripheral blood as a diagnostic test for endometriosis. *Reprod. Sci.* **2008**, *15*, 906–911. [CrossRef] [PubMed]
63. Vodolazkaia, A.; El-Aalamat, Y.; Popovic, D. Evaluation of a panel of 28 biomarkers for the non-invasive diagnosis of endometriosis. *Hum. Reprod.* **2012**, *27*, 2698–2711. [CrossRef] [PubMed]
64. Ozhan, E.; Kokcu, A.; Yanik, K.; Gunaydin, M. Investigation of diagnostic potentials of nine different biomarkers in endometriosis. *Eur. J. Obstet. Gynecol.* **2014**, *178*, 128–133. [CrossRef] [PubMed]
65. Mosbah, A.; Nabiel, Y.; Khashaba, E. Interleukin-6, intracellular adhesion molecule-1, and glycodelin A levels in serum and peritoneal fluid as biomarkers for endometriosis. *Obstet. Gynecol.* **2016**, *134*, 247–251. [CrossRef] [PubMed]
66. Kocbek, V.; Vouk, K.; Bersinger, N.A.; Mueller, M.D.; Lanišnik Rižner, T. Panels of Cytokines and Other Secretory Proteins as Potential Biomarkers of Ovarian Endometriosis. *J. Mol. Diagn.* **2015**, *17*, 325–334. [CrossRef]
67. Pretice Crapper, E. Clinical Biomarkers for the Noninvasive Diagnosis of Endometriosis. 2016. Available online: http://hdl.handle.net/11375/20495 (accessed on 26 February 2020).
68. Reis, F.M.; Luisi, S.; Abrão, M.S.; Rocha, A.L.L.; Viganò, P.; Rezende, C.P.; Florio, P.; Petraglia, F. Diagnostic value of serum activin A and follistatin levels in women with peritoneal, ovarian and deep infiltrating endometriosis. *Hum. Reprod.* **2012**, *27*, 1445–1450. [CrossRef]
69. Vigano, P.; Infantino, M.; Lattuada, D.; Lauletta, R.; Ponti, E.; Somigliana, E.; Vignali, M.; DiBlasio, A.M. Intercellular adhesion molecule-1 (ICAM-1) gene polymorphisms in endometriosis. *Mol. Hum. Reprod.* **2003**, *9*, 47–52. [CrossRef]
70. Othman, E.E.R.; Hornung, D.; Salem, H.T.; Kalifa, E.A.; El-Metwally, T.H.; Al-Hendy, A. Serum cytokines as biomarkers for nonsurgical prediction of endometriosis. *Eur. J. Obstet. Gynecol. Repd. Biol.* **2008**, *137*, 240–246. [CrossRef]
71. Borrelli, G.M.; Abrão, M.S.; Mechsner, S. Can chemokines be used as biomarkers for endometriosis? A systematic review. *Hum. Reprod.* **2014**, *29*, 253–266. [CrossRef]
72. Martinez, S.; Garrido, N.; Coperias, J.L.; Pardo, F.; Desco, J.; Garcia-Velasco, J.A.; Simon, C.; Pellicer, A. Serum interleukin-6 levels are elevated in women with minimal-mild endometriosis. *Hum. Reprod.* **2007**, *22*, 836–842. [CrossRef]
73. Socolov, R.; Butureanu, S.; Angioni, S.; Sindilar, A.; Boiculese, V.L.; Cozma, L.; Socolov, D. The value of serological markers in the diagnosis and prognosis of endometriosis: A prospective case-control study. *Eur. J. Obstet. Gynecol. Reprod. Biol.* **2010**, *154*, 215–217. [CrossRef] [PubMed]
74. Kalu, E.; Sumar, N.; Giannopoulos, T.; Patel, P.; Croucher, C.; Sherriff, E.; Bansal, A. Cytokine profiles in serum and peritoneal fluid from infertile women with and without endometriosis. *J. Obstet. Gynaecol. Res.* **2007**, *33*, 490–495. [CrossRef] [PubMed]

75. Pizzo, A.; Salmeri, F.M.; Ardita, F.V.; Sofo, V.; Tripepi, M.; Marsico, S. Behaviour of cytokine levels in serum and peritoneal fluid of women with endometriosis. *Gynecol. Obstet. Investig.* **2002**, *54*, 82–87. [CrossRef] [PubMed]
76. Ohata, Y.; Harada, T.; Miyakoda, H.; Taniguchi, F.; Iwabe, T.; Terakawa, N. Serum interleukin-8 levels are elevated in patients with ovarian endometrioma. *Fertil. Steril.* **2008**, *90*, 994–999. [CrossRef]
77. Darai, E.; Detchev, R.; Hugol, D.; Quang, N.T. Serum and cyst fluid levels of interleukin (IL) -6, IL-8 and tumour necrosis factor-alpha in women with endometriomas and benign and malignant cystic ovarian tumours. *Hum. Reprod.* **2003**, *18*, 1681–1685. [CrossRef] [PubMed]
78. Xavier, P.; Belo, L.; Beires, J.; Rebelo, I.; Martinez-de-Oliveira, J.; Lunet, N.; Barros, H. Serum levels of VEGF and TNF-a and their association with C-reactive protein in patients with endometriosis. *Arch. Gynecol. Obstet.* **2006**, *273*, 227–231. [CrossRef]
79. Cho, S.H.; Oh, Y.J.; Nam, A.; Kim, H.Y.; Park, J.H.; Kim, J.H.; Cho, D.J.; Lee, B.S. Evaluation of Serum and Urinary Angiogenic Factors in Patients with Endometriosis. *Am. J. Reprod. Immunol.* **2007**, *58*, 497–504. [CrossRef]
80. Seeber, B.; Sammel, M.D.; Fan, X.; Gerton, G.L.; Shaunik, A.; Chittams, J.; Barnhart, K.T. Panel of markers can accurately predict endometriosis in a subset of patients. *Fertil. Steril.* **2008**, *89*, 1073–1081. [CrossRef]
81. Steff, A.M.; Gagné, D.; Pagé, M.; Rioux, A.; Hugo, P.; Gosselin, D. Insulin-like growth factor-1, soluble tumor necrosis factor receptor-1 and angiogenin in endometriosis patients. *Am. J. Reprod. Immunol.* **2004**, *51*, 166–173. [CrossRef]
82. Choi, Y.S.; Kim, S.; Oh, Y.S.; Cho, S.; Hoon Kim, S. Elevated serum interleukin-32 levels in patients with endometriosis: A cross-sectional study. *Am. J. Reprod. Immunol.* **2019**, *82*, e13149. [CrossRef]
83. Kikuchi, Y.; Ishikawa, N.; Hirata, J.; Imaizumi, E.; Sasa, H.; Nagata, I. Changes of peripheral blood lymphocyte subsets before and after operation of patients with endometriosis. *Acta Obstet. Gynecol. Scand.* **1993**, *72*, 157–161. [CrossRef] [PubMed]
84. Tuten, A.; Kucur, M.; Imamoglu, M.; Kaya, B.; Acikgoz, A.S.; Yilmaz, N.; Ozturk, Z.; Oncul, M. Copeptin is associated with the severity of endometriosis. *Arch. Gynecol. Obstet.* **2014**, *290*, 75–82. [CrossRef] [PubMed]
85. Carvalho, L.F.; Samadder, A.N.; Agarwal, A.; Fernandes, L.F.; Abrao, M.S. Oxidative stress biomarkers in patients with endometriosis: Systematic review. *Arch. Gynecol. Obstet.* **2012**, *286*, 1033–1040. [CrossRef] [PubMed]
86. Scutiero, G.; Iannone, P.; Bernardi, G.; Bonaccorsi, G.; Spadaro, S.; Volta, C.A.; Greco, P.; Nappi, L. Oxidative stress and endometriosis: A systematic review of the literature. *Oxidative Med. Cell Longev.* **2017**, *2017*, 7265238. [CrossRef] [PubMed]
87. Nasiri, N.; Moini, A.; Eftekhari-Yazdi, P.; Karimian, L.; Salman-Yazdi, R.; Arabipoor, A. Oxidative stress statues in serum and follicular fluid of women with endometriosis. *Cell. J.* **2017**, *18*, 582–587. [PubMed]
88. Verit, F.F.; Erel, O.; Celik, N. Serum paraoxonase-1 activity in women with endometriosis and its relationship with the stage of the disease. *Hum. Reprod.* **2008**, 100–104. [CrossRef]
89. Jackson, L.W.; Schisterman, E.F.; Dey-Rao, R.; Browne, R.; Armstrong, D. Oxidative stress and endometriosis. *Hum. Reprod.* **2005**, *20*, 2014–2020. [CrossRef]
90. Turkyilmaz, E.; Yildirim, M.; Cendek, B.D.; Baran, P.; Alisik, M.; Dalgaci, F.; Yavuz, A.F. Evaluation of oxidative stress markers and intra-extracellular antioxidant activities in patients with endometriosis. *Eur. J. Obstet. Gynecol. Reprod. Biol.* **2016**, *199*, 164–168. [CrossRef]
91. Prieto, L.; Quesada, J.F.; Cambero, O.; Pacheco, A.; Pellicer, A.; Codoceo, R.; Garcia-Velasco, J.A. Analysis of follicular fluid and serum markers of oxidative stress in women with infertility related to endometriosis. *Fertil. Steril.* **2012**, *98*, 126–130. [CrossRef]
92. Andrisani, A.; Dona, G.; Brunati, A.M.; Clari, G.; Armanini, D.; Ragazzi, E.; Ambrosini, G.; Bordin, L. Increased oxidation-related glutathionylation and carbonic anhydrase activity in endometriosis. *Reprod. Biomed. Online* **2014**, *28*, 773–779. [CrossRef]
93. Gurgan, T.; Bukulmez, O.; Yarali, H.; Tanir, M.; Akyildiz, S. Serum and peritoneal fluid levels of IGF I and II and insulin-like growth binding protein-3 in endometriosis. *J. Reprod. Med.* **1999**, *44*, 450–454. [CrossRef] [PubMed]
94. Steff, A.M.; Gagne, D.; Page, M.; Hugo, P.; Gosselin, D. Concentration of soluble intercellular adhesion molecule-1 in serum samples from patients with endometriosis collected during the luteal phase of the menstrual cycle. *Hum. Reprod.* **2004**, *19*, 172–178. [CrossRef] [PubMed]

95. Philippoussis, F.; Gagne, D.; Hugo, P.; Gosselin, D. Concentrations of alpha-fetoprotein, insulin-like growth factor binding protein-3, c-erbB-2, and epidermal growth factor in serum of patients with endometriosis. *J. Soc. Gynecol. Investig.* **2004**, *11*, 175–181. [CrossRef] [PubMed]
96. Garcia-Galiano, D.; Navarro, V.M.; Gaytan, F.; Tena-Sempere, M. Expanding roles of NUCB2/nesfatin-1 in neuroendocrine regulation. *J. Mol. Endocrinol.* **2010**, *45*, 281–290. [CrossRef]
97. Sengul, O.; Dilbaz, B.; Halici, Z.; Ferah, I.; Cadirci, E.; Yilmaz, F. Decreased serum nesfatin-1 levels in endometriosis. *Eur. J. Obstet. Gynecol. Reprod. Biol.* **2014**, *177*, 34–37. [CrossRef]
98. Tokmak, A.; Ugur, M.; Tonguc, E.; Var, T.; Moraloglu, O.; Ozaksit, G. The value of urocortin and CA-125 in the diagnosis of endometrioma. *Arch. Gynecol. Obstet.* **2011**, *283*, 1075–1079. [CrossRef]
99. Chmaj-Wierzchowska, K.; Kampioni, M.; Wilczak, M.; Sajdak, S.; Opala, T. Novel markers in the diagnostics of endometriomas: Urocortin, ghrelin and leptin or leukocytes, fibrinogen, and CA-125? *Taiwan. J. Obstet. Gynecol.* **2015**, *54*, 126–130. [CrossRef]
100. Florio, P.; Reis, F.M.; Torres, P.B.; Calonaci, F.; Toti, P.; Bocchi, C.; Linton, E.A.; Petraglia, F. Plasma urocortin levels in the diagnosis of ovarian endometriosis. *Obstet. Gynecol.* **2007**, *110*, 594–600. [CrossRef]
101. Mohamed, M.L.; El Behery, M.M.; Mansour, S.A.E.-A. Comparative study between VEGF-A and CA-125 in diagnosis and follow-up of advanced endometriosis after conservative laparoscopic surgery. *Arch. Gynecol. Obstet.* **2013**, *287*, 77–82. [CrossRef]
102. Bourlev, V.; Iljasova, N.; Adamyan, L.; Larsson, A.; Olovsson, M. Signs of reduced angiogenic activity after surgical removal of deeply infiltrating endometriosis. *Fertil. Steril.* **2010**, *94*, 52–57. [CrossRef]
103. Szubert, M.; Suzin, J.; Duechler, M.; Szuławska, A.; Czyz, M.; Kowalczyk-Amico, K. Evaluation of selected angiogenic and inflammatory markers in endometriosis before and after danazol treatment. *Reprod. Fertil. Dev.* **2014**, *26*, 414–420. [CrossRef] [PubMed]
104. Chen, L.; Fan, R.; Huang, X.; Xu, H.; Zhang, X. Reduced levels of serum pigment epithelium-derived factor in women with endometriosis. *Reprod. Sci.* **2012**, *19*, 64–69. [CrossRef]
105. Ozhan, E.; Kokcu, A.; Yanik, K.; Gunaydin, M. Investigation of diagnostic potentials of nine different biomarkers in endometriosis. *Eur. J. Obstet. Gynecol. Reprod. Biol.* **2014**, *178*, 128–133. [CrossRef] [PubMed]
106. Gajbhiye, R.; Sonawani, A.; Khan, S.; Suryawanshi, A.; Kadam, S.; Warty, N.; Raut, V.; Khole, V. Identification and validation of novel serum markers for early diagnosis of endometriosis. *Hum. Reprod.* **2012**, *27*, 408–417. [CrossRef] [PubMed]
107. Yi, Y.-C.; Wang, S.-C.; Chao, C.-C.; Su, C.-L.; Lee, Y.-L.; Chen, L.-Y. Evaluation of serum autoantibody levels in the diagnosis of ovarian endometrioma. *J. Clin. Lab Anal.* **2010**, *24*, 357–362. [CrossRef] [PubMed]
108. Nabeta, M.; Abe, Y.; Kagawa, L.; Haraguchi, R.; Kito, K.; Ueda, N.; Sugita, A.; Yokoyama, M.; Kusanagi, Y.; Ito, M. Identification of anti-α-enolase autoantibody as a novel serum marker for endometriosis. *Proteom. Clin. Appl.* **2009**, *3*, 1201–1210. [CrossRef]
109. Inagaki, J.; Matsuura, E.; Kaihara, K.; Kobayashi, K.; Yasuda, T.; Nomizu, M.; Sugiura-Ogasawara, M.; Katano, K.; Aoki, K. IgG antilaminin-1 autoantibody and recurrent miscarriages. *Am. J. Reprod. Immunol.* **2001**, *45*, 232–238. [CrossRef]
110. Inagaki, J.; Sugiura-Ogasawara, M.; Nomizu, M.; Nakatsuka, M.; Ikuta, K.; Suzuki, N.; Kaihara, K.; Kobayashi, K.; Yasuda, T.; Shoenfeld, Y.; et al. An association of IgG anti-laminin-1 autoantibodies with endometriosis in infertile patients. *Hum. Reprod.* **2003**, *18*, 544–549. [CrossRef]
111. Mathur, S.; Garza, D.E.; Smith, L.F. Endometrial autoantigens eliciting immunoglobulin (Ig) G, IgA, and IgM responses in endometriosis. *Fertil. Steril.* **1990**, *54*, 56–63. [CrossRef]
112. Odukoya, O.A.; Wheatcroft, N.; Weetman, A.P.; Cooke, I.D. The prevalence of endometrial immunoglobulin G antibodies in patients with endometriosis. *Hum. Reprod.* **1995**, *10*, 1214–1219. [CrossRef]
113. Long, X.; Jinag, P.; Zhou, L.; Zhang, W. Evaluation of novel serum biomarkers and the proteomic differences of endometriosis and adenomyosis using MALDI-TOF–MS. *Arch. Gynecol Obstet.* **2013**, *288*, 201–205. [CrossRef] [PubMed]
114. Wölfler, M.M.; Schwamborn, C.; Otten, D.; Hornung, D.; Liu, H.; Rath, W. Mass spectrometry and serum pattern profiling for analyzing the individual risk for endometriosis: Promising insights? *Fertil. Steril.* **2009**, *91*, 2331–2337. [CrossRef]
115. Zheng, N.; Pan, C.; Liu, W. New serum biomarkers for detection of endometriosis using matrix-assisted laser desorption/ionization time-of-flight mass spectrometry. *J. Int. Med. Res.* **2011**, *39*, 1184–1192. [CrossRef] [PubMed]

116. Wang, L.; Zheng, W.; Mu, L.; Zhang, S.-Z. Identifying biomarkers of endometriosis using serum protein fingerprinting and artificial neural networks. *Int. J. Gynaecol. Obstet.* **2008**, *101*, 253–258. [CrossRef]
117. Jing, J.; Qiao, Y.; Suginami, H.; Taniguchi, F.; Shi, H.; Wang, S. Two novel serum biomarkers for endometriosis screened by surface-enhanced laser desorption/ionization time-of-flight mass spectrometry and their change after laparoscopic removal of endometriosis. *Fertil. Steril.* **2008**, *92*, 1221–1227. [CrossRef]
118. Malin, E.; Bodil, R.; Gunnar, E.; Bodil, O. AXIN1 in Plasma or Serum Is a Potential New Biomarker for Endometriosis. *Int. J. Mol. Sci.* **2019**, *20*, 189. [CrossRef]
119. Signorile, P.G.; Baldi, A. Supporting evidences for potential biomarkers of endometriosis detected in peripheral blood. *Data Brief.* **2015**, *5*, 971–974. [CrossRef]
120. Signorile, P.G.; Baldi, A. Serum Biomarker of Endometriosis. *J. Cell Physiol.* **2014**, *229*, 1731–1735. [CrossRef]
121. Dutta, M.; Joshi, M.; Srivastava, S.; Lodh, I.; Chakravarty, B.; Chaudhury, K. A metabonomics approach as a means for identification of potential biomarkers for early diagnosis of endometriosis. *Mol. Biosyst.* **2012**, *8*, 3281–3287. [CrossRef]
122. Vouk, K.; Hevir, N.; Ribic-Pucelj, M.; Haarpaintner, G.; Scherb, H.; Osredkar, J.; Moller, G.; Prehn, C.; Lanisnik Rizner, T.; Adamski, J. Discovery of phosphatidylcholines and sphingomyelins as biomarkers for ovarian endometriosis. *Hum. Reprod.* **2012**, *27*, 2955–2965. [CrossRef]
123. Zachariah, R.; Schmid, S.; Radpour, R.; Buerki, N.; Fan, A.X.-C.; Hahn, S.; Holzgreve, W.; Zhong, X.Y. Circulating cell free DNA as a potential biomarker for minimal and mild endometriosis. *Reprod. Biomed. Online* **2009**, *18*, 407–411. [CrossRef]
124. Creed, J.; Maggrah, A.; Reguly, B.; Harbottle, A. Mitochondrial DNA deletions accurately detect endometriosis in symptomatic females of child-bearing age. *Biomark. Med.* **2019**, *13*, 291–306. [CrossRef] [PubMed]
125. Bartel, D.P. MicroRNAs: Genomics, biogenesis, mechanism, and function. *Cell* **2004**, *116*, 281–297. [CrossRef]
126. Weber, J.A.; Baxter, D.H.; Zhang, S.; Huang, D.Y.; Huang, K.H.; Lee, M.J.; Galas, D.J.; Wang, K. The microRNA spectrum in 12 body fluids. *Clin. Chem.* **2010**, *56*, 1733–1741. [CrossRef] [PubMed]
127. Ohlsson Teague, E.M.C.; Print, C.G.; Hull, M.L. The role of microRNAs in endometriosis and associated reproductive conditions. *Hum. Reprod. Update* **2009**, *16*, 142–165. [CrossRef] [PubMed]
128. Zhao, M.; Tang, Q.; Wu, W.; Xia, Y.; Chen, D.; Wang, X. miR-20a contributes to endometriosis by regulating NTN4 expression. *Mol. Biol. Rep.* **2014**, *41*, 5793–5797. [CrossRef]
129. Wang, W.T.; Zhao, Y.N.; Han, B.W.; Hong, S.J.; Chen, Y.Q. CirculatingMicroRNAsIdentifiedinaGenome-Wide Serum MicroRNA Expression Analysis as Noninvasive Biomarkers for Endometriosis. *J. Clin. Endocrinol. Metab.* **2013**, *98*, 281–289. [CrossRef]
130. Kozomara, A.; Birgaoanu, M.; Griffiths-Jones, S. miRBase: From microRNA sequences to function. *Nucleic Acids Res.* **2019**, *47*, D155–D162. [CrossRef]
131. Rekker, K.; Saare, M.; Roost, A.M.; Kaart, T.; Sõritsa, D.; Karro, H.; Sõritsa, A.; Simón, C.; Salumets, A.; Peters, M. Circulating miR-200-family micro-RNAs have altered plasma levels in patients with endometriosis and vary with blood collection time. *Fertil. Steril.* **2015**, *104*, 938–946. [CrossRef]
132. Nisenblat, V.; Sharkey, D.J.; Wang, Z.; Evans, S.F.; Healey, M.; Ohlsson Teague, E.M.C.; Print, C.G.; Robertson, S.A.; Hull, M.L. Plasma miRNAs display limited potential as diagnostic tools for endometriosis. *Clin. Endocrinol. Metab.* **2019**, *104*, 1999–2022. [CrossRef]
133. Vanhie, A.; Peterse, D.O.D.; Beckers, A.; Cuellar, A.; Fassbender, A.; Meuleman, C.; Mestdagh, P.; D'Hooghe, T. Plasma miRNAs as biomarkers for endometriosis. *Hum. Reprod.* **2019**, *34*, 1650–1660. [CrossRef]
134. Jia, S.Z.; Yang, Y.; Lang, J.; Sun, P.; Leng, J. Plasma miR-17-5p, miR-20a and miR-22 are down-regulated in women with endometriosis. *Hum. Reprod.* **2013**, *28*, 322–330. [CrossRef] [PubMed]
135. Suryawanshi, S.; Vlad, A.M.; Lin, H.M.; Mantia-Smaldone, G.; Laskey, R.; Lee, M.; Lin, Y.; Donnellan, N.; Klein-Patel, M.; Lee, T.; et al. Plasma MicroRNAs as novel biomarkers for endometriosis and endometriosis-associated ovarian cancer. *Clin. Cancer Res.* **2013**, *19*, 1213–1224. [CrossRef] [PubMed]
136. Cosar, E.; Mamillapalli, R.; Ersoy, G.S.; Cho, S.; Seifer, B.; Taylor, H.S. Serum microRNAs as diagnostic markers of endometriosis: A comprehensive array-based analysis. *Fertil. Steril.* **2016**, *106*, 402–409. [CrossRef] [PubMed]
137. Zhang, X.-Y.; Zheng, L.-W.; Li, C.-J.; Xu, Y.; Zhou, X.; Fu, L.-I.; Li, D.-D.; Sun, L.-T.; Zhang, D.; Cui, M.-H.; et al. Dysregulated Expression of Long Noncoding RNAs in Endometriosis. *Crit. Rev. Eukaryot. Expr.* **2019**, *29*, 113–121. [CrossRef]

138. Wang, W.-T.; Sun, Y.-M.; Huang, W.; He, B.; Zhao, Y.-N.; Chen, Y.-Q. Genome-wide long non-coding RNA Analysis identified circulating LncRNAs as novel non-invasive diagnostic biomarkers for gynecological disease. *Sci. Rep.* **2016**, *6*, 23343. [CrossRef]
139. Qiu, J.; Zhang, X.; Ding, Y.; Hua, K. 1856 circulating exosomal long noncoding RNA-TC0101441 as a non-invasive biomarker for the prediction of endometriosis severity and recurrence. *J. Minim. Invasive Gynecol.* **2019**, *26*, S170–S171. [CrossRef]
140. Gueye, N.A.; Stanhiser, J.; Valentine, L.; Kotlyar, A.; Goodman, L.; Falcone, T. Biomarkers for Endometriosis in saliva, urine, and peritoneal fluid. *Biomark. endometr.* **2017**, 141–163. [CrossRef]
141. Kuessel, C.; Jaeger-Lamsky, A.; Pateisky, P.; Rossberg, N.; Schulz, A.; Schmitz, A.A.P.; Staudigl, C.; Wenzl, R. Cytokeratin-19 as a biomarker in urine and in serum for the diagnosis of endometriosis—A prospective study. *Gynecol. Endocrinol.* **2014**, *30*, 38–41. [CrossRef]
142. Hawkins, S.M.; Creighton, C.J.; Han, D.Y.; Zariff, A.; Anderson, M.L.; Gunaratne, P.H.; Matzuk, M.M. Functional microRNA involved in endometriosis. *Molec Endocrinol.* **2011**, *25*, 821–832. [CrossRef]
143. Becker, C.M.; Louis, G.; Exarhopoulos, A.; Mechsner, S.; Ebert, A.D.; Zurakowski, D.; Moses, M.A. Matrix metalloproteinases are elevated in the urine of patients with endometriosis. *Fertil. Steril.* **2010**, *94*, 2343–2346. [CrossRef] [PubMed]
144. Tokushige, N.; Markham, R.; Crossett, B.; Ahn, S.B.; Nelaturi, V.L.; Khan, A.; Fraser, I.S. Discovery of a novel biomarker in the urine in women with endometriosis. *Fertil. Steril.* **2011**, *95*, 46–49. [CrossRef]
145. El-Kasti, M.M.; Wright, C.; Fye, H.K.S.; Roseman, F.; Kessler, B.M.; Becker, C.M. Urinary peptide profiling identifies a panel of putative biomarkers for diagnosing and staging endometriosis. *Fertil. Steril.* **2011**, *95*, 1261–1266. [CrossRef] [PubMed]
146. Cho, S.; Choi, Y.S.; Yim, S.Y.; Yang, H.I.; Jeon, Y.E.; Lee, K.E.; Kim, H.Y.; Seo, S.K.; Lee, B.S. Urinary vitamin D-binding protein is elevated in patients with endometriosis. *Hum. Reprod.* **2012**, *27*, 515–522. [CrossRef] [PubMed]
147. Potlog-Nahari, C.; Stratton, P.; Winkel, C.; Widra, E.; Sinaii, N.; Connors, S.; Nieman, L.K. Urine vascular endothelial growth factor-A is not a useful marker for endometriosis. *Fertil. Steril.* **2004**, *81*, 1507–1512. [CrossRef] [PubMed]
148. Chen, X.; Liu, H.; Sun, W.; Guo, Z.; Lang, J. Elevated urine histone 4 levels in women with ovarian endometriosis revealed by discovery and parallel reaction monitoring proteomics. *J. Proteom.* **2019**, *204*, 103398. [CrossRef]
149. Gmyrek, G.B.; Sozanski, R.; Jerzak, M.; Chrobak, A.; Wickiewicz, D.; Skupnik, A.; Sierazka, U.; Fortuna, W.; Gabrys, M.; Chelmonska-Syta, A. Evaluation of monocyte chemotactic protein-1 levels in peripheral blood of infertile women with endometriosis. *Eur. J. Obstet. Gynecol. Reprod. Biol.* **2005**, *122*, 199–205. [CrossRef]
150. Gungor, T.; Kanat-Pektas, M.; Karayalcin, R.; Mollamahmutoglu, L. Peritoneal fluid and serum leptin concentrations in women with primary infertility. *Arch. Gynecol. Obstet.* **2009**, *279*, 361–364. [CrossRef]
151. Huang, H.; Hong, H.; Tan, Y.; Sheng, J. Matrix metalloproteinase 2 is associated with changes in steroids hormones in the sera and peritoneal fluid of patients with endometriosis. *Fertil. Steril.* **2004**, *81*, 1235–1239. [CrossRef]
152. Morin, M.; Bellehumeur, C.; Therriault, M.J.; Metz, C.; Maheux, R.; Akoum, A. Elevated levels of macrophage migration inhibitory factor in the peripheral blood of women with endometriosis. *Fertil. Steril.* **2005**, *83*, 865–872. [CrossRef]

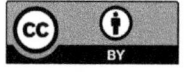

© 2020 by the authors. Licensee MDPI, Basel, Switzerland. This article is an open access article distributed under the terms and conditions of the Creative Commons Attribution (CC BY) license (http://creativecommons.org/licenses/by/4.0/).

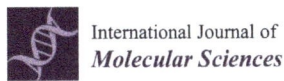

Article

Genetic Characterization of Endometriosis Patients: Review of the Literature and a Prospective Cohort Study on a Mediterranean Population

Stefano Angioni [1,*], Maurizio Nicola D'Alterio [1,*], Alessandra Coiana [2], Franco Anni [3], Stefano Gessa [4] and Danilo Deiana [1]

[1] Department of Surgical Science, University of Cagliari, Cittadella Universitaria Blocco I, Asse Didattico Medicna P2, Monserrato, 09042 Cagliari, Italy; danideiana82@gmail.com
[2] Department of Medical Science and Public Health, University of Cagliari, Laboratory of Genetics and Genomics, Pediatric Hospital Microcitemico "A. Cao", Via Edward Jenner, 09121 Cagliari, Italy; acoiana@unica.it
[3] Department of Medical Science and Public Health, University of Cagliari, Cittadella Universitaria di Monserrato, Asse Didattico E, Monserrato, 09042 Cagliari, Italy; francoanni@gmail.com
[4] Laboratory of Molecular Genetics, Service of Forensic Medicine, AOU Cagliari, Via Ospedale 54, 09124 Cagliari, Italy; stefagessa@libero.it
* Correspondence: sangioni@yahoo.it (S.A.); mauridalte84@gmail.com (M.N.D.); Tel.: +39-07051093399 (S.A.)

Received: 31 January 2020; Accepted: 2 March 2020; Published: 4 March 2020

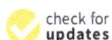

Abstract: The pathogenesis of endometriosis is unknown, but some evidence supports a genetic predisposition. The purpose of this study was to evaluate the recent literature on the genetic characterization of women affected by endometriosis and to evaluate the influence of polymorphisms of the wingless-type mammalian mouse tumour virus integration site family member 4 (WNT4), vezatin (VEZT), and follicle stimulating hormone beta polypeptide (FSHB) genes, already known to be involved in molecular mechanisms associated with the proliferation and development of endometriotic lesions in the Sardinian population. **Materials and Methods:** In order to provide a comprehensive and systematic tool for those approaching the genetics of endometriosis, the most cited review, observational, cohort and case-control studies that have evaluated the genetics of endometriosis in the last 20 years were collected. Moreover, 72 women were recruited for a molecular biology analysis of whole-blood samples—41 patients affected by symptomatic endometriosis and 31 controls. The molecular typing of three single nucleotide polymorphisms (SNPs) was evaluated in patients and controls: rs7521902, rs10859871 and rs11031006, mapped respectively in the WNT4, VEZT and FSHB genes. In this work, the frequency of alleles, genotypes and haplotypes of these SNPs in Sardinian women is described. **Results:** From the initial search, a total of 73 articles were chosen. An analysis of the literature showed that in endometriosis pathogenesis, the contribution of genetics has been well supported by many studies. The frequency of genotypes observed in the groups of the study population of 72 women was globally coherent with the law of the Hardy–Weinberg equilibrium. For the SNP rs11031006 (FSHB), the endometriosis group did not show an increase in genotypic or allelic frequency due to this polymorphism compared to the control group ($p = 0.9999$, odds ratio (OR) = 0.000, 95% confidence interval (CI), 0.000–15.000 and $p = 0.731$, OR = 1639, 95% CI, 0.39–683, respectively, for the heterozygous genotype and the polymorphic minor allele). For the SNP rs10859871 (VEZT), we found a significant difference in the frequency of the homozygous genotype in the control group compared to the affected women ($p = 0.0111$, OR = 0.0602, 95% CI, 0.005–0.501). For the SNP rs7521902 (WNT4), no increase in genotypic or allelic frequency between the two groups was shown ($p = 0.3088$, OR = 0.4133, 95% CI, 0.10–1.8 and $p = 0.3297$, OR = 2257, 95% CI, 0.55–914, respectively, for the heterozygous genotype and the polymorphic minor allele). **Conclusion:** An analysis of recent publications on the genetics of endometriosis showed a discrepancy in the results obtained in different populations. In the Sardinian population, the results obtained do not show a significant association between the investigated variants of the genes and a greater risk of developing endometriosis, although several other studies in the literature have shown the opposite. Anyway, the data underline the importance of evaluating genetic variants in different populations. In fact, in different ethnic groups, it is possible that specific risk alleles could act differently in the pathogenesis of the disease.

Keywords: endometriosis; genetic polymorphisms; SNPs; pathogenesis; aetiology; Mediterranean population; Sardinian population

1. Introduction

Endometriosis is a chronic disease of the reproductive age with a prevalence of 5%, reaching its peak between 25 and 35 years of age [1]. The scientific community agrees in recognizing a multifactorial aetiology of endometriosis, with possible genetic, hormonal, immunological and environmental factors as causes. Studies on family aggregation and twins have emphasized the genetic component, demonstrating how predisposition generated by certain susceptibility genes plays an important role in the development, maintenance and recurrence of the disease [2–5]. Nonetheless, studies on the genetics of endometriosis are complicated by various factors: the phenotypic heterogeneity of the disease; the still unknown prevalence in the population, burdened by the absence of registries and diagnostic underestimation; the invasiveness of diagnostic methods; and various co-morbidities that can generate bias [3]. In the field of research on the genetic basis of endometriosis, Simpson is considered a pioneer. In 1980, he verified in a sample of 123 women with histological diagnosis of endometriosis that 6.9% of first-degree relatives (mother and sisters) were affected, while the disease prevalence in controls (first-degree female relatives of the corresponding "husbands") was less than 1% [6]. In 1999, Treloar's work on an Australian population demonstrated a concordance ratio of 2:1 between monozygotic and dizygotic twins and a correspondent genetic risk of 2.34 to affect a sister. The study results show that 51% of genetic influence is responsible for developing endometriosis [7]. There is therefore enough evidence on how endometriosis is clearly heritable, although in what manner is not yet clear. The increased genetic risk in first-degree relatives (5–8%) suggests polygenic and multifactorial inheritance rather than monogenic. However, this recurrence risk is higher than the expected risk for a polygenic pathology (2–5%). The other, more likely, hypothesis is that phenotypic heterogeneity reflects genetic heterogeneity and that therefore not all forms of endometriosis are the same disease; in fact, some forms of endometriosis, due to their characteristics, behave almost like Mendelian pathologies [2]. The aim of this study was to evaluate the recent literature on the genetic characterization of women affected by endometriosis and to evaluate the influence of polymorphisms of the WNT4, VEZT and FSHB genes, known to be involved in molecular mechanisms associated with proliferation and development of endometriotic lesions in a particular Mediterranean population, the Sardinian population. The people of the Mediterranean island of Sardinia are particularly well suited for genetic studies, as is evident from a number of successes in complex trait and disease mapping [8].

The wingless-type mammalian mouse tumour virus integration site family member 4 (WNT4) gene is positioned on chromosome 1p36.23-p35 and codifies a protein which is essential in developing the female reproductive system [9–14]. It critically regulates the appropriate postnatal uterine maturation, as well as ovarian antral follicle growth [10]. The WNT class is an extensive group of secreted glycoproteins, codified through 19 different genes implicated in the WNT signalling pathway [9]. WNT-mediated signal transduction pathways address the specific mobilization of groups of genes which are responsible for managing several cellular responses, including cell growth, differentiation, movement, migration, polarity, cell survival and immune response [9]. A study published by Jordan et al. [15] demonstrated that WNT4 is the first signalling molecule causing the chain of events which ends with sex determination, through local secernment of growth factors. Imperfections in WNT4 activity play a role in the development of three important organs deriving from the primordial urogenital ridge—the kidneys, adrenal glands and gonads [9]. This may demonstrate the significant position of WNT4 at an early embryological stage of development. The loss of WNT4 in knockout mice determines the total absence of the Mullerian duct and its derivatives [11]. Apart from being crucial for epithelial–stromal cell communication in the endometrium, WNT signalling is likely important for endometrial maturation and differentiation and embryonic implantation [16]. An association between endometriosis and markers located in or near WNT4 has been highlighted in a number of extensive studies on gene mapping [17,18]. The expression of WNT4 has also been detected at the level of the peritoneum, leading to the consideration of a possible metaplastic hypothesis in promoting the transformation of peritoneal cells into endometriosic cells, through pathways with a role in the development of the female genital tract [12]. Pagliardini et al. demonstrated that a single nucleotide polymorphism (SNP), rs7521902, located 21 kb up/downstream of the WNT4 region, has a susceptibility locus for endometriosis. The functional significance of this SNP in endometriosis remains to be explained [10]. While the SNP rs7521902 was connected to endometriosis susceptibility in British, Australian, Italian and Japanese women [10,18,19], in Belgian [13] and Brazilian women this association was not found [9]. The different genetic backgrounds of the cohorts may be identified as the reason for the lack of association between this polymorphism and endometriosis.

The vezatin (VEZT) gene is located on chromosome 12 locus 12q22; it codifies vezatin, a significant element of the cadherin–catenin complex, which plays a crucial role in the formation and sustenance of adherent joints [20–24]. According to Kussel-Andermann et al., vezatin was found to be a plasma membrane component with a short extracellular domain, a transmembrane domain and an extended intracellular domain. Its intracellular domain connects to myosin VIIA as part of the adherens junctional complex in epithelial cells [21]. Furthermore, several studies on co-immunoprecipitation showed that the system between vezatin and myosin VIIA is able to interact with the system between E-cadherin and catenin, although the specificity of this interaction remains to be determined [21,22]. Also, VEZT is fundamental for implantation; embryos from mice with silenced VEZT cannot develop after the blastocyst stage, because of a loss of adhesion between cells [25]. It has been highlighted that VEZT protein is extensively expressed in human endometrium and myometrium. During the secretory phase of the menstrual cycle, VEZT expression increases in the glandular epithelium in a significant way. The mRNA expression of adherens junction members (E-cadherin and A- and B-catenin) is also enhanced in the secretory phase with respect to the proliferative phase. This indicates that progesterone could be responsible for activating cell-to-cell adhesion [20]. The VEZT promoter does not contain a reaction point for the progesterone receptor (PR), but it contains a nuclear factor kappa B (NF-kB) binding site. As a pro-inflammatory transcription factor, NF-kB is involved in the pathogenesis of endometriosis, showing cycle control in the endometrium and reciprocal management with PR [26]. Therefore, variations in VEZT levels in endometrial glandular cells are likely to occur in response to the dynamic oscillation in progesterone and associated NF-kB changes [20]. Considering the studied physiological roles of VEZT, its potential for a functional role in endometriosis is a likely option, since VEZT has been demonstrated to be upregulated in ectopic endometrium with respect to eutopic endometrium in patients suffering from endometriosis [20,23,24].

The follicle-stimulating hormone beta polypeptide (FSHB) gene, positioned on chromosome 11 locus 11p14.1, codifies subunit b of the hormone-specific follicle-stimulating hormone (FSH), with a crucial role in the growth of ovarian follicles and production of oestrogens [27–29]. Recently, some evidence for an association between endometriosis and SNPs of FSHB was reported in independent targets from the UK Biobank, firmly supporting this result [28]. FSH and luteinizing hormone (LH) are related gonadotropin hormones sharing the same alpha subunit. A connection between these SNPs on chromosome 11 with concentrations of both hormones indicates a common mechanism of regulation, with both being key elements in managing follicle development in the ovary, influencing oestradiol release during the proliferative phase of the cycle and contributing to a role for oestradiol in endometriosis risk [27]. Data from the ENCODE project [30] show that the SNP rs11031006 modifies the sequence of 11 protein-binding motifs, including that of oestrogen receptor α, with a possible effect on hormonal feedback inhibition. Recently, allele G of this SNP has been proven to be significantly associated with higher levels of serum FSH [29].

1.1. Review of the Literature

This review aims to provide a comprehensive and systematic tool for those approaching the genetics of endometriosis. Computerized literature searches were conducted using the Medline/PubMed database and a manual search of relevant and frequently cited publications in the English language from 1999 to 2019. Additional articles were identified by manually searching references from the retrieved eligible articles. Keywords included: endometriosis combined with genes, genetics, SNPs, genome-wide association study (GWAS), WNT4, VEZT, FSHB, next-generation sequencing (NGS) and epigenetics. Review, observational, cohort and case-control studies that evaluated the genetics of endometriosis are herein described.

1.2. Cohort Study

The study was carried out through molecular typing of the following single nucleotide polymorphisms (SNPs): rs7521902, rs10859871 and rs11031006, mapped, respectively, in the WNT4, VEZT and FSHB genes. In this work, we set out to describe the frequency of alleles and genotypes of these SNPs among Sardinian women, and to evaluate their impact on the susceptibility to develop endometriosis. The choice of which polymorphisms were to be analysed fell to WNT4, VEZT and FSHB genes because of their hypothetical correlation with endometriosis, according to recent findings in the literature. Several GWAS meta-analyses have reported a possible pathogenetic role [16,27]. In particular, an association study published in 2017 analysed these SNPs in a Greek population, highlighting a significant connection with the disease [29]. The molecular biological examinations of single-substitution polymorphisms in our study were carried out from whole blood drawn exclusively from Sardinian patients, upon their informed consent. We chose to limit the study to only patients of Sardinian origin, considering the peculiarity of this island, which can be seen as a genetic macro-isolate. The choice of limiting the selection of the target population to patients of Sardinian origin for at least three generations was not intended to exclude the possible influence of genetic features from non-Sardinian distant ancestors. It was, rather, an attempt to make the target more homogeneous.

The genetic analysis of complex traits is simplified in isolated populations such as this one, in which inbreeding and the "founder effect" reduce the genetic diversity of complex and polygenic diseases such as endometriosis. The goal was to identify a genetic characterization of the disease in the Sardinian population, to shed light on the etiopathogenetic mechanisms of endometriosis, and to provide predictive markers for a non-invasive diagnosis of the disease.

Patients and Study Design

The present clinical study represents the initial application, on a small scale, of a study protocol conducted at the Department of Obstetrics and Gynaecology of the Hospital "Duilio Casula" of Monserrato, University of Cagliari, in collaboration with the Laboratory of Genetics and Genomics of the Pediatric Hospital Microcitemico "A. Cao" of Cagliari. Written consent was obtained from the local ethics committee (EndoSNPs, Prot. PG/2019/13157). In line with the Declaration of Helsinki 1975, revised in Hong Kong in 1989, the clinical trial was registered (ClinicalTrials.gov ID: NCT02388854). This study involved a total of 72 women who underwent surgery, 41 representing the cases with clinical and histological diagnosis of endometriosis, and 31 representing the corresponding controls—women without a diagnosis of endometriosis who underwent surgery for benign indications different from endometriosis and chronic pelvic pain. For each patient, a data collection folder was prepared in a database elaborated for the purpose. Apart from personal records, data on geographic origin and anthropometric measurements (weight, height, body mass index (BMI)), the data collection form contained data on habits such as cigarette smoking and alcohol intake, and clinical data on possible co-morbidities or previous surgical interventions. In patients with a diagnosis of endometriosis, data on this pathology were obviously included (familiarity, staging, location of lesions, transvaginal ultrasound data, gynaecological examination, symptomatology, number and type of surgical operations, histological data), type and duration of drug therapy (nonsteroidal anti-inflammatory drugs (NSAIDs), hormone therapy and antibiotics). The diagnosis of endometriosis was clinical, related to ultrasound and histology reports. The staging used was the revised classification proposed by the American Fertility Society/American Society for Reproductive Medicine (AFS/ASRM) [30], which is still the most widespread and widely used, in clinical and academic fields, to describe the severity of endometriosis in a standardized format. Localizations of deep infiltrating endometriosis (DIE) infiltrating the bladder or bowel were classified as severe. For each main symptom (dysmenorrhea, chronic pelvic pain, dyspareunia, intestinal symptoms, urinary symptoms), a score was assigned based on the intensity perceived by the patient (visual analogue scale (VAS) 0–3: mild; 4–7: moderate; 8–10: severe). For the controls, women who had never had a diagnosis or a suspicion of endometriosis were selected. The close and remote pathological medical history of these patients was also negative for dysmenorrhea, dyspareunia, chronic pelvic pain and infertility/sub-fertility, as one of the inclusion criteria was to have given birth to at least 2 children. A common criterion to be included in the study was geographic origin. All participants had an exclusively Sardinian origin for at least 3 generations (maternal and paternal grandparents from Sardinia).

2. Results

2.1. Review of the Literature

2.1.1. Gene Polymorphisms

Single nucleotide polymorphisms are present in the population with an allelic frequency >1%, and represent the most common type of genetic variation in humans (90% of polymorphisms). They are present with alternative allelic variants and follow a Mendelian inheritance. Their wide dissemination in the genetic makeup (one in every 100–300 base pairs) makes them interesting in studies on allelic association and usable as molecular markers. Single nucleotide polymorphisms (SNPs) can generate synonymous or non-synonymous mutations if present in coding regions of genes, or lead to alterations of the gene product if present in intronic or intergenic regions [2]. Variations in the genome may determine different individual susceptibilities to a disease, or different pharmacological responses. SNPs are therefore useful to identify "disease genes" through association studies based on population screening [2]. Technological advances in the field of molecular biology, especially through polymerase chain reaction (PCR) techniques, have stimulated interest in identifying certain gene polymorphisms and their influence on susceptibility in developing endometriosis. The choice of candidate genes falls to those genes whose polymorphic variants are hypothesized to be involved in the pathophysiological molecular mechanisms underlying the disease: genes involved in steroidogenesis and in receptorial activity of sex hormones, genes involved in inflammatory and immune response processes, genes regulating metabolism, genes affecting the processes of tissue remodelling and neoangiogenesis, and DNA repair genes [31,32].

2.1.2. Genes Involved in Stereidogenesis and Receptorial Activity of Sex Hormones

Endometriosic and endometrial tissues are responsive to the effect of sexual steroid hormones, especially oestrogens. It is no coincidence that the risk factors of this disease include early menarche and late-onset menopause, conditions that notoriously involve extended exposure to endogenous oestrogens throughout life. Therefore, among the most common pathogenetic hypotheses is that there is possible dysregulation of the ligand-receptorial signalling involving the main sex hormones, oestrogens and progesterone [33,34]. The choice of candidate genes for various association studies is based on this mechanism. The two estrogenic receptor (ER) isoforms (ER-beta and ER-alpha) are codified by two genes (ESR2 and ESR1) with tissue-specific distributions, and have different capacities in connecting ligands (oestrogen and antioestrogen) and starting the transcription of target genes. The influence of ESR1 gene polymorphisms was studied in women affected by endometriosis in different populations, both European and Asian, but with inconsistent results. For the ESR2 gene, the studied polymorphism is localized in region 3′UTR of the gene, on nucleotide 1730 (1730 adenine (A) → guanine (G)), and it is recognized by the restriction enzyme AluI. This polymorphism has been related to a risk of severe stage IV endometriosis in women of Japanese origin [35], but no significant association with the development of the disease in Italian and Korean women was seen [36]. The pathogenetic hypothesis that there is involvement of the corresponding receptors and their malfunctioning in determining those phenomena involved in the development of endometriosis is based on the dysregulation of tissue sensitivity influenced by progesterone. In particular, as an object of numerous studies on their role in the onset and development of ovarian carcinoma, the polymorphism of progesterone receptor (PR) gene, called PROGINS, seems to compromise the perfect receptor–ligand functionality in target tissues, making them less sensitive to progesterone and altering the hormonal balance in favour of oestrogenic activity. The PROGINS polymorphism was found more frequently in women suffering from endometriosis. A statistically significant association was found in affected women from Italy [37], Austria [38] and Brazil [39], while similar studies on women from India [40], Australia [41] and Germany [42] came to exactly opposite conclusions. Other more or less recent studies focused their research on gene polymorphisms of the androgen receptor (AR). Androgens play an important role, although not sufficiently clarified, in endometrial physiology and physiopathology, counteracting the effect of oestrogen on cell proliferation [43–46]. The AR gene is localized on the Xq11.2-q12 chromosome; the corresponding protein has eight domains with transactivation function, all distributed in exon 1. Here, we find a polymorphic microsatellite consisting of a cytosine–adenine–guanine (CAG) sequence, variously repeated in individuals, on which the length of glutamine residues in the amino-terminal end of the AR protein depends, with repercussions on its functionality [47,48]. In this case, the results are very different regarding the ethnic group used as a sample. Shaik's work on a female Indian population concluded that the presence of 19–21 CAG repeats of the AR gene could be considered a susceptibility marker for endometriosis and uterine leiomyoma [49], confirming the results obtained from a previous work on Taiwanese women [50], but in stark contrast to Lattuada's results on Italian women [51].

2.1.3. Genes Involved in Inflammation and Immune Response

The development of the inflammatory process is an integral part of the pathophysiology of endometriosis. Polymorphisms of numerous cytokines have become the objects of many studies, but with conflicting results. In their work on a female Taiwanese population, Hsieh et al. demonstrated an association between susceptibility to endometriosis and the presence of gene polymorphisms: −509C/T in the region promoter of the transforming growth factor-β1 (TGF-β1) gene, −627A/C in the region promoter of the interleukin 10 (IL-10) gene, and 881T/C in the IL2 beta receptor gene [52]. A 2017 study focused on TGF-β1, in particular on how it affects the development and progression of the disease with regard to hypoxia. The results support the hypothesis that TGF-β1 is involved in the pathogenesis of endometriosis through the regulation of vascular endothelial growth factor (VEGF) expression. TGF-β not only increased its levels, but also had an additive effect at the transcriptional level on hypoxia itself, increasing the expression of VEGF up to 87% [53]. The polymorphisms of the gene coding for cytokine TNF-α, with regard to its key role in the development of the acute phase of inflammatory processes and regulation of the immune response, have also been at the centre of several works: variations in promoter regions do not appear to be associated with an increased risk of endometriosis in Korean, Taiwanese and Caucasian women [54]. Several lines of evidence prove that endometriosis is characterized by specific modifications of the immune system, in particular endowing endometriosic cells with the ability to elude the mechanisms of immunosurveillance and thus guarantee easier implantation and development in ectopic sites. Among these mechanisms, we can hypothesize changes in the expression of human leukocyte antigens (HLAs), important for immunological recognition, secretion of circulating antigens competing with surface antigens, critical for self/non-self-recognition, and production of immunosuppressive or proapoptotic factors against T cell effector [55]. The HLA system or major histocompatibility complex (MHC) is the gene complex which boasts the largest number of polymorphisms in the human genome. Wang's study of 2001 on Chinese women reported the influence of polymorphisms of the HLA-B gene, but not the HLA-A gene, on the susceptibility to the development of endometriosis [56], whereas Ishi in 2003 reported a significant association with HLA-DRB1*1403 and HLA-DQB1*03031 alleles in Japanese women, but not with HLADPB1 [57]. In this case, too, we detect conflicting results. PTPN22 is a coding gene for a protein involved in the responsiveness of B and T lymphocyte receptors, whose mutations may be responsible for the onset of autoimmune diseases. The associations observed between PTPN22 (C1858T) and the risk of endometriosis suggest that this polymorphism could be a useful marker of susceptibility to the disease [58].

2.1.4. Genes Involved in the Processes of Tissue Remodeling and Neoangiogenesis

Vascular endothelial growth factor (VEGF) and endothelial growth factor receptor (EGFR) are molecular factors known to be involved in the regulation of neoangiogenesis, tissue remodelling and proliferation, phenomena also necessary for the growth of ectopic foci of endometrial tissue. Specifically, VEGF induces the proliferation, migration and differentiation of endothelial cells and capillary formation. Several studies have shown high levels of VEGF in peritoneal fluid and serum, and increased expression of mRNA and proteins in patients with endometriosis [59]. Furthermore, VEGF causes an increase in vascular permeability and a release of proteases such as metalloproteases (MMPs), enzymes able to "cut" the proteins of matrix and basement membrane, important for cellular invasion and tissue remodelling. It can also prevent apoptosis of different cell types. Perini's group study in 2014 on Brazilian women indicated a risk association with –1154G> polymorphism A of the VEGF gene [59]. EGFR is a transmembrane glycoprotein which plays an important role in the control of growth, differentiation and cell motility. The EGFR +2073A/T polymorphism, a candidate as a susceptibility gene, was studied by Hsieh et al. in 122 Taiwanese women and 139 controls, showing an association with a high risk of disease. These results were subsequently denied when reported to the Japanese population [60].

2.1.5. Genes Regulating Metabolism

Glutathione S-transferase mu M1 (GSTM1), glutathione S-transferase P1 (GSTP1), glutathione S-transferase theta T1 (GSTT1), N-acetyltransferase 1 (NAT1) and N-acetyltransferase 2 (NAT2) genes all encode phase II enzymes involved in the metabolism of xenobiotics, including toxic compounds such as dioxin and polycyclic aromatic hydrocarbons. In particular, a 2015 meta-analysis by Guo on the association between variants of GST, GSTM1 and GSTT1 genes, which encode for glutathione S transferase, and the development of endometriosis showed a significant increase in risk. Women with GSTM1-null genotype compared to other genotypes recorded a summary OR of 1.96, demonstrating an approximately double risk of endometriosis. Women with GSTT1-null genotype compared to other genotypes recorded a summary OR of 1.77, showing an 80% risk of endometriosis. Nevertheless, the existence of bias in this meta-analysis indicates that the magnitude of risk could be smaller or even non-existent [61]. Many gene polymorphisms corresponding to phase I enzymes involved in, among other things, oestrogen metabolism were investigated as variants associated with a greater susceptibility to disease, for example CYP1A1 6235T/C, CYP17A1 –34T/C and CYP19A1 microsatellite TTTA repeat [62,63].

2.1.6. Genes Related to the Process of DNA Repair

Many studies have proposed oxidative stress as a factor involved in the pathophysiology of endometriosis [64]. An excess of reactive oxygen species causes DNA damage, base modifications and chromosomal aberrations, which would justify the metaplastic features of the disease. The DNA repair system from oxidative stress involves the intervention of enzymes encoded by genes including X-ray repair cross-complementing 1 and 3 (XRCC1 and XRCC3) and XPD (also known as excision repair cross-complementing (ERCC)), whose defective functioning decisively contributes to develop endometriosic lesions. Attar et al. in 2010 reported no significant differences between the frequency of genotypes and polymorphic alleles of APE1, XRCC1, XPD, XPG and HOGG1 genes in patients with and without endometriosis, whilst a significant increase in disease frequency would appear to be associated with the XRCC3 Thr/Thr genotype [65].

2.1.7. Genome-Wide Association Study (GWAS) and Next-Generation Sequencing (NGS)

So far, we have discussed works adopting an investigative approach based on the a priori selection of polymorphisms of candidate genes known to have hypothetical biological roles in the pathogenesis of endometriosis, and their subsequent research on DNA samples. A radical change in perspective was applied in the so-called hypothesis-free methods, such as the analysis of family linkage, association studies on the genomic scale, or genome-wide studies (GWASs), up to the most recent new generation sequencing technique, next-generation sequencing (NGS), which targets the entire genome, without pre-selecting a particular gene or gene region, therefore with no initial pathogenetic hypothesis. Among its main advantages, this type of approach can detect alterations of unexpected molecular pathways perhaps shared by apparently very different pathologies. Analyses of family linkage and genome-wide association studies are different though complementary approaches to the identification of genetic risk variants across the whole spectrum of allele frequencies. A linkage analysis aims to identify those genetic variants which are rare in the general population, but are responsible for the family aggregation of a given pathology, while a GWAS aims to identify genetic common variants in the general population associated with the risk of the disease [66]. Studies of family linkage have analysed the association between a known marker and the unknown gene/disease, assuming their proximity to the chromosome and the consequent co-segregation in affected families. In 2005, an impressive linkage study was carried out by Treloar's group on 1176 English and Australian families, each with at least two members, mainly sister pairs, with a surgical diagnosis of endometriosis, for a total of 4985 genotyped individuals, 2709 of them women with endometriosis. This study found a strongly significant linkage on chromosome 10q26 and another region suggestive of linkage on chromosome 20p13 [67]. The fine-mapping of the 10q26 region using 11,984 SNPs in 1144 affected families and 1190 controls was described in a study by Painter's group in 2011, which identified three signs of significant association with endometriosis [68]. Among them, the only one to be replicated in an independent cohort was rs11592737, located in the CYP2C19 gene, an important candidate gene involved in oestrogenic metabolism, particularly in the conversion of oestradiol to oestrone [69]. However, despite the valuable contribution of this method to the study of monogenic pathologies, this technique was shown to be less accurate when applied to multifactorial diseases such as endometriosis, able to identify extensive chromosome regions containing hundreds of genes with too large and inaccurate linkage peaks. This fact, together with the lack of sensitivity and the difficulty of independently replicating the positive results related to the need for a large number of affected families with more generations available to test, has made this method obsolete, opening the way to the more promising GWAS. A GWAS is a survey on all, or almost all, genes of an individual of a particular species to determine the gene variations between them. Later, attempts are made to associate the observed differences with some specific traits, such as a disease. In these cases, samples from hundreds or thousands of individuals are evaluated, usually looking for single nucleotide polymorphisms (SNPs). Instead of reading whole gene sequences, these systems usually identify SNP markers of groups of gene variations (haplotypes). If some gene variations are significantly more frequent in sick individuals, then the variations are said to be associated with the disease. These variations are then considered indicative of the region where the disease-causing mutation is likely to be found. The first GWAS on endometriosis was carried out on a Japanese population in 2010, on a sample of 1432 cases and 1318 controls. The study identified a significant association ($p = 5.6 \times 10^{-12}$; OR 1.44 (1.30–1.59)) with the SNP rs10965235 located on the CDKN2B-AS1 gene on chromosome 9 and with the SNP rs16826658 ($p = 1.7 \times 10^{-6}$ OR 1.2 (1.11–1.29)) located on the WNT4 gene on chromosome 1 [18]. The first gene regulates some onco-suppressors such as CDKN2B, CDKN2A and ARF; its inactivation has been correlated with the development of endometriosic foci and endometrial carcinoma [70]. The second one is a very important gene involved in the development of the female genital apparatus, indispensable for the formation of Müllerian ducts [12]. It has a sequence that regulates ESR1 and ESR2 genes, and it is still among the main candidate genes for endometriosis and ovarian cancer. A subsequent GWAS of 2016 also focused on this gene. Using a sample of 7090 individuals (2594 cases and 4496 controls), the study found the marker in the region of the WNT4 gene, with the strongest association with the risk of endometriosis: the SNP rs3820282 [71]. In 2011, a subsequent GWAS was conducted through the International Endogene Consortium (IEC) by Painter's group on British and Australian women, analysing 3194 cases of surgically diagnosed endometriosis and 7060 controls [19]. The study divided the sample of affected individuals into two categories based on the severity of the pathology (stage I–II and stage III–IV), and detected a strongly significant linkage, in particular in the "severe" subgroup, with two SNPs: rs1250248 ($p = 3.2 \times 10^{-8}$; OR 1.30 (1.19–1.43)), located on the FN1 gene on chromosome 2, involved in cell adhesion and migration, and rs12700667, ($p = 1.5 \times 10^{-9}$; OR 1.38 (1.24–1.53)), located on an intergenic region of chromosome 7p15 containing regulatory elements, located upstream of three candidate genes: miRNA148a (88kb), the closest, encoding a microRNA implicated in the important Wnt β-catenin signalling pathway for the homeostasis of sex hormones; NFE2L3 (331 kb), encoding a transcription factor involved in the processes of phlogosis, differentiation and carcinogenesis, highly expressed in the placenta; and the HOXA 10-11 genes, coding for homeobox A transcription factors, considered important in the spatial and temporal regulation of uterine development about 1.35 Mb downstream. Thanks to the data of this GWAS, it was also possible to refute the conclusions of later works, such as the study of Grechukhina in 2012, which reported a high frequency (31% vs. 5% case-control) of SNP rs61764370 in the 3'UTR region of the Kirsten rat sarcoma viral oncogene homolog (KRAS) gene in women with endometriosis [72]. The KRAS gene was considered a strong candidate gene; in fact, KRAS activation determined the development of peritoneal endometriosis in 47% of mice and endometriosis-like ovarian lesions in 100%. SNP rs61764370 interrupts the link between the LCS6 complementary site and let-7 miRNA, altering the expression of the KRAS gene and favouring the development of the disease. The analysis conducted in 2012 by Hien Luong and Painter denied this risk association [73]. A meta-analysis of the GWASs of the IEC and the Japanese group, carried out in 2012, confirmed the associations previously reported in the respective studies and identified further significant new loci of association localized on GREB1 genes, involved in estrogenic regulation; VEZT, involved in cell growth, migration and adhesion; and ID4, an ovarian tumour suppressor [17]. Another interesting GWAS of 2017 was a meta-analysis of 11 case-control datasets, for a total of 17,045 cases of endometriosis and 191,596 controls. Five additional new loci significantly associated with the risk of endometriosis ($p < 5 \times 10^{-8}$) of genes involved in sexual steroid hormone pathways (FN1, CCDC170, ESR1, SYNE1 and FSHB) were identified, for a total of 16 genomic regions associated with endometriosis risk in one or more populations [27]. At present, 19 independent single nucleotide polymorphisms (SNPs) have been validly associated with endometriosis, explaining 5.19% of disease variance [27]. In particular, a recent study investigated in a Greek population three of these SNPs: rs7521902, rs10859871 and rs11031006, mapped respectively on WNT4, VEZT and FSHB genes, highlighting a significant association with endometriosis [29]. In recent years, thanks above all to the reduction in cost and time of examination, an innovative DNA reading technique has come forward forcefully: next-generation sequencing (NGS). Through NGS, it is possible to analyse a large number of DNA fragments in parallel, until the sequences of many genes are obtained simultaneously, even the entire coding region (exome sequencing) or the whole genome (whole genome sequencing) of an individual. Instead of screening several variants, the most common ones, scattered throughout the genome as in the genome arrays of GWASs, with an NGS reading it is possible to search for the rarest variants in a population. A study of families affected by endometriosis using NGS was conducted in 2014 by Chettier et al.; out of 13 pairs of affected sisters, five shared genomic regions (in chromosomes 2, 5, 9 and 11) where rare gene variants associated with endometriosis are located [74]. In February 2016, Er's research group focused on the molecular characterization of endometriosis associated with ovarian cancer through targeted NGS of 409 cancer-related genes by identifying gene variants on the PIK3CA and ARID1A genes, related to endometriosis with a high risk of malignant transformation [75]. Most GWA variants associated with the risk of endometriosis are not codified and the genes responsible for association signals have not been identified. A direct approach to identifying target genes could be identifying variants encoding common proteins associated with the risk of endometriosis. Large international exon sequencing projects have identified exome variants modifying the coding of corresponding proteins (nonsynonymous codification, alternative splicing sites or stopping codon gain or loss), classifying them according to their frequency. The role of protein-coding variants associated with endometriosis risk was therefore directly tested by genotyping through a specific Illumina array (Illumina exome chip) designed to allow the simultaneous capture of rare, low-frequency and common frequency exonerated variants. In all, 7164 patients with endometriosis and 210,005 controls were analysed. The initial association between disease and variations in encoding the CUBN, CIITA and PARP4 genes was not confirmed when replicating the study [76]. There is therefore no clear evidence of the existence of codifying variants of common or low-frequency proteins which can influence the risk of endometriosis. Variants capable of directly modifying the sequence and function of protein amino acids would have provided immediate gene targets. The causal SNPs are probably located in non-codifying sequences, but are involved in functions regulating gene expression and are able to influence the development and progression of disease [77]. If GWASs have identified various susceptibility loci, the biggest challenge of the post-GWAS era is therefore to understand the functional consequences of these loci. Studying the association between genetic variations and gene expression offers a way to link risk variants with the corresponding target genes. Gene expression varies in different individuals, and the level of expression of certain genes is under the control of particular regulatory variants indicated as expression quantitative traits loci (eQTLs), which can influence the abundance of specific transcripts [78]. Various study groups have identified three eQTLs capable of altering the transcription of potential target genes: LINC0039 and CDC42 on chromosome 1, CDKN2A-AS1 on chromosome 9 and VEZT on chromosome 12. Further functional studies are needed to confirm the role of causal genes in different susceptibility loci [79].

2.1.8. Epigenetics

During the past five years, evidence has emerged that endometriosis may be an epigenetic disease. Epigenetics proves to be the common denominator of a pathology in which both genetic and environmental components play pathogenetic roles. Many large-scale profiling studies on gene expression have unequivocally demonstrated that many genes are deregulated in endometriosis [80]. Several aspects related to possible post-transcriptional interference that may result in changes in endometriosic tissues, compared to healthy ones, have been investigated. These modifications are expressed at different levels (transcriptional, post-transcriptional, post-translational) and through different mechanisms (methylation, histone modification, activators, repressors, miRNAs). In particular, changes in terms of hypermethylation and silencing of genes which are normally expressed during the proliferative phase of the cycle and regulate the modalities of cell adhesion have been studied, such as HOXA-10, E-cadherin, the GATA family of transcription factors and the group of nuclear receptors for steroids (SR), which includes the progesterone receptors in two isoforms, PR-A and PR-B. The opposite transcriptional activity of the two isoforms has been demonstrated to be due to binding of the Hic-5 differential co-regulator. This type of change affects the resistance of endometriosis to treatment with progesterone [81]. Expression by endometrial tissue of the two receptors for progesterone, PR-A and PR-B, and their relationship influences the reaction of tissue to exposure to progestins. A prevalence of PR-A results in resistance to therapy and loss of cell adhesion. In vitro studies have shown that deacetylase inhibitors show promise as therapies for the treatment of endometriosis. In particular, trichostatin A has been shown to reactivate the expression of E-cadherin, an intercellular adhesion protein, which is hypermethylated and therefore silenced in endometriotic cell lines, with a concomitant reduction in invasiveness [80]. MiRNAs are a class of endogenous NcRNAs of about 22 nucleotides, which play a key role in regulating gene expression. As well as DNA methylation and histone modification, they implement this regulation without any change in DNA sequence, but inhibit or induce miRNA degradation. A profiling study of miRNA expression identified 48 out of 287 miRNAs differentially expressed in healthy women and women with endometriosis. The target genes of these miRNAs include many genes involved in endometriosis (Erα, ERβ, PR, TGFβ), suggesting that miRNA deregulation may play a pathogenetic role [80]. Acetylation, methylation and phosphorylation are the most well-known and studied post-translational histone modifications. These changes alter the interaction of histone with DNA and nuclear proteins. In general, histone acetylation is associated with transcriptional activation and deacetylation with transcriptional repression [82,83]. Studies on animals seemed to suggest that HDAC2 is expressed aberrantly in ectopic endometrium. Furthermore, Sun et al. (2003) reported that treatment of endometriotic stromal cells with prostaglandin E2 (PGE2) resulted in increased acetylation of histone H3 bound to StAR promoter, with concomitant induction of co-activator CBP/p300, binding of CREB protein, and possible involvement in the pathogenesis of endometriosis [84]. So far, studies on epigenetics have barely scratched the surface of this area, and further research will allow us to shed light on the pathophysiology of endometriosis, and on the complex mechanisms regulating the activation or silencing of different genetic targets. Such knowledge will provide a basis for the identification of new drugs and diagnostic biomarkers.

2.2. Cohort Study

The patients' average age was 35 years (median 33 years in the group of cases, 36 years in the group of controls). The median values of body mass index (BMI) in the two groups were uniform (21 for cases vs. 22 for controls). Among the affected women, we found comorbidities in nine: two cases of haemorrhoidal disease, one of serous cystadenoma, borderline mucinous cystadenoma associated with breast cancer, mitral valve prolapse, umbilical hernia, anxiety disorder, hyperinsulinemia, and irritable colon. Among the controls, nine women had a pathological medical history: HashimotO's thyroiditis (5), type 2 diabetes mellitus, hypercholesterolaemia, uterine prolapse (1), renal ptosis (1), gastro-oesophageal reflux disease (1), breast fibroadenoma (1) (Table 1).

Table 1. Clinical and personal data of the study population. BMI, body mass index.

	Clinical and Personal Data of the Study Population		
Patients	Total (n = 72)	Endometriosis (n = 41)	No Endometriosis (n = 31)
Age (median, interval)	35 (20–68)	33 (20–45)	36 (26–68)
BMI (median, interval)	21 (15–30)	21 (17–30)	22 (15–30)
Comorbidity	18	9	9
Parity		0.25	2.3

In the sample of women diagnosed with endometriosis, six were at stage I (minimum disease), with superficial lesions; five were at stage II (mild disease), with extended foci (up to 4 cm) in different locations; 14 were at stage III (moderate disease), mostly cases of ovarian endometrioma; and 16 were at stage IV (severe disease), in which we included cases of deep endometriosis with extended nodular formations (5–6 cm) and infiltrating contiguous structures such as the rectum, pararectal spaces, ureters and retroperitoneum. Table 2 shows, for each stage, the data related to age and BMI at the time of diagnosis, which was almost uniform among the subgroups; number of term pregnancies; surgical interventions for the treatment of the disease, performed laparoscopically in all cases, two completed with intestinal resection; and extent and severity of symptoms (the percentage of symptoms perceived as severe (score 3) was higher in stage IV (94%) than in stage I (40%)). In stages II and III, the degree of symptom severity perceived by women showed similar scores (60% vs. 64%), proving that symptomatology is not always connected linearly to the surgical stage of the disease. None of the women in the group of affected patients reported a family medical history positive for endometriosis.

Table 2. Distribution of clinical anamnestic data of the group of affected women.

Stage	I	II	III	IV
Number of patients	6	5	14	16
Age (median)	35	22	37	31
Parity (number of patients with at least one pregnancy)	0	1	5	2
BMI (median)	21	20	20	20
Number of patients with previous surgical intervention for endometriosis	0	2	10	14
Dysmenorrhea				
Mild	2	0	0	1
Moderate	1	2	6	1
Severe	2	3	7	14
Chronic pelvic pain				
Mild	0	1	2	0
Moderate	2	2	3	6
Severe	0	0	3	6
Dyspareunia				
Mild	2	1	4	2
Moderate	1	2	2	6
Severe	0	1	3	6
Intestinal symptoms	2	0	7	10
Urinary symptoms	2	0	3	3
Severe symptomatology percentage *	40%	60%	64%	94%

* Percentage of women who attributed a maximum severity score (visual analogue scale (VAS) 7–10) to at least one symptom (dysmenorrhea, chronic pelvic pain, dyspareunia, intestinal or urinary symptoms); mild (0–3); moderate (4–7); severe (8–10).

The frequency of genotypes observed in the groups of the reference population, 72 individuals, was globally consistent with the Hardy–Weinberg equilibrium law (Table 3).

Table 3. Expected and observed frequencies and Hardy–Weinberg equilibrium (HWE) p-values for SNPs investigated in total population.

SNP	TEST	A1 Minor Allele	A2 Major Allele	GENO	Observed (HET)	Expected (HET)	P
SNP1(FSHB)G>A	ALL	A	G	1/7/62	0.1	0.1203	0.2396
SNP2(VEZT)A>C	ALL	C	A	8/27/32	0.403	0.4358	0.5766
SNP3(WNT4)C>A	ALL	A	C	0/10/55	0.1538	0.142	1

Applying the HWE test to all components of the study population (cases + controls), there are no consistent differences between expected and observed genotypic frequencies, as shown by the p-values calculated for each investigated SNP. The p-values obtained are equal to 0.2396 for rs11031006 (FSHB), 0.5766 for rs10859871 (VEZT) and 1 for rs7521902 (WNT4); they allow us to accept the starting hypothesis, according to which there is no difference among the examined groups concerning the considered parameters. For each SNP, checking the expected and observed genotypic/allelic frequencies in single groups of affected cases and healthy controls, a modest significance in deviation from the Hardy–Weinberg equilibrium is highlighted, regarding the group of positive controls for genotypes containing allele C of the polymorphism rs10859871 (VEZT) (HWE p-value = 0.0435.) This violation of the proportions of the Hardy–Weinberg equilibrium could constitute a bias selection (Table 4).

Table 4. Expected and observed frequencies and HWE *p*-values for SNPs investigated in groups of affected cases and healthy controls.

SNP	TEST	A1 Minor Allele	A2 Major Allele	GENO	Observed (HET)	Expected (HET)	P
SNP1(FSHB)G>A	AFF	A	G	1/4/34	0.1026	0.142	0.187
SNP1(FSHB)G>A	UNAFF	A	G	0/3/28	0.09677	0.09209	1
SNP2(VEZT)A>C	AFF	C	A	1/19/18	0.5	0.3999	0.2255
SNP2(VEZT)A>C	UNAFF	C	A	7/8/14	0.2759	0.4709	0.0435
SNP3(WNT4)C>A	AFF	A	C	0/7/27	0.2059	0.1847	1
SNP3(WNT4)C>A	UNAFF	A	C	0/3/28	0.09677	0.09209	1

The following data are related to the study on genetic association between the considered SNPs and endometriosis.

rs11031006 (FSHB): Patients with endometriosis did not have an increase in genotypic or allelic frequency for this polymorphism compared to the control group ($p = 0.9999$, OR = 0.000, 95% CI, 0.000–15.000 and $p = 0.731$, OR = 1639, 95% CI, 0.393–683, respectively, for heterozygous genotype GA and polymorphic minor allele A) (Table 5, Figure 1). We also verified whether, by stratifying the sample of cases based on the severity of the situation (considering only women with stage III and IV endometriosis), a possible association with the investigated polymorphism would emerge; however, no correlation was found.

Table 5. Genotypic and allelic frequencies of rs11031006 (FSHB).

Genotipic Test		Controls		Cases		P Value	Odds Ratio	95% CI
		N°	%	N°	%			
SNP1 (FSHB)	A A	0	0.000%	1	2.56%			1.00 Reference
	G A	3	9.68%	4	10.26%	>0.9999	0.000	0.000 to 15.000
	G G	28	90.32%	34	87.18%	>0.9999	0.91	0.215 to 3.631
	Total	31	100.00%	39	100.00%			
Allelic Test		Controls		Cases		P Value	Odds Ratio	95% CI
		N°	%	N°	%			
SNP1 (FSHB)	A	3	4.84%	6	7.69%	0.7311	1639	0.393 to 683
	G	59	95.16%	72	92.30%			
	Total	62	100.00%	78	100.00%			

rs10859871 (VEZT): In the case of the polymorphism of the VEZT gene, we found a significant difference in frequency of homozygous genotype CC in the healthy control group compared to the affected women ($p = 0.0111$, OR = 0.0602, 95% CI, 0.005–0.501) (Table 6).

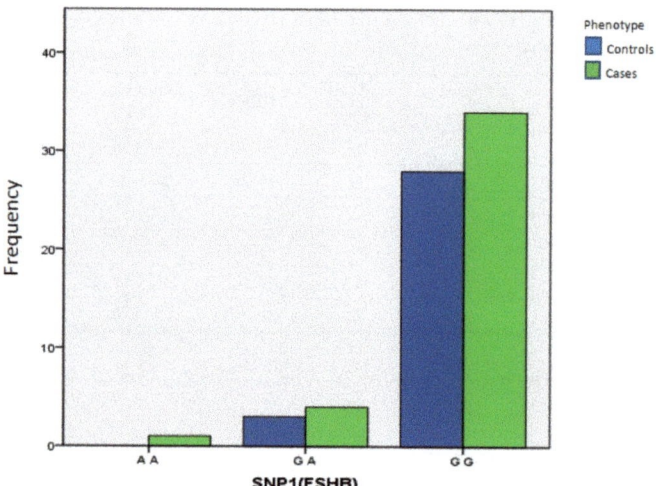

Figure 1. Distribution of AA, GA and GG genotypes obtained for the rs11031006 polymorphism (FSHB).

Table 6. Genotypic and allelic frequencies of rs10859871 (VEZT).

Genotipic Test		Controls		Cases		P Value	Odds Ratio	95% CI
		N°	%	N°	%			
SNP2 (VEZT)	A A	14	48.28%	18	47.37%			1.00 Reference
	A C	8	27.59%	19	50.00%	0.2931	1847.000	0.662 to 5.08
	C C	7	24.14%	1	2.63%	0.0111	0.06015	0.005 to 0.501
	Total	29	100.00%	38	100.00%			
Allelic Test		Controls		Cases		P Value	Odds Ratio	95% CI
		N°	%	N°	%			
SNP2 (VEZT)	C	22	37.93%	21	27.63%	0.2627	0.6248	0.300 to 129
	A	36	62.07%	55	72.36%			
	Total	58	100.00%	76	100.00%			

The same result was replicated by applying the analysis to the sub-group of affected women with moderate to severe endometriosis (stage III–IV) versus healthy controls, confirming a protective role for the homozygosity of the allelic variant ($p = 0.02703$). No significant differences between the groups concerning the allelic frequency of the minor allele C ($p = 0.2627$, OR = 0.6248, 95% CI, 0.300–129) were reported (Figure 2).

rs7521902 (WNT4): Patients with endometriosis did not have an increase in genotypic or allelic frequency of this polymorphism compared to the control group ($p = 0.3088$, OR = 0.4133, 95% CI, 0.10–1.8 and $p = 0.3297$, OR = 2257, 95% CI, 0.55–914, respectively, for heterozygous genotype CA and polymorphic minor allele A) (Table 7, Figure 3). No association was found between this SNP and the disease, even when limiting the analysis to the sample of severe surgical cases (stage III and IV).

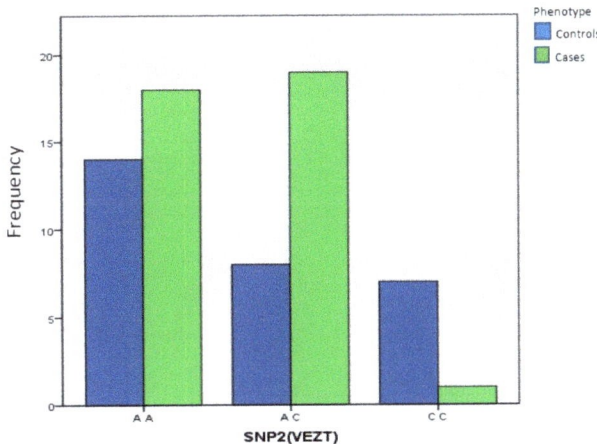

Figure 2. Distribution of AA, AC and CC genotypes obtained for polymorphism rs10859871 (VEZT).

Table 7. Genotypic and allelic frequencies of rs7521902 (WNT4).

Genotipic Test		Controls		Cases		P Value	Odds Ratio	95% CI
		N°	%	N°	%			
SNP3 (WNT4)	C A	3	9.68%	7	20.59%			1.00 Reference
	C C	28	90.32%	27	79.41%	0.3088	0.4133	0.108 to 1.811
	Total	31	100.00%	34	100.00%			

Allelic Test		Controls		Cases		P Value	Odds Ratio	95% CI
		N°	%	N°	%			
SNP3 (WNT4)	A	3	4.84%	7	10.29%			0.557 to 914
	C	59	95.16%	61	89.71%	0.3297	2257	
	Total	62	100.00%	68	100.00%			

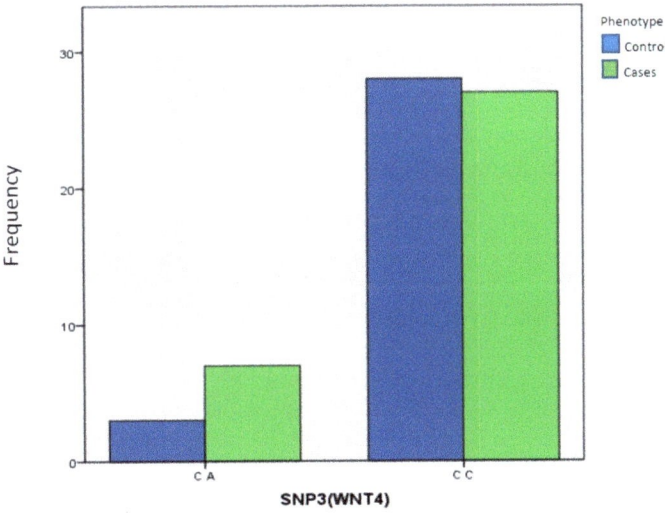

Figure 3. Distribution of CC and CA genotypes obtained for polymorphism rs7521902 (WNT4).

3. Discussion

Our analysis of the recent literature shows evidence of many genes possibly implicated in different pathogenetic mechanisms of endometriosis (Figure 4).

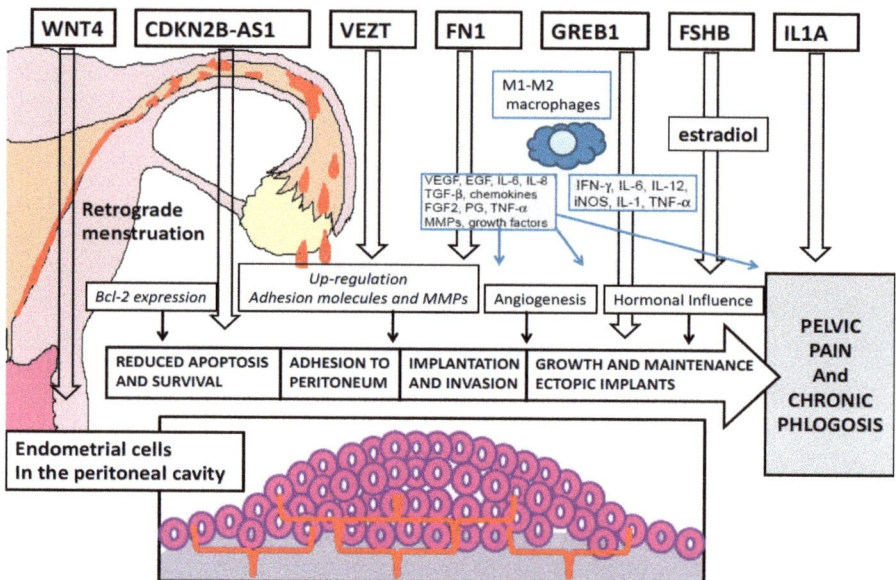

Figure 4. Pathogenetic targets of the most important genes related to endometriosis.

Nevertheless, it is clear that there are differences in genetic associations in endometriosis between different populations around the world. Therefore, it is important to study the genetic basis of this condition in several populations and to replicate the previous results, in order to define the role of significant variants of the risk of endometriosis. In this study, we specifically wanted to test the association between rs11031006 (FSHB), rs10859871 (VEZT) and rs7521902 (gene polymorphisms) and greater susceptibility to the development of endometriosis in a native Sardinian population. SNP rs7521902 WNT4 has been repeatedly associated in the literature with greater susceptibility to endometriosis in women of different ethnicities, including British, Australian, Italian and Japanese [10,16,17]. In the present study, no association between the risk C allele of this SNP and increased risk of endometriosis was detected. These data are consistent with those previously reported by Sundqvist et al. and Mafra et al. [9,13] in a Belgian population. Similarly, no association was detected in a study conducted on 800 Brazilian women (400 with and 400 without endometriosis) [9], or in another conducted on Chinese women (646 with and 766 without endometriosis) [14]. The SNP rs11031006 (FSHB) is another polymorphism candidate for a pathogenetic role, under its possible effect on the inhibition of hormonal feedback; although a significant association in a Greek population was reported, our results in a Sardinian population do not appear to be in line with the literature. The SNP rs10859871 is located in chromosomal region 12q22, 17 kb upstream of the VEZT 187 gene. VEZT is a transmembrane protein with a short extracellular and long intracellular domain, which clips on myosin VIIA as part of the adherent junctional complex in epithelial cells [21,22]. In the blood and endometrium, the C allele at risk of endometriosis of rs10859871 SNP in previous works was associated with increased expression of VEZT, and a pathogenetic role had been hypothetically attributed to this over-expression of VEZT [20]. In the case of gene polymorphism rs10859871 (VEZT), in our study, we instead show a significant and unexpected protective role in the pathology, in sharp contrast to the results obtained in other association studies conducted on populations with different ethnicities. We believe that this is the result of bias due to the small sample. As proof, the preliminary calculation of the Hardy–Weinberg equilibrium indeed signalled a significant deviation precisely in the group of positive controls for this polymorphism, compromising the validity of the results. Therefore, the obtained results did not highlight a significant association between the studied gene variants and a greater risk of developing the disease, although several other studies in the literature show the opposite. This is not surprising, if we consider that the obtained results refer to a Sardinian population known for its unique characteristics. The Sardinian population has always aroused considerable interest in human genetics, both for the peculiar distribution of different genetic variants and for the numerous genetically based diseases particularly frequent on the island. The Sardinian population, even if placed within European variability, shows singular characteristics: some frequent variants in Sardinia are rare or even absent in other populations, and vice versa. For example, the lack of significance of the SNP rs7521902 WNT4 as an endometriosis risk variant in the population of our study is largely due to a minimum allelic frequency (MAF), very low in the Sardinian population (0.0971). In other words, if a gene variant in a given ethnic population is quite rare, a large sample of individuals will be needed to test its frequency in terms relevant to the study. Similarly, the results in our study related to the SNP rs10859871 (VEZT), curiously not in line with what is highlighted in the literature, may have experienced interference because of the reduced size of the sample. It is equally true that most of the SNPs analysed in association studies or detected in GWASs do not fall within regions codifying the gene, and functional studies on them are insufficient. It is easy to hypothesize that the regulatory effect of these polymorphic variants on the expression of certain genes is in turn influenced by the modulation of other factors and co-factors expressed on other regions of the genome whose location and function we do not know. There is also more and more evidence for the role of epigenetic influences, which, through environmental, food-related and/or misunderstood factors and through methylation mechanisms of sequences and histone acetylation, can induce modifications in DNA gene expression without changing its sequence, but simply by turning on or off certain target genes. Since the pathogenesis of endometriosis is extremely complex, involving both genetic background and environmental conditions, studies with conflicting results in several cases have made it difficult to interpret these data. The lack of confirmation of the previous results is therefore largely attributed to an insufficient sample, to population differences and the interaction with genetic and/or non-genetic factors. For this reason, it appears mandatory to extend the case histories of the study in order to reveal or confirm the influence of these gene variants on the Sardinian population.

4. Materials and Methods

4.1. Sampling and Genotyping

After collecting their informed consent, we took a sample of whole blood from each patient (9mL EDTA tube) for genetic analysis. On each sample, a label indicating the date of acquisition and an alphanumeric code (single coding) was affixed, through which only authorized personnel could trace the patient's identity through a special data collection file. The samples were stored in a freezer at a temperature of $-30\ °C$, locked and accessible only by authorized personnel. Genomic DNA was extracted from whole blood with a Qiagen Extraction Kit (QIAmp ® DNA Mini Kit (QIAGEN GmbH, Hilden, Germany), according to the protocol illustrated in the kit manual. Subsequently, genomic DNA extracted from whole blood was read in a NanoDrop photometer 3300^{Tm} ThermoFisher Scientific (www.termofisher.com) at wavelengths of 260, 280 and 260nm/280nm, to assess its quality and quantity. The extracted nuclear DNA was subsequently aliquoted for the next phases of PCR. The analysis of rs7521902, rs10859871 and rs11031006 SNPs examined in the study was carried out by sequencing with the Sanger method. For each selected SNP, the minimum allelic frequency (MAF) in the Sardinian population was preliminarily verified, using the online PheWeb dataset (http://sardinia-pheweb.sph.umich.edu) (Table 8).

Table 8. Minimum allelic frequency (MAF) in Sardinian population of single nucleotide polymorphisms (SNPs) under investigation. WNT4, wingless-typemammalian mouse tumour virus integration site family member 4; VEZT, vezatin; FSHB, follicle stimulating hormone beta polypeptide.

Gene	SNP	MAF Sardinia
WNT4	rs7521902	0.0971
VEZT	rs10859871	0.407
FSHB	rs11031006	0.106

Each DNA sample was amplified with PCR (final volume 25 µL) according to the following protocol: to 75 ng of genomic DNA, 2.5 µL of the specific Taq Polymerase ThermoFisher Scientific (www.termofisher.com) 10× buffer and 1.5 µL of MgCl$_2$ solution (25 mM) was added 0.2 µL of a 2.5 mM dNTP solution, 0.125 µL of Taq Polymerase (5 U/µL), and the forward and reverse primers (25 pmol/µLeach) specific to each analysed region. For each fragment, the same amplification file was used in which initial denaturation was foreseen at 95 °C for 10 min, 30 amplification cycles at 95 °C for 30 min, 60 °C for 30 min, 72 °C for 40 min and a final extension at 72 °C for 10 min. The PCR products were then sequenced using a BigDye Terminator v3.1 Cycle Sequencing Kit ThermoFisher Scientific (www.termofisher.com), according to the manufacturer's instructions. The primers used for sequencing were the same ones used for the amplification of the fragments. Sequence reactions were subsequently subjected to electrophoresis with an ABI3130XL genetic analyser instrument (Applied Biosystems–ThermoFisher) and analysed with SeqScapev3.0 software (ThermoFisher).

4.2. Statistical Analysis

Data were tabulated in a specific database and analysed through specific software. For statistical analysis, Plink v.1.7, SPSS Statistics for Windows v.18 (IBM Corp., Armonk, NY, USA) and GraphPad Prism v.8 (GraphPad Software, La Jolla, CA, USA) software were used, applying addictive, allelic, dominant and recessive models. To examine the differences in frequency of genotypes and alleles among the groups of cases and controls, and to consider a possible association among the SNPs and the pathology under study, Fisher's exact test was used. All of the examined SNPs had a >98% callrate. We considered a 2-tailed p-value < 0.05 to be statistically significant. The odds ratio (OR) and 95% confidence interval (CI) were calculated. The studied genetic variants were evaluated in advance for deviation from the Hardy–Weinberg equilibrium (HWE), comparing the observed and expected genotype frequencies in the groups of the reference sample, through Fisher's exact test.

5. Conclusions

Our data underline the importance of evaluating genetic variants in different populations, in an attempt to define the genetic architecture of endometriosis and the extent of the effects of specific risk alleles in different ethnic groups. An important advantage of the analysis of genetic associations for different ethnic populations is that it can also shed light on the decomposition of the different disequilibrium linkage of populations. At the genomic level, this "trans-ethnic fine mapping" is an important method to restrict the signal to a causal variant [29]. To test this aspect further, exploration of the loci is needed, analysing the surrounding variants, for example through GWASs. GWASs allow the examination of a high number of SNPs and rare variants (up to 4.5 million) in a very large population, to find possible associations with a disease. Recent GWAS meta-analyses, identifying some genetic loci associated with endometriosis, have marked a starting point to define the molecular basis at the origin of the disease, representing the proverbial tip of the iceberg. Studies in very large populations are needed to identify new polymorphisms and to understand their molecular mechanisms. At the moment, the identified gene polymorphisms cannot be used in clinical practice to predict the risk of developing endometriosis or as diagnostic/prognostic markers, but this constitutes a concrete goal for the near future. In fact, defining the genetic alterations predisposing the onset of endometriosis has several potential benefits. First, it could allow us to identify patients at risk of developing endometriosic pathology during the pre-pubescent phase, and contribute to a non-invasive diagnosis in adulthood. Moreover, it could help to better define the molecular mechanisms responsible for its onset and, consequently, represent a rational basis for determining specific therapeutic molecules for this disease.

Author Contributions: Conceptualization, D.D. and S.A..; methodology, S.A..; software, F.A.; validation, S.A.; formal analysis, S.G. and A.C.; investigation, D.D.; data curation, F.A.; writing—original draft preparation, S.A., M.N.D. and D.D.; writing—review and editing, M.N.D., S.A. and D.D.; visualization, M.N.D.; supervision, S.A.; project administration, S.A.; funding acquisition, D.D. All authors have read and agreed to the published version of the manuscript.

Funding: This research received no external funding.

Acknowledgments: This publication was created as part of a research project financed with the resources of P.O.R. SARDEGNA F.S.E. 2014-2020-Asse III "Istruzione e Formazione, Obiettivo Tematico: 10, Obiettivo Specifico: 10.5, Azione dell'accordo fi Partenariato:10.5.12 "Avviso di chiamata per il finanziamento di Progetti di ricerca–Anno 2017.

Conflicts of Interest: The authors declare no conflict of interest.

Abbreviations

SNP	Single nucleotide polymorphism
PCR	Polymerase chain reaction
UTR	Untranslated region
AR	Androgen receptor
ER	Estrogenic receptor
PR	Progesterone receptor
A	Adenine
T	Thymine
C	Cytosine
G	Guanine
TGF-β	Transforming growth factor β
IL	Interleukin
VEGF	Vascular endothelial growth factor
TNF	Tumour necrosis factor
HLA	Human leukocyte antigen
MHC	Major histocompatibility complex
EGFR	Endothelial growth factor receptor
mRNA	Messenger ribonucleic acid
MMP	Matrix metalloproteinase
GSTM1	Glutathione S-transferase mu, M1
GSTP1	Glutathione S-transferase P1
GSTT1	Glutathione S-transferase theta, T1
NAT	N-acetyltransferase
CYP	Cytochrome P450
XRCC	X-ray repair cross-complementing
ERCC	Excision repair cross-complementing
GWAS	Genome-wide association study
NGS	Next-generation sequencing
KRAS	Kirsten rat sarcoma viral oncogene homolog
eQTLs	Expression quantitative traits loci
MiRNA	Micro RNA
NcRNA	Non-coding RNA

References

1. Alio, L.; Angioni, S.; Arena, S.; Bartiromo, L.; Bergamini, N.; Berlanda, N.; Bonanni, V.; Bonin, C.; Buggio, L.; Candiani, M.; et al. Endometriosis: Seeking optimal management in women approaching menopause. *Climacteric* **2019**, *22*, 329–338. [CrossRef] [PubMed]

2. Deiana, D.; Gessa, S.; Anardu, M.; Danilidis, A.; Nappi, L.; D'Alterio, M.N.; Pontis, A.; Angioni, S. Genetic of endometriosis: A comprehensive review. *Gynecol. Endocrinol.* **2019**, *35*, 553–558. [CrossRef] [PubMed]
3. Melis, I.; Agus, M.; Pluchino, N.; Sardo, A.D.S.; Litta, P.; Melis, G.B.; Angioni, S. Alexithymia in women with deep endometriosis? A pilot. Study. *J. Endometr. Pelvic. Pain Dis.* **2014**, *6*, 26–33.
4. Angioni, S. New insights on endometriosis. *Minerva Ginecol.* **2017**, *69*, 438–439. [PubMed]
5. Locci, R.; Nisolle, M.; Angioni, S.; Foidart, J.M.; Munat, C. Expression of the gamma 2 chain of laminin-332 in eutopic and ectopic endometrium of patients with endometriosis. *Rep. Biol. Endocrinol.* **2013**, *11*, 94. [CrossRef] [PubMed]
6. Simpson, J.L.; Elias, S.; Malinak, L.R.; Buttram, V.C., Jr. Heritable aspects of endometriosis. Genetic studies. *Am. J. Obstet. Gynecol.* **1980**, *137*, 327–331. [CrossRef]
7. Treloar, S.A.; O'Connor, D.T.; O'Connor, V.M.; Martin, N.G. Genetic influences on endometriosis in an Australian twin sample. *Fertil. Steril.* **1999**, *71*, 701–710. [CrossRef]
8. Lettre, G.; Hirschhorn, J.N. Small island, big genetic discoveries. *Nat. Genet.* **2015**, *47*, 1224–1225. [CrossRef]
9. Mafra, F.; Catto, M.; Bianco, B.; Barbosa, C.P.; Christofolini, D. Association of WNT4 polymorphisms with endometriosis in infertile patients. *J. Assist. Reprod. Genet.* **2015**, *32*, 1359–1364. [CrossRef]
10. Pagliardini, L.; Gentilini, D.; Vigano', P.; Panina-Bordignon, P.; Busacca, M.; Candiani, M.; Di Blasio, A.M. An Italian association study and meta-analysis with previous GWAS confirm WNT4, CDKN2BAS and FN1 as the first identified susceptibility loci for endometriosis. *J. Med. Genet.* **2013**, *50*, 43–46. [CrossRef]
11. Vainio, S.; Heikkilä, M.; Kispert, A.; Chin, N.; McMahon, A.P. Female development in mammals is regulated by Wnt-4 signalling. *Nature* **1999**, *397*, 405–409. [CrossRef] [PubMed]
12. Gaetje, R.; Holtrich, U.; Engels, K.; Kissler, S.; Rody, A.; Karn, T.; Kaufmann, M. Endometriosis may be generated by mimicking the ontogenetic development of the female genital tract. *Fertil. Steril.* **2007**, *87*, 651–656. [CrossRef] [PubMed]
13. Sundqvist, J.; Xu, H.; Vodolazkaia, A.; Fassbender, A.; Kyama, C.; Bokor, A.; Gemzell-Danielsson, K.; D'Hooghe, T.M.; Falconer, H. Replication of endometriosis-associated single-nucleotide polymorphisms from genome-wide association studies in a Caucasian population. *Hum. Reprod.* **2013**, *28*, 835–839. [CrossRef] [PubMed]
14. Wu, Z.; Yuan, M.; Li, Y.; Fu, F.; Ma, W.; Li, H.; Wang, W.; Wang, S. Analysis of WNT4 polymorphism in Chinese Han women with endometriosis. *Reprod. Biomed. Online* **2015**, *30*, 415–420. [CrossRef] [PubMed]
15. Jordan, B.K.; Mohammed, M.; Ching, S.T.; Délot, E.; Chen, X.N.; Dewing, P.; Swain, A.; Rao, P.N.; Elejalde, B.R.; Vilain, E. Up-regulation ofWNT-4 signaling and dosage-sensitive sex reversal in humans. *Am. J. Hum. Genet.* **2001**, *68*, 1102–1109. [CrossRef]
16. Rahmioglu, N.; Nyholt, D.R.; Morris, A.P.; Missmer, S.A.; Montgomery, G.W.; Zondervan, K.T. Genetic variants underlying risk of endometriosis: Insights from meta-analysis of eight genome-wide association and replication datasets. *Hum. Reprod. Update* **2014**, *20*, 702–716. [CrossRef]
17. Nyholt, D.R.; Low, S.K.; Anderson, C.A.; Painter, J.N.; Uno, S.; Morris, A.P.; MacGregor, S.; Gordon, S.D.; Henders, A.K.; Martin, N.G.; et al. Genome-wide association meta-analysis identified new endometriosis risk loci. *Nat. Genet.* **2012**, *44*, 1355–1359. [CrossRef]
18. Uno, S.; Zembutsu, H.; Hirasawa, A.; Takahashi, A.; Kubo, M.; Akahane, T.; Aoki, D.; Kamatani, N.; Hirata, K.; Nakamura, Y. A genome-wide association study identifies genetic variants in the CDKN2BAS locus associated with endometriosis in Japanese. *Nat. Genet.* **2010**, *42*, 707–710. [CrossRef]
19. Painter, J.N.; Anderson, C.A.; Nyholt, D.R.; Macgregor, S.; Lin, J.; Lee, S.H.; Lambert, A.; Zhao, Z.Z.; Roseman, F.; Guo, Q.; et al. Genome-wide association study identifies a locus at 7p15.2 associated with the development of endometriosis. *Nat. Genet.* **2011**, *43*, 51–54. [CrossRef]
20. Haldsworth-Carson, S.J.; Fung, J.N.; Luong, H.T.; Sapkota, Y.; Bowdler, L.M.; Wallace, L.; Teh, W.T.; Powell, J.E.; Girling, J.E.; Healey, M.; et al. Endometrial vezatin and it association with endometriosis risk. *Hum. Reprod.* **2016**, *31*, 999–1013. [CrossRef]
21. Küssel-Andermann, P.; El-Amraoui, A.; Safieddine, S.; Nouaille, S.; Perfettini, I.; Lecuit, M.; Cossart, P.; Wolfrum, U.; Petit, C. Vezatin, a novel transmembrane protein, bridges myosin VIIA to the cadherin-catenins complex. *Embo J.* **2000**, *19*, 6020–6029. [CrossRef] [PubMed]
22. Blaschuk, O.W.; Rowlands, T.M. Plasma membrane components of adherens junctions. *Mol. Membr. Biol.* **2002**, *19*, 75–80. [CrossRef] [PubMed]

23. Luong, H.T.T.; Painter, J.N.; Sapkota, Y.; Niholt, D.R.; Rogers, P.A.; Montgomery, G.W. Identifying the functional role of VEZT Gene for endometriosis risk. *Ann. Transl. Med.* **2015**, *3*, AB028.
24. Pagliardini, L.; Gentilini, D.; Sanchez, A.M.; Candiani, M.; Viganò, P.; Di Blasio, A.M. Replication and meta-analysis of previous genome-wide association studies confirm vezatin as the locus with the strongest evidence for association with endometriosis. *Hum. Reprod.* **2015**, *30*, 987–993. [CrossRef] [PubMed]
25. Meola, J.; Rosa, E.; Silva, J.C.; Dentillo, D.B.; Da Silva, W.A., Jr.; Veiga-Castelli, L.C.; Bernardes, L.A.; Ferriani, R.A.; De Paz, C.C.; Giuliatti, S.; et al. Differentially expressed genes in eutopic and ectopic endometrium of women with endometriosis. *Fertil. Steril.* **2010**, *93*, 1750–1773. [CrossRef]
26. Guo, S.-W. Nuclear factor-kappab (NF-κB): An unsuspected major culprit in the pathogenesis of endometriosis that is still at large? *Gynecol. Obstet. Investig.* **2007**, *63*, 71–97. [CrossRef]
27. Sapkota, Y.; Steinthorsdottir, V.; Morris, A.P.; Fassbender, A.; Rahmioglu, N.; De Vivo, I.; Buring, J.E.; Zhang, F.; Edwards, T.L.; Jones, S.; et al. Meta-analysis identifies five novel loci associated with endometriosis highlighting key genes involved in hormone metabolism. *Nat. Commun.* **2017**, *8*, 15539. [CrossRef]
28. Ruth, K.S.; Beaumont, R.N.; Tyrrell, J.; Jones, S.E.; Tuke, M.A.; Yaghootkar, H.; Wood, A.R.; Freathy, R.M.; Weedon, M.N.; Frayling, T.M.; et al. Genetic evidence that lower circulating FSH levels lengthen menstrual cycle, increase age at menopause and impact female reproductive health. *Hum. Reprod.* **2016**, *31*, 473–481. [CrossRef]
29. Matalliotakis, M.; Zervou, M.I.; Matalliotaki, C.; Ramhioglu, N.; Koumantakis, G.; Kalogiannidis, I.; Prapas, I.; Zondervan, K.; Spandidos, D.A.; Matalliotakis, I.; et al. The role of gene polymorphisms in endometriosis. *Molec. Med. Rep.* **2017**, *16*, 5881–5886. [CrossRef]
30. Revised American Society for Reproductive Medicine classification of endometriosis: 1996. *Fertil. Steril.* **1997**, *67*, 817–821. [CrossRef]
31. Vercellini, P.; Viganò, P.; Somigliana, E.; Fedele, L. Endometriosis: Pathogenesis and treatment. *Nat. Rev. Endocrinol.* **2014**, *10*, 261–275. [CrossRef] [PubMed]
32. Laganà, A.S.; Garzon, S.; Gotte, M.; Viganò, P.; Franchi, M.; Ghezzi, F.; Martin, D.C. Pathogenesis of Endometriosis: Molecular and Cell Biology Insights. *Int. J. Mol. Sci.* **2019**, *20*, 5615. [CrossRef] [PubMed]
33. Angioni, S.; Cofelice, V.; Pontis, A.; Tinelli, R.; Socolov, R. New trends of progestins treatment of endometriosis. *Gynecol. Endocrinol.* **2014**, *30*, 769–773. [CrossRef] [PubMed]
34. Angioni, S.; Cofelice, V.; Sedda, F.; Stochino Loi, E.; Multinu, F.; Pontis, A.; Melis, G.B. Progestins for symptomatic endometriosis: Results of clinical studies. *Curr. Drug. Ther.* **2015**, *10*, 91–104. [CrossRef]
35. Wang, Z.; Yoshida, S.; Negoro, K.; Kennedy, S.; Barlow, D.; Maruo, T. Polymorphisms in the estrogen receptor beta gene but not estrogen receptor alpha gene affect the risk of developing endometriosis in a Japanese population. *Fertil. Steril.* **2004**, *81*, 1650–1656. [CrossRef]
36. Lee, G.H.; Kim, S.H.; Choi, Y.M.; Suh, C.S.; Kim, J.G.; Moon, S.Y. Estrogen receptor beta gene +1730 G/A polymorphism in women with endometriosis. *Fertil. Steril.* **2007**, *88*, 785–788. [CrossRef]
37. Lattuada, D.; Somigliana, E.; Vigano, P.; Candiani, M.; Pardi, G.; Di Biasio, A.M. Genetics of endometriosis: A role for the progesterone receptor gene polymorphism PROGINS? *Clin. Endocrinol.* **2004**, *61*, 190–194. [CrossRef]
38. Wieser, F.; Schneeberger, C.; Tong, D.; Tempfer, C.; Huber, J.C.; Wenzl, R. PROGINS receptor gene polymorphism is associated with endometriosis. *Fertil. Steril.* **2002**, *77*, 309–312. [CrossRef]
39. De Carvalho, C.V.; Nogueira-De-Souza, N.C.; Costa, A.M.; Baracat, E.C.; Girao, M.J.; D'Amora, P.; Schor, E.; da Silva, I.D. Genetic polymorphisms of cytochrome P450cl7alpha (CYP17) and progesterone receptor gene (PROGINS) in the assessment of endometriosis risk. *Gynecol. Endocrinol.* **2007**, *23*, 29–33. [CrossRef]
40. Govindan, S.; Ahmad, S.N.; Vedicherla, B.; Kodati, V.; Jahan, P.; Rao, K.P.; Ahuja, Y.R.; Hasan, Q. Association of progesterone receptor gene (PROGINS) with endometriosis, uterine fibroids and breast cancer. *Cancer Biomark.* **2007**, *3*, 73–77. [CrossRef]
41. Treloar, S.A.; Zhao, Z.Z.; Armitage, T.; Duffy, D.L.; Wicks, J.; O'Connor, D.T.; Martin, N.G.; Montgomery, G.W. Association between polymorphisms in the progesterone receptor gene and endometriosis. *Mol. Hum. Reprod.* **2005**, *11*, 641–647. [CrossRef] [PubMed]
42. Van Kaam, K.J.; Romano, A.; Schouten, J.P.; Dunselman, G.A.; Groothuis, P.G. Progesterone receptor polymorphism +331G/A is associated with a decreased risk of deep infiltrating endometriosis. *Hum. Reprod.* **2007**, *22*, 129–135. [CrossRef] [PubMed]

43. Slayden, O.D.; Nayak, N.R.; Burton, K.A.; Chwalisz, K.; Cameron, S.T.; Critchley, H.O.; Baird, D.T.; Brenner, R.M. Progesterone antagonist increase androgen receptor expression in the rhesus macaque and human endometrium. *J. Clin. Endocrinol. Metab.* **2001**, *86*, 2668–2679. [CrossRef] [PubMed]
44. Mertens, H.J.; Heinemann, M.J.; Theunissen, P.H.; de Jong, F.H.; Evers, J.L. Androgen, estrogen and progesterone receptor expression in the human uterus during the mestrual cycle. *Eur. J. Obstet. Gynecol. Reprod. Biol.* **2001**, *98*, 58–65. [CrossRef]
45. Tuckermann, E.M.; Okon, M.A.; Li, T.; Laird, S.M. Do androgens have a direct effect on endometrial function? An in vitro study. *Fertil. Steril.* **2000**, *74*, 771–779. [CrossRef]
46. Carneiro, M.M.; Morsch, D.M.; Camargos, A.F.; Reis, F.M.; Spritzer, P.M. Androgen receptor and 5α-reductase are expressed in pelvic endometriosis. *Int. J. Obstet. Gynaecol.* **2008**, *115*, 113–117. [CrossRef]
47. Gelmann, P.E. Molecular Biology of the AR. *J. Clin. Oncol.* **2002**, *20*, 3001–3015. [CrossRef]
48. Rajender, S.; Singh, L.; Thangaraj, K. Phenotypic heterogeneity of mutations in androgen receptor gene. *Asian J. Androl.* **2007**, *9*, 147–179.
49. Shaik, N.A.; Govindan, S.; Kodati, V.; Rao, K.P.; Hasan, Q. Polymorphic (CAG) repeats in the androgen receptor gene: A risk marker for endometriosis and uterine leiomyomas. *Hematol. Oncol. Stem Cel. Ther.* **2009**, *2*, 289–293. [CrossRef]
50. Hsieh, Y.Y.; Chang, C.C.; Tsai, F.J.; Wu, J.Y.; Tsai, C.H.; Tsai, H.D. Androgen receptor trinucleotide polymorphism in endometriosis. *Fertil. Steril.* **2001**, *76*, 412–413. [CrossRef]
51. Lattuada, D.; Viganò, P.; Somigliana, E.; Odorizzi, M.P.; Vignali, M.; Di Biasio, A.M. Androgen receptor gene cytosine, adenine, and guanine trinucleotide repeats in patients with endometriosis. *J. Soc. Gynecol. Investig.* **2004**, *11*, 237–240. [CrossRef] [PubMed]
52. Hsieh, Y.Y.; Chang, C.C.; Tsai, F.J.; Hsu, Y.; Tsai, H.D.; Tsai, C.H. Polymorphisms for interleukin-4 (IL-4)—590 promoter, IL-4 intron3, and tumor necrosis factor alpha -308 promoter: Non-association with endometriosis. *J. Clin. Lab. Anal.* **2002**, *16*, 121–126. [CrossRef] [PubMed]
53. Yu, Y.X.; Xiu, Y.L.; Chen, X.; Li, Y.L. Transforming Growth Factor-beta 1 involved in the pathogenesis of endometriosis through regulating expression of vascular endothelial growth factor under hypoxia. *Chin. Med. J.* **2017**, *130*, 950–956. [CrossRef] [PubMed]
54. Wieser, F.; Fabjani, G.; Tempfer, C.; Schneeberger, C.; Zeillinger, R.; Huber, J.C.; Wenzl, R. Tumor necrosis factor–alpha promoter polymorphisms and endometriosis. *J. Soc. Gynecol. Investig.* **2002**, *9*, 313–318. [CrossRef]
55. Somigliana, E.; Viganò, P.; Vignali, M. Endometriosis and unexplained recurrent spontaneous abortion: Pathological states resulting from aberrant modulation of natural killer cell function? *Hum. Reprod. Update* **1999**, *5*, 41–52. [CrossRef] [PubMed]
56. Wang, X.; Lin, Q.; Guo, S. Study on polymorphism of human leukocyte antigen I in patients with endometriosis. *Zhanghua Fu Chan Ke Za Zhi* **2001**, *36*, 150–152.
57. Ishii, K.; Takakuwa, K.; Kashima, K.; Tamura, M.; Tanaka, K. Associations between patients with endometriosis and HLA class II; the analysis of HLA-DQB1 and HLA- DPB1 genotypes. *Hum. Reprod.* **2003**, *18*, 985–989. [CrossRef]
58. Pabalan, N.; Jarjanazi, H.; Christofolini, D.M.; Bianco, B.; Barbosa, C.P. Association of the protein tyrosine phosphatase non receptor 22 polymorphism (PNTN22) with endometriosis: A meta-analysis. *Rev. Artic. Einstein* **2017**, *15*, 105–111. [CrossRef]
59. Perini, J.A.; Cardoso, J.V.; Berardo, P.T.; Vianna-Jorge, R.; Nasciutti, L.E.; Bellodi-Privato, M.; Machado, D.E.; Abrao, M.S. Role of vascular endothelial growth factor polymorphisms (−2578C > A, −460T > C, −1154G > A, +405G > C and + 936C > T) in endometriosis: A case-control study with Brazilians. *BMC Womens Health* **2014**, *14*, 117. [CrossRef]
60. Hsieh, Y.Y.; Chang, C.C.; Tsai, F.J.; Lin, C.C.; Tsai, C.H. T homozygote and allele of epidermal growth factor receptor 2073 gene polymorphism are associated with higher susceptibility to endometriosis and leiomyomas. *Fertil. Steril.* **2005**, *83*, 796–799. [CrossRef]
61. Guo, S.W. Glutathione S-transferases M1/T1 gene polymorphism and endometriosis: A meta-analysis of genetic association studies. *Mol. Hum. Reprod.* **2005**, *11*, 729–743. [CrossRef] [PubMed]
62. Arvanatis, D.A.; Koumantakis, G.E.; Gouemenou, A.G.; Metalliokatis, E.E.; Spandidos, D.A. CYP1A1, CYP19, and GSTM1 polymorphisms increase the risk of endometriosis. *Fertil. Steril.* **2003**, *79*, 707–709. [CrossRef]

63. Hsieh, Y.Y.; Chang, C.C.; Tsai, F.J.; Lin, C.C.; Tsai, C.H. Cytochrome P450c17alpha 5'- untranslated region *T/C polymorphism in endometriosis. *J. Genet.* **2004**, *83*, 189–192. [CrossRef] [PubMed]
64. Lambrinoudaki, I.V.; Augoulea, A.; Christodoulakos, G.E.; Economou, E.V.; Kaparos, G.; Kontoravdis, A.; Papadias, C.; Creatsas, G. Measurable serum markers of oxidative stress response in women with endometriosis. *Fertil. Steril.* **2009**, *91*, 46–50. [CrossRef]
65. Attar, R.; Cacina, C.; Sozen, S.; Attar, E.; Agachan, B. DNA repair genes in endometriosis. *Gen. Mol. Res.* **2010**, *9*, 629–636. [CrossRef]
66. Rahmioglu, N.; Montgomery, G.W.; Zondervan, K.T. Genetics of endometriosis. *Womens Health* **2015**, *11*, 577–586. [CrossRef]
67. Treloar, S.A.; Wicks, J.; Nyholt, D.R.; Montgomery, G.W.; Bahlo, M.; Smith, V.; Dawson, G.; Mackay, I.J.; Weeks, D.E.; Bennett, S.T.; et al. Genome-wide Linkage Study in 1,176 affected sister pair families identifies a significant susceptibility locus for endometriosis on chromosome 10q26. *Am. J. Hum. Genet.* **2005**, *77*, 365–376. [CrossRef]
68. Painter, J.N.; Nyholt, D.R.; Morris, A.; Zhao, Z.Z.; Henders, A.K.; Lambert, A.; Wallace, L.; Martin, N.G.; Kennedy, S.H.; Treloar, S.A.; et al. High-density fine-mapping of a chromosome 10q26 linkage peak suggests association between endometriosis and variants close to CYP2C19. *Fertil. Steril.* **2011**, *95*, 2236–2240. [CrossRef]
69. Cribb, A.E.; Knight, M.J.; Dryer, D.; Guernsey, J.; Hender, K.; Tesch, M.; Saleh, T.M. Role of a polymorphic human CYP450 enzymes in estrone oxidation. *Cancer Epidemiol. Biomark. Prev.* **2006**, *15*, 551–558. [CrossRef]
70. Martini, M.; Ciccarone, M.; Garganese, G.; Maggiore, C.; Evangelista, A.; Rahimi, S.; Zannoni, G.; Vittori, G.; Larocca, L.M. Possible involvement of hMLH1, p16INK4a and PTEN in the malignant transformation of endometriosis. *Int. J. Cancer* **2002**, *102*, 398–406. [CrossRef]
71. Powell, J.E.; Fung, J.N.; Shakhbazov, K.; Sapkota, Y.; Cloonan, N.; Hemani, G.; Hillman, K.M.; Kaufmann, S.; Luong, H.T.; Bowdler, L.; et al. Endometriosis risk alleles at 1p36.12 act through inverse regulation of CDC42 and LINC00339. *Hum. Mol. Genet.* **2016**, *25*, 5046–5058. [PubMed]
72. Grechukhina, O.; Petracco, R.; Popkhadze, S.; Massasa, E.; Paranjape, T.; Chan, E.; Flores, I.; Weidhaas, J.B.; Taylor, H.S. A polymorphism in a let-7 microRNA binding site of KRAS in women with endometriosis. *EMBO Mol. Med.* **2012**, *4*, 202–217. [CrossRef] [PubMed]
73. Luong, H.T.; Nyholt, D.R.; Painter, J.N.; Chapman, B.; Kennedy, S.; Treloar, S.A.; Zondervan, K.T.; Montgomery, G.W. No evidence for genetic association with the let-7 microRNA-binding site or the common KRAS variants in risk of endometriosis. *Hum. Reprod.* **2012**, *12*, 3616–3621. [CrossRef] [PubMed]
74. Chettier, R.; Albertsen, H.M.; Ward, K. Next Generation Sequencing of families with endometriosis identifies new genomic regions likely to contribute to heritability. *Fertil. Steril.* **2014**, *102*, 76–77. [CrossRef]
75. Er, T.K.; Su, Y.F.; Wu, C.C.; Chen, C.C.; Wang, J.; Hsieh, T.H.; Herreros-Villanueva, M.; Chen, W.T.; Chen, Y.T.; Liu, T.C.; et al. Targeted next-generation sequencing for molecular diagnosis of endometriosis-associated ovarian cancer. *J. Mol. Med.* **2016**, *94*, 835–847. [CrossRef]
76. Sapkota, Y.; Vivo, I.; Steinthorsdottir, V.; Fassbender, A.; Bowdler, L.; Buring, J.E.; Edwards, T.L.; Jones, S.; Dorien, O.; Peterse, D.; et al. Analysis of potential protein-modifying variants in 9000 endometriosis patients and 150000 controls of European ancestry. *Sci. Rep.* **2017**, *7*, 11380. [CrossRef]
77. Fung, J.N.; Montgomery, G.W. Genetics of endometriosis: State of art on genetic risk factors for endometriosis. *Best. Pract. Res. Clin. Obstetr. Gynecol.* **2018**, *50*, 61–71. [CrossRef]
78. Freedman, M.L.; Monteiro, A.N.; Gayther, S.A.; Coetzee, G.A.; Risch, A.; Plass, C.; Casey, G.; De Biasi, M.; Carlson, C.; Duggan, D.; et al. Principles for the post- GWAS functional characterization of cancer risk. *Nat. Genet.* **2011**, *43*, 513–518. [CrossRef]
79. Westra, H.J.; Peters, M.J.; Esko, T.; Yaghootkar, H.; Schurmann, C.; Kettunen, J.; Christiansen, M.W.; Fairfax, B.P.; Schramm, K.; Powell, J.E.; et al. Systematic identification of trans eQTLs as putative drivers of known disease associations. *Nat. Genet.* **2013**, *45*, 1238–1243. [CrossRef]
80. Guo, S.W. Epigenetics of endometriosis. *Mol. Hum. Reprod.* **2009**, *15*, 587–607. [CrossRef]
81. Wu, Y.; Starzinski-Powitz, A.; Guo, S.W. Trichostatin A, a histone deacetylase inhibitor, attenuates invasiveness and reactivates E-cadherin expression in immortalized endometriotic cells. *Reprod. Sci.* **2007**, *14*, 374–382. [CrossRef] [PubMed]
82. Jenuwein, T.; Allis, C.D. Translating the histone code. *Science* **2001**, *293*, 1074–1080. [CrossRef] [PubMed]

83. Bernstein, B.E.; Meissner, A.; Lander, E.S. The mammalian epigenome. *Cell* **2007**, *128*, 669–681. [CrossRef] [PubMed]
84. Sun, H.S.; Hsiao, K.Y.; Hsu, C.C.; Wu, M.H.; Tsai, S.J. Transactivation of steroidogenic acute regulatory protein in human endometriotic stromalcells is mediated by the prostaglandin EP2 receptor. *Endocrinology* **2003**, *144*, 3934–3942. [CrossRef] [PubMed]

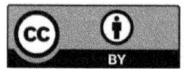

© 2020 by the authors. Licensee MDPI, Basel, Switzerland. This article is an open access article distributed under the terms and conditions of the Creative Commons Attribution (CC BY) license (http://creativecommons.org/licenses/by/4.0/).

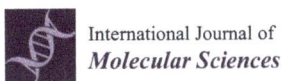

Article

Peritoneal Fluid Cytokines Reveal New Insights of Endometriosis Subphenotypes

Jieliang Zhou [1,†], Bernard Su Min Chern [2,3,†], Peter Barton-Smith [4,‡], Jessie Wai Leng Phoon [3,5], Tse Yeun Tan [5], Veronique Viardot-Foucault [5], Chee Wai Ku [2,3], Heng Hao Tan [3,5], Jerry Kok Yen Chan [3,5] and Yie Hou Lee [1,3,*,§]

1. Translational 'Omics and Biomarkers group, KK Research Centre, KK Women's and Children's Hospital, Singapore 229899, Singapore; zhou.jieliang@kkh.com.sg
2. Division of Obstetrics and Gynaecology, KK Women's and Children's Hospital, Singapore 229899, Singapore; bernard.chern.s.m@singhealth.com.sg (B.S.M.C.); gmskcw@nus.edu.sg (C.W.K.)
3. OBGYN-Academic Clinical Program, Duke-NUS Medical School, Singapore 169857, Singapore; jessie.phoon.w.l@singhealth.com.sg (J.W.L.P.); tan.heng.hao@singhealth.com.sg (H.H.T.); jerry.chan.k.y@singhealth.com.sg (J.K.Y.C.)
4. Department of Obstetrics and Gynaecology, Singapore General Hospital, Singapore 169608, Singapore; pcbartonsmith@gmail.com
5. Department of Reproductive Medicine, KKH, Singapore 229899, Singapore; tan.tse.yeun@singhealth.com.sg (T.Y.T.); veronique.viardot@singhealth.com.sg (V.V.-F.)
* Correspondence: yiehou.lee@smart.mit.edu; Tel.: +65-6238-4013
† These authors contributed equally to this work.
‡ Current address: The Princess Grace Hospital, 42-52 Nottingham Place, London W1U 5NY, UK.
§ Current address: Singapore-MIT Alliance for Research and Technology, 1 CREATE Way, Singapore 138602, Singapore.

Received: 20 April 2020; Accepted: 10 May 2020; Published: 15 May 2020

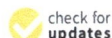

Abstract: Endometriosis is a common inflammatory gynecological disorder which causes pelvic scarring, pain, and infertility, characterized by the implantation of endometrial-like lesions outside the uterus. The peritoneum, ovaries, and deep soft tissues are the commonly involved sites, and endometriotic lesions can be classified into three subphenotypes: superficial peritoneal endometriosis (PE), ovarian endometrioma (OE), and deep infiltrating endometriosis (DIE). In 132 women diagnosed laparoscopically with and without endometriosis (n = 73, 59 respectively), and stratified into PE, OE, and DIE, peritoneal fluids (PF) were characterized for 48 cytokines by using multiplex immunoassays. Partial-least-squares-regression analysis revealed distinct subphenotype cytokine signatures—a six-cytokine signature distinguishing PE from OE, a seven-cytokine signature distinguishing OE from DIE, and a six-cytokine-signature distinguishing PE from DIE—each associated with different patterns of biological processes, signaling events, and immunology. These signatures describe endometriosis better than disease stages (p < 0.0001). Pathway analysis revealed the association of ERK1 and 2, AKT, MAPK, and STAT4 linked to angiogenesis, cell proliferation, migration, and inflammation in the subphenotypes. These data shed new insights on the pathophysiology of endometriosis subphenotypes, with the potential to exploit the cytokine signatures to stratify endometriosis patients for targeted therapies and biomarker discovery.

Keywords: endometriosis; cytokines; peritoneal fluid; microenvironment; precision medicine

1. Introduction

Endometriosis inflicts 6–10% of women of reproductive age, with affected women suffering from debilitating pelvic pain, dysmenorrhea, dyspareunia, and painful defecation. The prevalence of subfertility or infertility is higher in the endometriosis population, with up to half of endometriotic women suffering from reduced fecundity [1]. Endometriotic lesions can be classified into three subphenotypes: superficial peritoneal endometriosis (PE), ovarian cysts (ovarian endometrioma; OE), and deep infiltrating endometriosis (DIE) [2]. Superficial peritoneal lesions refer to implants found on the pelvic organs or pelvic peritoneum. They are typically white, red, or blue–black power burns and may be phenotypically progressive over time [3–5]. Endometriomas are formed when endometrial tissue implants on the ovary surface or penetrate into the ovary [6–8]. By contrast, DIE involves nodular lesions which invade the surrounding organs beneath the peritoneum [9]. They are commonly found on the uterosacral ligaments, bladder, vagina, and intestine and are more aggressive in nature [10]. The endometriosis subphenotypes are being recognized as clinicopathologically different from one another and are thought to be separate entities [3,10,11].

Many theories and hypotheses have been proposed to explain the pathogenesis and development of endometriosis [12,13]. The most widely accepted theory to explain the etiology of endometriosis is the retrograde menstrual hypothesis. During menses, viable menstrual fragments of eutopic endometrial origin back-traverse through the fallopian tubes, into the peritoneal cavity, which subsequently leads to these cells being implanted onto extra-uterine ectopic sites. However, this theory is insufficient to explain the presence of the disease in early puberty and in adolescents [14], and it does not address why endometriosis only occurs in a certain subset of the female population. Other theories have been put forth, including the coelomic metaplasia theory, endometrial stem/progenitor cells theory, and Müllerianosis theory. These complementary theories and hypotheses help to generally frame our understanding of plausible mechanisms of the endometriosis pathogenesis and allow for the testing of hypotheses and improvement of the currently existing treatment options and the introduction of new treatments. Recent advances had been made with respect to elucidating partial progestin response based on the progesterone receptor status of endometriosis patients [15], which infers the prospect of precision or targeted medicine for treating endometriosis. In addition, key non-hormonal inflammation or signaling pathways associated with endometriosis subphenotypes could be exploited for therapeutic advantage, particularly in the era of targeted treatment and precision medicine [16].

Ectopic endometriotic lesions secrete chemokines into their surrounding tissues, recruiting immune cells, which in turn secrete cytokines and growth factors, such as TNF-α, IL-1β, IL-6, IL-8, IL-17, EGF, FGF, and VEGF, creating locally specific microenvironments that develop a reciprocal interaction with the peritoneal fluid (PF) [17–19]. The interaction of cytokines constitutes molecular signatures that are used to orchestrate immune and other complex responses in endometriosis development, plausibly in the evolution of lesion subphenotypes [14,20]. With increased appreciation that immunomodulatory proteins are part of an overall signaling network [21,22], significant discoveries of pro-angiogenic, macrophage-derived, and endometriosis-associated infertility cytokine signatures have been made in recent years [23–27]. While these studies provide insight into major pathways involved in disease stages, several outstanding gaps remain in terms of the cytokine relationship with endometriosis subphenotypes [28] and their implications in stratified treatment. Here, in this study, we investigated PF cytokines and their association with the three endometriosis subphenotypes. This allowed us to assemble cytokine signatures, which revealed dysregulated biological processes associated with the pathogenesis/pathophysiology of the three endometriosis subphenotypes. These results might direct new endometriosis therapeutic and diagnostic efforts toward subphenotype clinically relevant cytokine targets.

2. Results

2.1. Peritoneal Fluid Cytokines Inadequately Describe Endometriosis Stages and Their Heterogeneity

PF samples from 132 women (without endometriosis, EM− = 59; with endometriosis, EM+ = 73) (Table 1) were analyzed for 48 cytokines, using a validated multiplex immunoassay platform. Among the cytokines analyzed, 38 (79%) cytokines were detected and compared using univariate analysis

(Tables S1 and S2). Because inflammatory cascades are brought about by the interaction of pro-inflammatory and anti-inflammatory cytokines [21], multivariate analysis such as PLSR provides a powerful way to obtain cytokine signatures to molecularly distinguish the patient groups in relation to disease presence and stages. Using partial least squares regression (PLSR), we identified a cytokine signature comprising IFN-α2, IL-12p70, IL-18, SCGF-β, VEGF-A, IL-3, and HGF that distinguished EM- from EM+ (Figure 1A). Notably, IFN-α2, IL-12p70, IL-18, SCGF-β, and VEGF-A are cytokines previously identified to be significantly altered between EM- from EM+ individuals [29–31]. However, a significant overlap between the EM- and EM+ clusters was observed (cumulative principal component (PC) score: 43%; Figure 1B), congruent with other studies [32]. We used the cumulative PC score as a measure of how well the cytokines could distinguish between EM-, EM+, EM+$_{Mild}$, and EM+$_{Severe}$ patients (perfect separation of patient clusters at 100% cumulative PC score). When EM+$_{Mild}$ and EM+$_{Severe}$ individuals were compared to EM-, the PLSR separations improved slightly, as indicated by higher cumulative PC scores of 51% and 49% (Figure 1C and Figure S1A,B). PLSR modeling of PF cytokines in EM+$_{Mild}$ from EM+$_{Severe}$ separated at 59%, but remains relatively poor as observed in the other models of disease stages (EM- versus EM+$_{Mild}$, EM- versus EM+$_{Severe}$), suggesting heterogeneity of disease stages and subsequent incompleteness to distinguish endometriosis (Figure S1A–F).

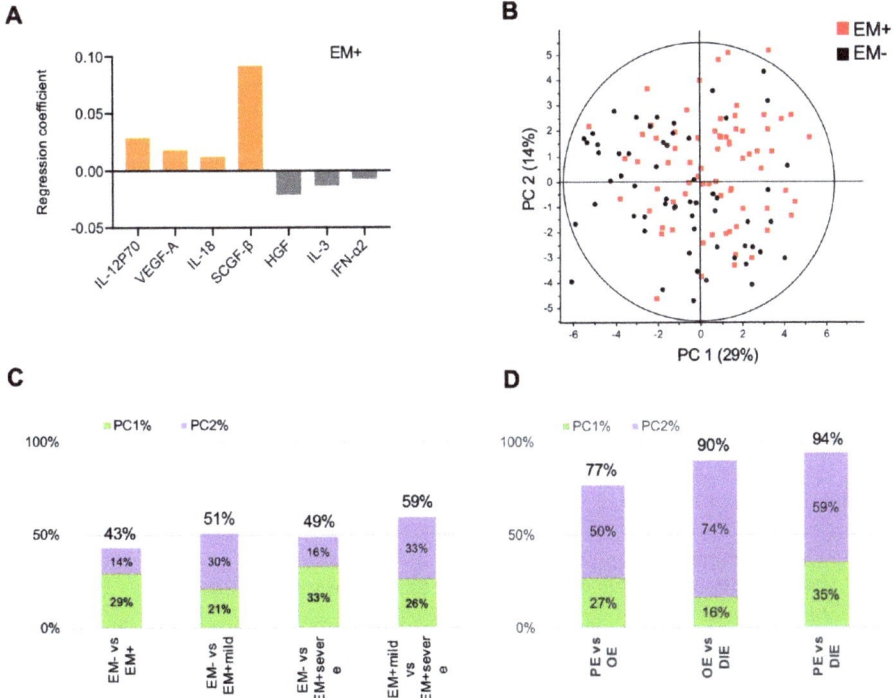

Figure 1. Peritoneal fluid cytokines associate with endometriosis stages. (**A**) Partial least squares regression (PLSR) coefficient analysis revealed a signature comprising elevated IL-12p70, IL-18, VEGF-A, and SCGF-β and decreased IFN-α2, IL-3, and HGF that distinguished women with endometriosis (EM+) from women without (EM-). (**B**) Modeling by PLSR scores plot reveals overlap of EM- and EM+, suggesting heterogeneity in the peritoneal fluid environment. PLSR-derived principal component scores of principal component 1 (PC1) and principal component 2 (PC2) of (**C**) stages and (**D**) subphenotypes. Cumulative principal-component scores are shown at the top of each bar.

Table 1. Patient characteristics.

Characteristics	EM- (n = 59)	EM+ (n = 73)	p-Value [†]
Age, y			0.844
Mean	35	35	
Range	22–51	25–45	
ASRM Stage			
I–II	NA	31	
III–IV	NA	42	
Subtype			
Peritoneal	NA	17	
Endometrioma	NA	30	
Deep infiltrating	NA	14	
Undetermined	NA	12	
Preoperative pain symptoms [a]			<0.0001
Dysmenorrhea	20	56	
Dyspareunia [b]	5	20	
Menstrual phase			0.290
Proliferative	27	41	
Secretory	32	32	
Race			0.650
Chinese	36	46	
Malay	14	13	
Others [c]	9	14	

[†] Student's t-test was performed for age, and Chi square for categorical data in pain, menstrual phase, and race.
[a] 18 patients present with both dysmenorrhea and dyspareunia. [b] 10 patients did not have coitus at time of surgery.
[c] Includes Indians and Filipinos

2.2. Peritoneal Fluid Cytokine Signatures Delineate Endometriosis Subphenotypes

The three subphenotypes of endometriosis, OE, PE, and DIE, present peculiar clinicopathological characteristics, which prompted us to hypothesize that PF cytokines might describe endometriosis better, viz-a-viz capturing molecular variations of the subphenotypes. Based on PF cytokines, PLSR modeling of endometriosis subphenotypes resulted in better models than disease stages (cumulative PC scores: 77% to 92%, $p < 0.0001$; Figures 1D and 2A–C; Table S3). PLSR scores plots revealed clear delineation of OE, PE, and DIE (Figure S2A), suggesting their distinct molecular makeups. In addition, analysis of the subphenotypes with controls showed significant moderate separation (cumulative PC score = 55–69%, $p < 0.001$; Table S4).

DIE has been considered a specific entity in which lesions penetrate more than 5 mm underneath the peritoneum [9,33]. Indeed, PC scores from comparisons of PE with OE (Figure 2A) was smaller than PC scores comparing PE or OE with DIE (Figure 2B,C), suggesting greater distinction of DIE from the superficial subphenotypes. A six-cytokine signature comprising IL-1α, IL-7, IL-8, MCP-1, MIF, and TNF-α distinguished OE from PE was identified (Figure 2D). Comparing OE to DIE, a seven-cytokine signature comprising IL-1α, IL-1RA, IL-8, IL-12p40, IL-12p70, IL-16, and TNF-α was identified (Figure 2E). Comparing DIE to PE, an all-upregulated six-cytokine signature of IL-8, IL-12p70, IL-16, IL-18, MCP-1, and MIP-1α that correlated to DIE was identified (Figure 2F). Cross-correlation and hierarchical clustering of cytokines showed not only intercorrelated inflammatory cytokines (e.g., TNFα, IL-1β, IL-10, and IL-1RA), but also cytokines that are anti-correlated (e.g., IL-12p40 and IL-12p70) [34], affirming the underlying biological information embedded within the PLSR-derived cytokine signatures (Figure 3. Table S3 shows the univariate statistical analysis.

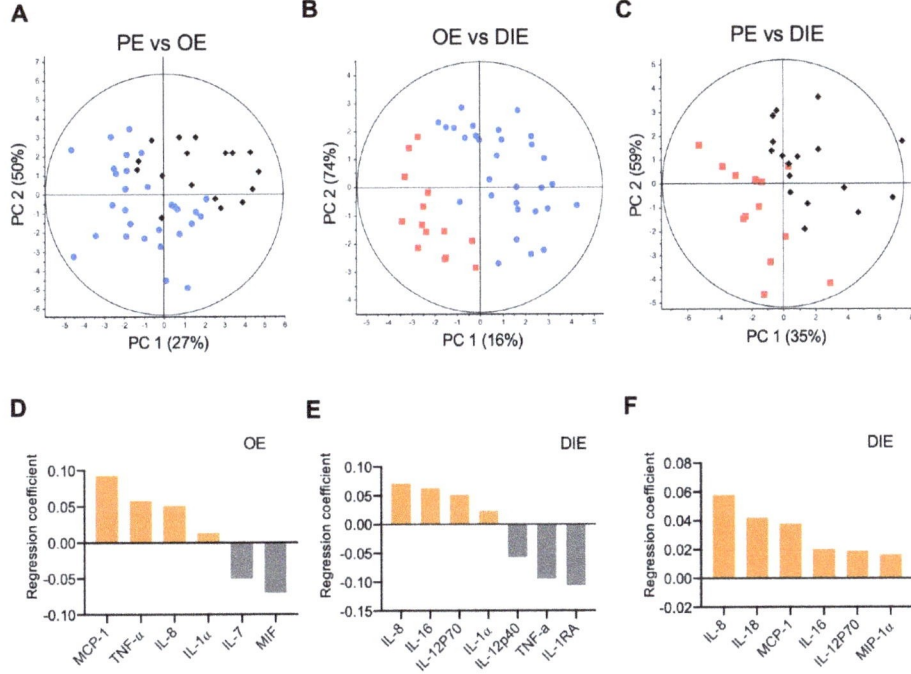

Figure 2. Peritoneal fluid cytokines show distinct delineation of endometriosis subphenotypes. Partial least squares regression (PLSR) models separated (**A**) ovarian endometriomas from peritoneal endometriosis, (**B**) ovarian endometriomas from deep infiltrating endometriosis, and (**C**) peritoneal endometriosis from deep infiltrating endometriosis. The principal component (PC) scores show good separation of endometriosis subphenotypes by using PF cytokines. (**D–F**). Corresponding PLSR coefficient analyses reveal cytokine signatures delineating the various subphenotypes. Elevated cytokines associated with a particular endometriosis subphenotype (OE, PE, or DIE) relative to its comparator appear in the same upper or lower half of the plot.

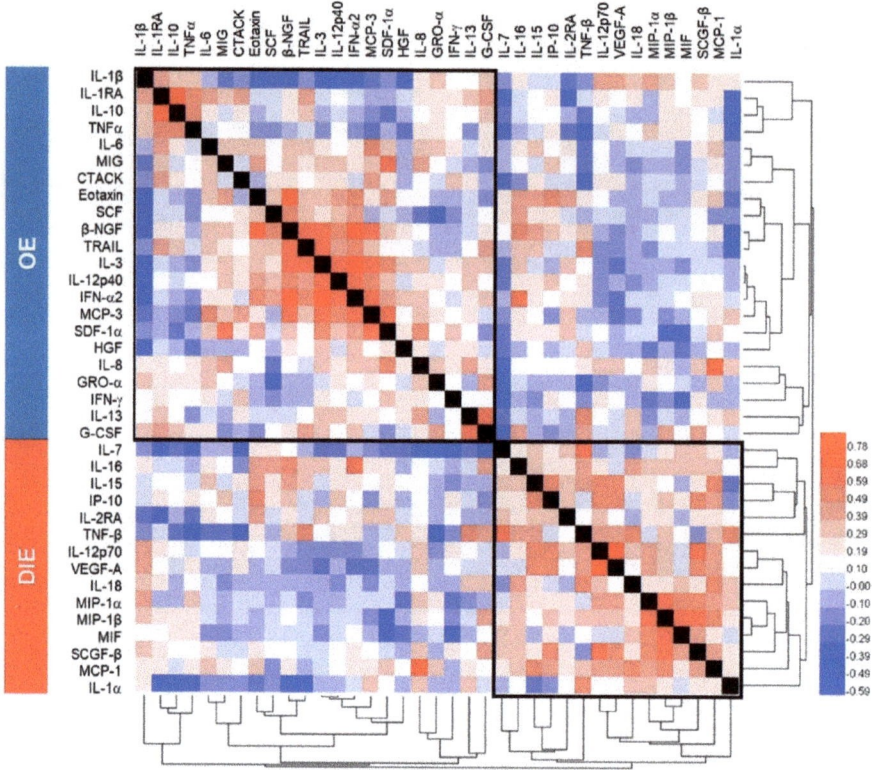

Figure 3. Correlation matrix of peritoneal fluid cytokines. Hierarchical clustering was performed on Spearman *r*-values between the subphenotypes ovarian endometriosis, and deep infiltrating endometriosis revealed consistency in PLSR-derived cytokine signatures that segregated OE from DIE.

2.3. Subphenotype Cytokine Signatures Are Associated with Different Biological Processes.

To examine whether the cytokine signatures associated with different endometriosis subphenotypes showed themes of functional categorization, each signature was investigated by using the gene ontology (GO) classification system (Table 2). In OE relative to PE, enriched biological processes include the following: negative regulation of extrinsic apoptotic signaling pathway; positive regulation of B-cell proliferation; positive regulation of angiogenesis; and positive regulation of ERK1 and ERK2 cascade. In OE relative to DIE, natural-killer-cell-mediated cytotoxicity is directed against tumor-cell target, cell-cycle arrest, and cell migration, and tyrosine phosphorylation of Stat4 protein. Smooth muscle cell metaplasia that is associated with DIE was also identified in our pathway enrichment analysis [35], providing assurance that our cytokine-signature-derived identified meaningful subphenotype biological characteristics. In PE versus DIE, enriched biological processes include the following: positive regulation of interferon-gamma production, protein kinase B (also known as AKT) signaling, and MAPK cascade.

Table 2. Functional enrichment analysis of endometriosis subphenotype cytokine signatures.

(A) OE vs. PE		
Term Identifier	Fold Enrichment	p-Value
immune response	29.9	1.90×10^{-3}
positive regulation of B-cell proliferation	215.3	7.00×10^{-3}
inflammatory response	33.2	1.50×10^{-3}
negative regulation of extrinsic apoptotic signaling pathway in absence of ligand	226.9	6.60×10^{-3}
positive regulation of angiogenesis	73	2.00×10^{-2}
positive regulation of ERK1 and ERK2 cascade	48	3.10×10^{-2}
cell proliferation	22.9	6.40×10^{-2}
negative regulation of apoptotic process	18.5	7.90×10^{-2}
(B) OE vs. DIE		
Term Identifier	Fold Enrichment	p-Value
immune response	31.9	6.10×10^{-5}
positive regulation of natural killer cell activation	1343.4	1.20×10^{-3}
positive regulation of NK T-cell activation	1343.4	1.20×10^{-3}
positive regulation of tyrosine phosphorylation of Stat4 protein	1679.2	9.50×10^{-4}
positive regulation of lymphocyte proliferation	959.5	1.70×10^{-3}
positive regulation of natural killer cell mediated cytotoxicity directed against tumor cell target	959.5	1.70×10^{-3}
positive regulation of mononuclear cell proliferation	2238.9	7.10×10^{-4}
response to UV-B	746.3	2.10×10^{-3}
positive regulation of smooth muscle cell apoptotic process	746.3	2.10×10^{-3}
negative regulation of interleukin-17 production	610.6	2.60×10^{-3}
positive regulation of T-cell-mediated cytotoxicity	516.7	3.10×10^{-3}
defense response to protozoan	353.5	4.50×10^{-3}
negative regulation of smooth muscle cell proliferation	231.6	6.90×10^{-3}
positive regulation of interferon-gamma production	146	1.10×10^{-2}
positive regulation of cell adhesion	156.2	1.00×10^{-2}
positive regulation of T-cell proliferation	111.9	1.40×10^{-2}
cellular response to lipopolysaccharide	59.4	2.70×10^{-2}
cytokine-mediated signaling pathway	51.3	3.10×10^{-2}
cell cycle arrest	47.6	3.30×10^{-2}
cell migration	39.1	4.00×10^{-2}
(C) PE vs. DIE		
Term Identifier	Fold Enrichment	p-Value
immune response	39.9	1.60×10^{-5}
positive regulation of protein kinase B signaling	100	1.50×10^{-2}
positive regulation of inflammatory response	115	1.30×10^{-2}
cellular response to organic cyclic compound	142.3	1.10×10^{-2}
positive regulation of interferon-gamma production	182.5	8.20×10^{-3}
lipopolysaccharide-mediated signaling pathway	262.4	5.70×10^{-3}
MAPK cascade	32	4.60×10^{-2}
cell–cell signaling	33.1	4.50×10^{-2}
inflammatory response	22.2	6.60×10^{-2}

3. Discussion

Reports have long recognized endometriotic lesion heterogeneity in characteristics such as color, size, and location [3–5]. There is increasing evidence that there is marked variation in lesion subphenotypes at the molecular level [36]. Santulli et al. reported that DIE is associated with higher PF advanced oxidation protein products than PE and OE [37]. Immunohistochemical analyses showed a higher prevalence of cyclooxygenase-2 protein expression in OE (78.5%) compared to 11.1% and 13.3% in PE and DIE [38], whereas nerve growth factor is expressed higher in DIE compared to PE and OE [39]. Methylation promotor sites in ectopic lesions are potentially different between the subphenotypes [40]. These reports, collectively, are in strong agreement with our results shown herein, in that OE, PE, and DIE are associated with unique cytokine signatures and corresponding enriched biological pathways.

Our study is likely to have implications for endometriosis therapeutics and biomarker discovery, particularly in the era of targeted treatment and precision medicine [41]. Further interpretation of our observations raises the potentiality of different therapies needed for treating patients with different endometriosis subphenotypes. It is apparent that broad, untargeted usage of therapeutics does not bring about clear clinical benefit across all endometriosis patients [2]. Endometriosis subphenotypes may partly explain these clinical phenomena. While targeted therapies have not been investigated in endometriosis, data from our study offer the possibility of exploiting each subphenotype's unique dependence on critical non-hormonal signaling or inflammation pathways to tailor therapy. Drug side-effect profile and efficacy are two main considerations of treatment choices [42]. Our findings, along with those of others, warrant further deep characterization of cytokine profiles and targeted use of immunomodulators, given the centrality of cytokines cells in the process of establishment and maintenance of this peritoneal disease. Due to often described elevation of peritoneal TNFα in endometriosis by us and others, blockers of TNFα, such as etanercept, leflunomide, and infliximab, were evaluated in preclinical models and in small randomized clinical trials [43–46]. Other immunomodulators, such as levamisole, and IL-12 inhibitors, have also been investigated in experimental models of endometriosis, with certain success [47]. In approved drugs such as infliximab, levamisole, and leflunomide, where safety profiles are established, monotherapeutic efficacy in humans remains untested or uncertain. While larger and more clinical trials are certainly required to test drug efficacy, immunomodulators are not always effective alone and require further development, along with new combination strategies, in order to enhance their efficacy, such as the use of combinatorial therapy or immunotherapy. These combination therapies can be classified based on their strategic targets: firstly, blockage of multiple cytokines based on the abovementioned signatures; secondly, to promote T- or NK-cell priming by enhancing lesion-associated antigen presentation; and thirdly, to target the immunosuppressive environment [48,49]. In the first strategy, choosing the key cytokines is critical, as cytokines are also required physiologically for endometrial growth, decidualization, and implantation [50]. In the second and third strategies, deep phenotyping of peritoneal immune cells and lesion microenvironments in endometriosis is needed before [51,52]. These strategies and their corresponding challenges must be overcome before the promise of an efficacious immunomodulatory therapy can be realized. Our study also has clinical implications on the biomarkers of endometriosis and biomarkers that are predictive of response to treatment. Heterogeneity in endometriosis has had a negative impact on the discovery and validation of predictive biomarkers, insofar that the lack of robust biomarkers is a critical area the community is working toward surmounting [53–55]. While this is not addressed in our study, our study creates the background for future investigations of stratifying patients according to their subphenotypes, prior to investigation of biomarkers.

During endometriosis development, cytokines develop a reciprocal interaction between the lesions and their surroundings, which constitute the modular microenvironment, influencing the evolution of lesion subphenotypes [14,20,56]. In this study, we opted to study the PF as a reflection of the spatial heterogeneity in endometriosis subphenotypes. By doing so, we were able to investigate the dynamic crosstalk between the secreted cytokines of lesions and their juxtaposed microenvironments, and their reciprocal adaptations. Indeed, ovarian endometriomas by growing near or at ovarian tissues with elevated CYP19A1 expressions are exposed to estrogen levels higher than that experienced by lesions implanted in the peritoneum or deep areas [57], creating an ovarian-specific microenvironment. Similarly, the transcriptome of the peritoneum in EM+ women is fundamentally different from that of EM- women [58–60]. The different expressions of inflammatory and adhesion molecules such as ICAM-1, matrix metalloproteases, and IL-6 confer a preferentially adhesive microenvironment for lesion implantation [61]. Elevated peritoneal reactive oxygen species acting through various signaling pathways, such as MAPK, ERK, and AKT, regulate gene expression of cytokines and cell adhesion molecules, which create microenvironments that promote various aspects of endometriosis development and its deleterious effects [62–64]. In DIE, significant fibrotic accumulation and smooth muscle differentiation secondary to the proliferation of stromal cells and inflammation are commonly noted and present yet another kind of microenvironment plausibly enhancing chronic inflammation [65,66]. In addition, the lesion microenvironment and its secreted cytokines plausibly play a key role in therapeutic approach of endometriosis, noting the elicitation of drug resistance by stromal microenvironment surrounding tumors in cancer [67]. Transcriptomic studies, such as those by Suryawanshi et al. [68], would be especially illuminating, had an analysis of the three endometriosis subphenotypes been performed in terms of elucidating each subphenotype's underlying pathogenic/pathophysiological mechanisms and potential "druggability". While additional experiments comparing transcriptome, epigenome, and proteome in PE, OE, and DIE are needed, our results suggest heterogeneity in the subphenotypes, at least in their cytokine levels, is associated with their microenvironments.

We used the GO database to analyze the cytokine signatures for enriched biological processes pertaining to the subphenotypes. Several key themes emerged: OE cytokines centered on proliferation/apoptosis regulation linked to ERK1 and ERK2 signaling, compared to PE; PE cytokines were implicated in MAPK and AKT signaling and highly inflammatory environments, compared to DIE; DIE cytokines were associated with cytotoxicity directed against "tumor cell target" and smooth muscle cell metaplasia, consistent with known outcomes associated with DIE [35]. Further, our analysis identified STAT4 regulation, and so it is congruent with studies by Zamani et al. and Bianco et al., showing *STAT4* polymorphism and susceptibility to endometriosis [69,70]. Increased angiogenesis is linked to the development of maintenance of endometriotic lesions, and our analysis suggests stronger angiogenesis in ovarian endometriomas [71,72], plausibly due to the strong induction of angiogenesis under high levels of ovarian estrogen. The GO analysis also revealed perturbations in immune cells. The positive regulation of natural killer cell activation could be construed as a compensatory mechanism consistent with reduced natural killer cell cytotoxicity [73], facilitating survival of regurgitated menstrual tissues at ectopic sites, probably more so in OE than DIE, as suggested. The combination of reduced IL-17 production and T-cell proliferation suggests exacerbated T-regulatory cells or Tregs activity [74].

Strengths of this study include the use of a carefully phenotyped clinical study population, use of a large, unbiased multiplexed cytokine approach, and advanced biostatistics. Additionally, this study, which was conducted in Singapore, represents a unique strength, as the study population pertains to Asians (Chinese, Malays, Indians, and Filipinos), providing a defined patient background for educated comparison and generalizability of the results when required. Limitations of this study include its observational nature, lack of longitudinal data, and the difficulty in dissecting the specific roles of cytokines within the molecular signatures. It is recognized that findings from this study are preliminary and will need to be validated in other populations, given that cytokine signatures may differ in other study populations. The cellular and molecular mechanisms of endometriosis development are likely to be overlapping (as observed in IL-8) and manifold, and many cytokines are able to induce the pathways. Thus, it is likely that multiple inflammatory pathways induced by a variety of stimuli might lead to endometriosis subphenotype development and endocrine failure. Further experiments will be necessary to define the precise roles of cytokines in the immune regulation of endometriosis. Taken together, the clustering of cytokines into functional groups hints at different pathogenic/pathophysiological mechanisms defining endometriosis subphenotypes. This would have important clinical ramifications, with the prediction that the endometriosis subphenotypes might require different treatment strategies and meet the need of a more personalized approach for endometriosis management [75].

4. Materials and Methods

4.1. Subjects and Sample Collection

Peritoneal fluids (PF) were collected from women participants ($n = 132$), comprising 59 women who are endometriosis-free (EM-) and 73 with endometriosis (EM+) undergoing laparoscopic procedures for suspected endometriosis, infertility, sterilization procedures, and/or pelvic pain recruited in KK Women's and Children's Hospital, Singapore, and Singapore General Hospital, Singapore, under

Centralized Institutional Research Board approval (CIRB 2010-167-D, approved 15 January 2016). Diagnostic laparoscopy was performed on all patients, with careful inspection of the uterus, fallopian tubes, ovaries, pouch of Douglas, and the pelvic peritoneum by gynecologists subspecializing in reproductive endocrinology and infertility. PFs were prepared as previously described [18], in line with Endometriosis Phenome and Biobanking Harmonisation Project Standard Operating Procedures [76]. Presence of endometriosis was systematically recorded and scored according to the revised American Fertility Society classification (rAFS) of endometriosis [77,78]. All patients gave written informed consent. Exclusion criteria included menstruating patients, post-menopausal patients, patients on hormonal therapy (e.g., norethisterone and microgynon) for at least three months before laparoscopy, and other confounding diseases, such as diabetes, adenomyosis, or any other chronic inflammatory diseases (rheumatoid arthritis, inflammatory bowel disease, systemic sclerosis, etc.). Patient characteristics are shown in Table 1. For the subjects undergoing robot-assisted excision of DIE at Singapore General Hospital, all women were preoperatively assessed for pelvic pain, bleeding, or fertility problems by trans-vaginal or trans-rectal ultrasound (if *virgo intacta*), using Voluson ultrasound machines (GE Healthcare). All sonographers were trained in the identification of DIE. All cases had pelvic DIE lesions of >5 mm, as well as evidence of partial or complete obliteration of the POD. In our unit, POD obliteration was taken to be the evidence of bowel involvement, and the use of robot-assisted technology for surgical excision was triggered due to suspected increased surgical complexity. Robot-assisted excision was performed by using the da Vinci Surgical Si™ system (Intuitive Surgical). The possible overlapping of the three lesion subphenotypes led us to classify the patients according to the worst lesion found in each subject, based on endometriosis subphenotype grouping by Chapron et al. [66,79]. Subjects who did not have endometriosis or have benign gynecological presentations, such as uterine fibroids and benign ovarian cysts, were taken as the endometriosis-free control group (EM-). All PFs were stored at −80 °C, until further analysis.

4.2. Multiplex Immunoassay Analysis

Cytokines were detected and measured by using multiplex immunoassay (BioRad, Hercules, CA, USA; Table S1), as previously described [50]. Briefly, 10 µL of PF was mixed with 10 µL of primary antibody-conjugated magnetic beads on in a 96 DropArray plate (Curiox Biosystems, Singapore) and rotated at 450 rpm on a plate shaker for 120 min at 25 °C, while protected from light. Subsequently, the plate was washed three times with wash buffer on the LT210 Washing Station (Curiox), before adding 5 µL of secondary antibody and rotating at 450 rpm for 30 min at 25 °C, protected from light. The plate was washed three times with wash buffer, and 10 µL of streptavidin-phycoerythrin was added and rotated at 450 rpm for 30 min at 25 °C, protected from light. The plate was again washed thrice with wash buffer. Then, 60 µL of reading buffer was added and transferred to a 96-conical-well microtiter plate, and the samples were read by using the Bio-Plex Luminex 200 (BioRad). The beads are classified by the red classification laser (635 nm) into its distinct sets, while a green reporter laser (532 nm) excites the phycoerythrin, a fluorescent reporter tag bound to the detection antibody. Quantitation of the 48 cytokines in each sample was then determined by extrapolation to a six- or seven-point standard curve, using five-parameter logistic regression modeling. Assay CV averaged <12%. When samples were detected in less than 50% of patients or below the lower limit of quantitation, they were considered undetected. Calibrations and validations were performed prior to runs and on a monthly basis, respectively.

4.3. Sample Size Calculation

We estimated the sample size before commencing the study: We assumed a 95% sensitivity of the cytokine signatures in distinguishing the subphenotypes, and a 95% confidence interval (CI) of approximately ±10.0% would need 18 cases of one endometriosis subphenotype and the same number of another subphenotype. This statistical analysis, assuming the sensitivity of the signature cutoff is $p =$ # test positive/N, where the sample size (n), number of women diagnosed with a particular endometriosis subtype (DIE, OE, PE), necessary to estimate p with precision ± L is given by the formula $n = Z^{*}Zp(1-p)/(L^{*}L)$, where Z corresponds to the correct percentile of the standard normal distribution [80]. Our clinical experience noted a 1:2:1 PE:OE:DIE ratio, and hence we targeted 36 OE cases, and the patient numbers were rounded to fall within the estimated sensitivity.

4.4. Statistical Analysis

GraphPad Prism 6 (GraphPad Software Inc., San Diego, CA, USA) was used for statistical analyses. Data were checked for normal distribution, using the Kolmogorov–Smirnov test. Unpaired or paired Student's *t*-test was performed, as appropriate, to determine statistical significance between groups for normally distributed data. Mann–Whitney U test was used for non-normally distributed data. For comparing three or more groups, the data were analyzed by using one-way ANOVA, followed by the Student's *t*-test with Bonferroni adjustment for pairwise comparisons. A *p*-value <0.05 was deemed to be statistically significant. A two-tailed Pearson correlation matrix was first performed with a confidence interval of 95%, followed by hierarchical clustering and the results plotted as heatmap 1.0 (GPS HemI 1.0 Heatmap Illustrator), using the clustering method of Average linkage and similarity metric of Pearson distance. Cytokines were further analyzed and signatures obtained by partial least squares regression (PLSR) modeling (Unscrambler X version 10.1) after the normalization of data by performing log2 transformation. Full cross-validation was applied in PLSR to increase model performance and for the calculation of coefficient regression values. PLSR models were compared by using Q-residuals obtained from the best principal components.

4.5. Pathway Enrichment Analysis

PLSR coefficient-derived cytokines were imputed into the Database for Annotation, Visualization and Integrated Discovery (DAVID) and cross-referenced against Gene Ontology (GO), for biological-process-enrichment analysis [81]. The *p*-values <0.05, based on Fisher Exact analysis and fold change >10 were imposed as enriched pathways. Bonferroni and Benjamini adjusted *p*-values are reported in Table S5. As a result of these corrections, the adjusted *p*-values get larger, and it could hurt the sensitivity of discovery if overemphasizing them [81,82]. Furthermore, these commonly used multiple testing-adjustment methods assume independence of tests, which in cytokines studies translates to a questionable assumption that all cytokines operate independently; instead, cytokines form biological networks [21,22].

5. Conclusions

Taken together, this study suggests that women with endometriosis subphenotypes can be stratified molecularly. Although the determination of lesion heterogeneity has not yet formed part of the clinical decision-making process in endometriosis, subphenotype-specific cytokine signatures suggest that suitable targeted therapeutic approaches specific to each individual patient's lesion and peritoneal heterogeneity composition may be tailored, and also the consideration of endometriosis subphenotypes for biomarker discovery studies. We anticipate our results to stimulate further studies, with accompanying detailed anatomical locations, and the use of genomic, proteomic, and metabolomic studies to evaluate the subphenotype molecular characteristics.

Supplementary Materials: Supplementary materials can be found at http://www.mdpi.com/1422-0067/21/10/3515/s1.

Author Contributions: P.B.-S., V.V.-F., J.K.Y.C., H.H.T., T.Y.T., and J.W.L.P. recruited patients and provided patient samples. J.Z. performed cytokine analysis and analyzed data. Y.H.L., C.W.K., and J.Z. wrote and revised the paper. Y.H.L. conceived of the study and supervised the study. Y.H.L., B.S.M.C., and J.K.Y.C. provided research resources. All authors have read and agreed to the published version of the manuscript.

Funding: This study was funded by Singapore Ministry of Health's National Medical Research Council (NMRC-OFYIRG16may012 and NMRC/CG/M003/2017 to Y.H. Lee) and Duke-NUS Academic Clinical Program Grant for Clinical and Translational Research in Endometriosis (to B.S.M.C.).

Conflicts of Interest: The authors declare no conflict of interest.

Abbreviations

ASRM	American Society for Reproductive Medicine
DIE	Deep infiltrating endometriosis
EM-	Control without endometriosis
EM+	Case with endometriosis
OE	Ovarian endometriosis
PC	Principal Component
PE	Peritoneal endometriosis
PF	Peritoneal fluid
PLSR	Partial least squares regression

References

1. Practice Committee of the American Society for Reproductive Medicine. Endometriosis and infertility. *Fertil. Steril.* **2006**, *86*, S156–S160. [CrossRef] [PubMed]
2. Bulun, S.E. Endometriosis. *N. Engl. J. Med.* **2009**, *360*, 268–279. [CrossRef] [PubMed]
3. Nisolle, M.; Donnez, J. Peritoneal endometriosis, ovarian endometriosis, and adenomyotic nodules of the rectovaginal septum are three different entities. *Fertil. Steril.* **1997**, *68*, 585–596. [CrossRef]
4. Stegmann, B.J.; Sinaii, N.; Liu, S.; Segars, J.; Merino, M.; Nieman, L.K.; Stratton, P. Using location, color, size, and depth to characterize and identify endometriosis lesions in a cohort of 133 women. *Fertil. Steril.* **2008**, *89*, 1632–1636. [CrossRef] [PubMed]
5. Burney, R.O.; Giudice, L.C. Pathogenesis and pathophysiology of endometriosis. *Fertil. Steril.* **2012**, *98*, 511–519. [CrossRef] [PubMed]
6. van Langendonckt, A.; Casanas-Roux, F.; Donnez, J. Oxidative stress and peritoneal endometriosis. *Fertil. Steril.* **2002**, *77*, 861–870. [CrossRef]
7. Yamaguchi, K.; Mandai, M.; Toyokuni, S.; Hamanishi, J.; Higuchi, T.; Takakura, K.; Fujii, S. Contents of endometriotic cysts, especially the high concentration of free iron, are a possible cause of carcinogenesis in the cysts through the iron-induced persistent oxidative stress. *Clin. Cancer Res.* **2008**, *14*. [CrossRef]
8. Guo, S.W.; Ding, D.; Shen, M.; Liu, X. Dating endometriotic ovarian cysts based on the content of cyst fluid and its potential clinical implications. *Reprod. Sci.* **2015**, *22*, 873–883. [CrossRef]
9. Koninckx, P.R.; Meuleman, C.; Demeyere, S.; Lesaffre, E.; Cornillie, F.J. Suggestive evidence that pelvic endometriosis is a progressive disease, whereas deeply infiltrating endometriosis is associated with pelvic pain. *Fertil. Steril.* **1991**, *55*, 759–765. [CrossRef]
10. Chapron, C.; Fauconnier, A.; Vieira, M.; Barakat, H.; Dousset, B.; Pansini, V.; Vacher-Lavenu, M.C.; Dubuisson, J.B. Anatomical distribution of deeply infiltrating endometriosis: Surgical implications and proposition for a classification. *Hum. Reprod.* **2003**, *18*, 157–161. [CrossRef]
11. Koninckx, P.R.; Kennedy, S.H.; Barlow, D.H. Endometriotic disease: The role of peritoneal fluid. *Hum. Reprod. Update* **1998**, *4*, 741–751. [CrossRef] [PubMed]
12. Laganà, A.S.; Garzon, S.; Götte, M.; Viganò, P.; Franchi, M.; Ghezzi, F.; Martin, D.C. The Pathogenesis of Endometriosis: Molecular and Cell Biology Insights. *Int. J. Mol. Sci.* **2019**, *20*, 5615. [CrossRef] [PubMed]
13. Riemma, G.; Laganà, A.S.; Schiattarella, A.; Garzon, S.; Cobellis, L.; Autiero, R.; Licciardi, F.; della Corte, L.; la Verde, M.; de Franciscis, P. Ion Channels in The Pathogenesis of Endometriosis: A Cutting-Edge Point of View. *Int. J. Mol. Sci.* **2020**, *21*, 1114. [CrossRef] [PubMed]
14. Gordts, S.; Koninckx, P.; Brosens, I. Pathogenesis of deep endometriosis. *Fertil. Steril.* **2017**, *108*, 872–885. [CrossRef]
15. Flores, V.A.; Vanhie, A.; Dang, T.; Taylor, H.S. Progesterone Receptor Status Predicts Response to Progestin Therapy in Endometriosis. *J. Clin. Endocrinol. Metab.* **2018**, *103*, 4561–4568. [CrossRef]
16. Zondervan, K.T.; Becker, C.M.; Missmer, S.A. Endometriosis. *N. Engl. J. Med.* **2020**, *382*, 1244–1256. [CrossRef]
17. Herington, J.L.; Bruner-Tran, K.L.; Lucas, J.A.; Osteen, K.G. Immune interactions in endometriosis. *Expert Rev. Clin. Immunol.* **2011**, *7*, 611–626. [CrossRef]

18. Lee, Y.H.; Tan, C.W.; Venkatratnam, A.; Tan, C.S.; Cui, L.; Loh, S.F.; Griffith, L.; Tannenbaum, S.R.; Chan, J.K.Y. Dysregulated sphingolipid metabolism in endometriosis. *J. Clin. Endocrinol. Metab.* **2014**, *99*, E1913–E1921. [CrossRef]
19. Lee, Y.H.; Cui, L.; Fang, J.; Chern, B.S.M.; Tan, H.H.; Chan, J.K.Y. Limited value of pro-inflammatory oxylipins and cytokines as circulating biomarkers in endometriosis—A targeted 'omics study. *Sci. Rep.* **2016**, *6*, 26117. [CrossRef]
20. Bhat, R.; Bissell, M.J. Of plasticity and specificity: Dialectics of the microenvironment and macroenvironment and the organ phenotype, Wiley Interdiscip. *Rev. Dev. Biol.* **2014**, *3*, 147–163. [CrossRef]
21. Schmitz, M.L.; Weber, A.; Roxlau, T.; Gaestel, M.; Kracht, M. Signal integration, crosstalk mechanisms and networks in the function of inflammatory cytokines. *Biochim. Biophys. Acta Mol. Cell Res.* **2011**, *1813*, 2165–2175. [CrossRef] [PubMed]
22. Pinheiro, M.B.; Martins-Filho, O.A.; Mota, A.P.L.; Alpoim, P.N.; Godoi, L.C.; Silveira, A.C.O.; Teixeira-Carvalho, A.; Gomes, K.B.; Dusse, L.M. Severe preeclampsia goes along with a cytokine network disturbance towards a systemic inflammatory state. *Cytokine* **2013**, *62*, 165–173. [CrossRef] [PubMed]
23. Siedentopf, F.; Tariverdian, N.; Rücke, M.; Kentenich, H.; Arck, P.C. Immune Status, Psychosocial Distress and Reduced Quality of Life in Infertile Patients with Endometriosis. *Am. J. Reprod. Immunol.* **2008**, *60*, 449–461. [CrossRef] [PubMed]
24. Khan, K.N.; Masuzaki, H.; Fujishita, A.; Kitajima, M.; Sekine, I.; Ishimaru, T. Differential macrophage infiltration in early and advanced endometriosis and adjacent peritoneum. *Fertil. Steril.* **2004**, *81*, 652–661. [CrossRef]
25. Beste, M.T.; Pfäffle-Doyle, N.; Prentice, E.A.; Morris, S.N.; Lauffenburger, D.A.; Isaacson, K.B.; Griffith, L.G. Molecular network analysis of endometriosis reveals a role for c-Jun-regulated macrophage activation. *Sci. Transl. Med.* **2014**, *6*, 222ra16. [CrossRef]
26. Gottschalk, P.G.; Dunn, J.R. The five-parameter logistic: A characterization and comparison with the four-parameter logistic. *Anal. Biochem.* **2005**, *343*, 54–65. [CrossRef]
27. Rakhila, H.; Al-Akoum, M.; Bergeron, M.-E.; Leboeuf, M.; Lemyre, M.; Akoum, A.; Pouliot, M. Promotion of angiogenesis and proliferation cytokines patterns in peritoneal fluid from women with endometriosis. *J. Reprod. Immunol.* **2016**, *116*, 1–6. [CrossRef]
28. Vercellini, P.; Viganò, P.; Somigliana, E.; Fedele, L. Endometriosis: Pathogenesis and treatment. *Nat. Rev. Endocrinol.* **2013**, *10*, 261–275. [CrossRef]
29. Bersinger, N.A.; Dechaud, H.; McKinnon, B.; Mueller, M.D. Analysis of cytokines in the peritoneal fluid of endometriosis patients as a function of the menstrual cycle stage using the Bio-Plex® platform. *Arch. Physiol. Biochem.* **2012**, *118*, 210–218. [CrossRef]
30. Jørgensen, H.; Hill, A.S.; Beste, M.T.; Kumar, M.P.; Chiswick, E.; Fedorcsak, P.; Isaacson, K.B.; Lauffenburger, D.A.; Griffith, L.G.; Qvigstad, E. Peritoneal fluid cytokines related to endometriosis in patients evaluated for infertility. *Fertil. Steril.* **2017**, *107*, 1191–1199. [CrossRef]
31. Mahnke, J.L.; Dawood, M.Y.; Huang, J.C. Vascular endothelial growth factor and interleukin-6 in peritoneal fluid of women with endometriosis. *Fertil. Steril.* **2000**, *73*, 166–170. [CrossRef]
32. Knific, T.; Fishman, D.; Vogler, A.; Gstöttner, M.; Wenzl, R.; Peterson, H.; Rižner, T.L. Multiplex analysis of 40 cytokines do not allow separation between endometriosis patients and controls. *Sci. Rep.* **2019**, *9*, 16738. [CrossRef] [PubMed]
33. Cornillie, F.J.; Oosterlynck, D.; Lauweryns, J.M.; Koninckx, P.R. Deeply infiltrating pelvic endometriosis: Histology and clinical significance. *Fertil. Steril.* **1990**, *53*, 978–983. [CrossRef]
34. Sun, L.; He, C.; Nair, L.; Yeung, J.; Egwuagu, C.E. Interleukin 12 (IL-12) family cytokines: Role in immune pathogenesis and treatment of CNS autoimmune disease. *Cytokine* **2015**, *75*, 249–255. [CrossRef]
35. van Kaam, K.J.A.F.; Schouten, J.P.; Nap, A.W.; Dunselman, G.A.J.; Groothuis, P.G. Fibromuscular differentiation in deeply infiltrating endometriosis is a reaction of resident fibroblasts to the presence of ectopic endometrium. *Hum. Reprod.* **2008**, *23*, 2692–2700. [CrossRef]
36. Carmona, F.; Chapron, C.; Martínez-Zamora, M.-Á.; Santulli, P.; Rabanal, A.; Martínez-Florensa, M.; Lozano, F.; Balasch, J. Ovarian endometrioma but not deep infiltrating endometriosis is associated with increased serum levels of interleukin-8 and interleukin-6. *J. Reprod. Immunol.* **2012**, *95*, 80–86. [CrossRef]

37. Santulli, P.; Chouzenoux, S.; Fiorese, M.; Marcellin, L.; Lemarechal, H.; Millischer, A.E.; Batteux, F.; Borderie, D.; Chapron, C. Protein oxidative stress markers in peritoneal fluids of women with deep infiltrating endometriosis are increased. *Hum. Reprod.* **2015**, *30*, 49–60. [CrossRef]
38. Fagotti, A. Analysis of cyclooxygenase-2 (COX-2) expression in different sites of endometriosis and correlation with clinico-pathological parameters. *Hum. Reprod.* **2004**, *19*, 393–397. [CrossRef]
39. Anaf, V.; Simon, P.; el Nakadi, I.; Fayt, I.; Simonart, T.; Buxant, F.; Noel, J.-C. Hyperalgesia, nerve infiltration and nerve growth factor expression in deep adenomyotic nodules, peritoneal and ovarian endometriosis. *Hum. Reprod.* **2002**, *17*, 1895–1900. [CrossRef]
40. Borghese, B.; Barbaux, S.; Mondon, F.; Santulli, P.; Pierre, G.; Vinci, G.; Chapron, C.; Vaiman, D. Research Resource: Genome-Wide Profiling of Methylated Promoters in Endometriosis Reveals a Subtelomeric Location of Hypermethylation. *Mol. Endocrinol.* **2010**, *24*, 1872–1885. [CrossRef]
41. Bedaiwy, M.A.; Alfaraj, S.; Yong, P.; Casper, R. New developments in the medical treatment of endometriosis. *Fertil. Steril.* **2017**, *107*, 555–565. [CrossRef] [PubMed]
42. Dunselman, G.A.J.; Vermeulen, N.; Becker, C.; Calhaz-Jorge, C.; D'Hooghe, T.; de Bie, B.; Heikinheimo, O.; Horne, A.W.; Kiesel, L.; Nap, A.; et al. ESHRE guideline: Management of women with endometriosis. *Hum. Reprod.* **2014**, *29*, 400–412. [CrossRef] [PubMed]
43. Altintas, D.; Kokcu, A.; Kandemir, B.; Cetinkaya, M.B.; Tosun, M. Efficacy of imiquimod, an immunomodulatory agent, on experimental endometriosis. *Fertil. Steril.* **2008**, *90*, 401–405. [CrossRef] [PubMed]
44. Uygur, D.; Aytan, H.; Zergeroglu, S.; Batioglu, S. Leflunomide—An Immunomodulator—Induces Regression of Endometrial Explants in a Rat Model of Endometriosis. *J. Soc. Gynecol. Investig.* **2006**, *13*, 378–383. [CrossRef]
45. Barrier, B.F.; Bates, G.W.; Leland, M.M.; Leach, D.A.; Robinson, R.D.; Propst, A.M. Efficacy of anti-tumor necrosis factor therapy in the treatment of spontaneous endometriosis in baboons. *Fertil. Steril.* **2004**, *81*, 775–779. [CrossRef]
46. Koninckx, P.R.; Craessaerts, M.; Timmerman, D.; Cornillie, F.; Kennedy, S. Anti-TNF-treatment for deep endometriosis-associated pain: A randomized placebo-controlled trial. *Hum. Reprod.* **2008**, *23*, 2017–2023. [CrossRef]
47. Itoh, H.; Sashihara, T.; Hosono, A.; Kaminogawa, S.; Uchida, M. Interleukin-12 inhibits development of ectopic endometriotic tissues in peritoneal cavity via activation of NK cells in a murine endometriosis model. *Cytotechnology* **2011**, *63*, 133–141. [CrossRef]
48. Oosterlynck, D.J.; Meuleman, C.; Waer, M.; Koninckx, P.R.; Vandeputte, M. Immunosuppressive activity of peritoneal fluid in women with endometriosis. *Obstet. Gynecol.* **1993**, *82*, 206–212.
49. Ścieżyńska, A.; Komorowski, M.; Soszyńska, M.; Malejczyk, J. NK Cells as Potential Targets for Immunotherapy in Endometriosis. *J. Clin. Med.* **2019**, *8*, 1468. [CrossRef]
50. Durairaj, R.R.P.; Aberkane, A.; Polanski, L.; Maruyama, Y.; Baumgarten, M.; Lucas, E.S.; Quenby, S.; Chan, J.K.Y.; Raine-Fenning, N.; Brosens, J.J.; et al. Deregulation of the endometrial stromal cell secretome precedes embryo implantation failure. *MHR Basic Sci. Reprod. Med.* **2017**, *23*, 478–487. [CrossRef]
51. Symons, L.K.; Miller, J.E.; Kay, V.R.; Marks, R.M.; Liblik, K.; Koti, M.; Tayade, C. The Immunopathophysiology of Endometriosis. *Trends Mol. Med.* **2018**, *24*, 748–762. [CrossRef] [PubMed]
52. Vallvé-Juanico, J.; Houshdaran, S.; Giudice, L.C. The endometrial immune environment of women with endometriosis. *Hum. Reprod. Update* **2019**, *25*, 565–592. [CrossRef] [PubMed]
53. Ahn, S.H.; Singh, V.; Tayade, C. Biomarkers in endometriosis: Challenges and opportunities. *Fertil. Steril.* **2017**, *107*, 523–532. [CrossRef] [PubMed]
54. May, K.E.; Villar, J.; Kirtley, S.; Kennedy, S.H.; Becker, C.M. Endometrial alterations in endometriosis: A systematic review of putative biomarkers. *Hum. Reprod. Update* **2011**, *17*, 637–653. [CrossRef] [PubMed]
55. Anastasiu, C.V.; Moga, M.A.; Neculau, A.E.; Bălan, A.; Scârneciu, I.; Dragomir, R.M.; Dull, A.-M.; Chicea, L.-M. Biomarkers for the Noninvasive Diagnosis of Endometriosis: State of the Art and Future Perspectives. *Int. J. Mol. Sci.* **2020**, *21*, 1750. [CrossRef]
56. Wimalachandra, D.; Yang, J.X.; Zhu, L.; Tan, E.; Asada, H.; Chan, J.Y.K. Lee, Y.H. Long-chain glucosylceramides crosstalk with LYN mediates endometrial cell migration. *Biochim. Biophys Acta. Mol. Cell Biol. Lipids.* **2018**, *1863*, 71–80. [CrossRef]

57. Huhtinen, K.; Desai, R.; Ståhle, M.; Salminen, A.; Handelsman, D.J.; Perheentupa, A.; Poutanen, M. Endometrial and Endometriotic Concentrations of Estrone and Estradiol Are Determined by Local Metabolism Rather than Circulating Levels. *J. Clin. Endocrinol. Metab.* **2012**, *97*, 4228–4235. [CrossRef]

58. Kyama, C.; Overbergh, L.; Debrock, S.; Valckx, D.; Vanderperre, S.; Meuleman, C.; Mihalyi, A.; Mwenda, J.; Mathieu, C.; Dhooghe, T. Increased peritoneal and endometrial gene expression of biologically relevant cytokines and growth factors during the menstrual phase in women with endometriosis. *Fertil. Steril.* **2006**, *85*, 1667–1675. [CrossRef]

59. Kyama, C.M.; Overbergh, L.; Mihalyi, A.; Meuleman, C.; Mwenda, J.M.; Mathieu, C.; D'Hooghe, T.M. Endometrial and peritoneal expression of aromatase, cytokines, and adhesion factors in women with endometriosis. *Fertil. Steril.* **2008**, *89*, 301–310. [CrossRef]

60. Young, V.J.; Brown, J.K.; Saunders, P.T.K.; Horne, A.W. The role of the peritoneum in the pathogenesis of endometriosis. *Hum. Reprod. Update* **2013**, *19*, 558–569. [CrossRef]

61. Tani, H.; Sato, Y.; Ueda, M.; Miyazaki, Y.; Suginami, K.; Horie, A.; Konishi, I.; Shinomura, T. Role of Versican in the Pathogenesis of Peritoneal Endometriosis. *J. Clin. Endocrinol. Metab.* **2016**, *101*, 4349–4356. [CrossRef] [PubMed]

62. Scutiero, G.; Iannone, P.; Bernardi, G.; Bonaccorsi, G.; Spadaro, S.; Volta, C.A.; Greco, P.; Nappi, L. Oxidative Stress and Endometriosis: A Systematic Review of the Literature. *Oxid. Med. Cell. Longev.* **2017**, *2017*, 1–7. [CrossRef] [PubMed]

63. Vitale, S.G.; Capriglione, S.; Peterlunger, I.; la Rosa, V.L.; Vitagliano, A.; Noventa, M.; Valenti, G.; Sapia, F.; Angioli, R.; Lopez, S.; et al. The Role of Oxidative Stress and Membrane Transport Systems during Endometriosis: A Fresh Look at a Busy Corner. *Oxid. Med. Cell. Longev.* **2018**, *2018*, 1–14. [CrossRef] [PubMed]

64. Lee, Y.H.; Yang, J.X.; Allen, J.C.; Tan, C.S.; Chern, B.S.M.; Tan, T.Y.; Tan, H.H.; Mattar, C.N.Z.; Chan, J.K.Y. Elevated peritoneal fluid ceramides in human endometriosis-associated infertility and their effects on mouse oocyte maturation. *Fertil. Steril.* **2018**, *110*, 767–777. [CrossRef]

65. Leconte, M.; Nicco, C.; Ngô, C.; Arkwright, S.; Chéreau, C.; Guibourdenche, J.; Weill, B.; Chapron, C.; Dousset, B.; Batteux, F. Antiproliferative Effects of Cannabinoid Agonists on Deep Infiltrating Endometriosis. *Am. J. Pathol.* **2010**, *177*, 2963–2970. [CrossRef]

66. Chapron, C.; Souza, C.; de Ziegler, D.; Lafay-Pillet, M.-C.; Ngô, C.; Bijaoui, G.; Goffinet, F.; Borghese, B. Smoking habits of 411 women with histologically proven endometriosis and 567 unaffected women. *Fertil. Steril.* **2010**, *94*, 2353–2355. [CrossRef]

67. Straussman, R.; Morikawa, T.; Shee, K.; Barzily-Rokni, M.; Qian, Z.R.; Du, J.; Davis, A.; Mongare, M.M.; Gould, J.; Frederick, D.T.; et al. Tumour micro-environment elicits innate resistance to RAF inhibitors through HGF secretion. *Nature* **2012**, *487*, 500–504. [CrossRef]

68. Suryawanshi, S.; Huang, X.; Elishaev, E.; Budiu, R.A.; Zhang, L.; Kim, S.; Donnellan, N.; Mantia-Smaldone, G.; Ma, T.; Tseng, G.; et al. Complement Pathway Is Frequently Altered in Endometriosis and Endometriosis-Associated Ovarian Cancer. *Clin. Cancer Res.* **2014**, *20*, 6163–6174. [CrossRef]

69. Zamani, M.R.; Salmaninejad, A.; Asbagh, F.A.; Masoud, A.; Rezaei, N. STAT4 single nucleotide gene polymorphisms and susceptibility to endometriosis-related infertility. *Eur. J. Obstet. Gynecol. Reprod. Biol.* **2016**, *203*, 20–24. [CrossRef]

70. Bianco, B.; Fernandes, R.F.M.; Trevisan, C.M.; Christofolini, D.M.; Sanz-Lomana, C.M.; Bernabe, J.V.; Barbosa, C.P. Influence of STAT4 gene polymorphisms in the pathogenesis of endometriosis. *Ann. Hum. Genet.* **2019**, *83*, 249–255. [CrossRef]

71. Fasciani, A. High concentrations of the vascular endothelial growth factor and interleukin-8 in ovarian endometriomata. *Mol. Hum. Reprod.* **2000**, *6*, 50–54. [CrossRef] [PubMed]

72. Jana, S.; Chatterjee, K.; Ray, A.K.; DasMahapatra, P.; Swarnakar, S. Regulation of Matrix Metalloproteinase-2 Activity by COX-2-PGE2-pAKT Axis Promotes Angiogenesis in Endometriosis. *PLoS ONE* **2016**, *11*, e0163540. [CrossRef] [PubMed]

73. Thiruchelvam, U.; Wingfield, M.; O'Farrelly, C. Natural Killer Cells: Key Players in Endometriosis. *Am. J. Reprod. Immunol.* **2015**, *74*, 291–301. [CrossRef] [PubMed]

74. Tanaka, Y.; Mori, T.; Ito, F.; Koshiba, A.; Takaoka, O.; Kataoka, H.; Maeda, E.; Okimura, H.; Mori, T.; Kitawaki, J. Exacerbation of Endometriosis Due to Regulatory T-Cell Dysfunction. *J. Clin. Endocrinol. Metab.* **2017**, *102*, 3206–3217. [CrossRef]

75. Ferrero, S.; Evangelisti, G.; Barra, F. Current and emerging treatment options for endometriosis. *Expert Opin. Pharmacother.* **2018**, *19*, 1109–1125. [CrossRef]
76. Rahmioglu, N.; Fassbender, A.; Vitonis, A.F.; Tworoger, S.S.; Hummelshoj, L.; D'Hooghe, T.M.; Adamson, G.D.; Giudice, L.C.; Becker, C.M.; Zondervan, K.T.; et al. World Endometriosis Research Foundation Endometriosis Phenome and Biobanking Harmonization Project: III. Fluid biospecimen collection, processing, and storage in endometriosis research. *Fertil. Steril.* **2014**, *102*, 1233–1243. [CrossRef]
77. ASRM. Revised American Society for Reproductive Medicine classification of endometriosis: 1996. *Fertil Steril.* **1997**, *67*, 817–821. [CrossRef]
78. AFS. Revised American Fertility Society classification of endometriosis: 1985. *Fertil. Steril.* **1985**, *43*, 351–352. [CrossRef]
79. Somigliana, E.; Infantino, M.; Candiani, M.; Vignali, M.; Chiodini, A.; Busacca, M.; Vignali, M. Association rate between deep peritoneal endometriosis and other forms of the disease: Pathogenetic implications. *Hum. Reprod.* **2004**, *19*, 168–171. [CrossRef]
80. Cochran, W.G. Methodological problems in the study of human populations. *Ann. N. Y. Acad. Sci.* **2006**, *107*, 476–489. [CrossRef]
81. Huang, D.W.; Sherman, B.T.; Lempicki, R.A. Systematic and integrative analysis of large gene lists using DAVID bioinformatics resources. *Nat. Protoc.* **2009**, *4*, 44–57. [CrossRef] [PubMed]
82. Yoav, B.; Daniel, Y. The control of the false discovery rate in multiple testing under dependency. *Ann. Stat.* **2001**, *29*, 1165–1188.

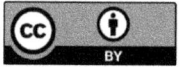

© 2020 by the authors. Licensee MDPI, Basel, Switzerland. This article is an open access article distributed under the terms and conditions of the Creative Commons Attribution (CC BY) license (http://creativecommons.org/licenses/by/4.0/).

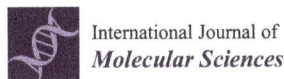

Review

Ion Channels in The Pathogenesis of Endometriosis: A Cutting-Edge Point of View

Gaetano Riemma [1,†], Antonio Simone Laganà [2,†], Antonio Schiattarella [1,*], Simone Garzon [2], Luigi Cobellis [1], Raffaele Autiero [1], Federico Licciardi [1], Luigi Della Corte [3], Marco La Verde [1] and Pasquale De Franciscis [1]

1. Department of Woman, Child and General and Specialized Surgery, University of Campania "Luigi Vanvitelli", 80138 Naples, Italy; Gaetano.riemma7@gmail.com (G.R.); luigi.cobellis@unicampania.it (L.C.); raffaele.autiero@libero.it (R.A.); licciardi.federico@gmail.com (F.L.); marco.laverde88@gmail.com (M.L.V.); pasquale.defranciscis@unicampania.it (P.D.F.)
2. Department of Obstetrics and Gynecology, "Filippo Del Ponte" Hospital, University of Insubria, 21100 Varese, Italy; antoniosimone.lagana@uninsubria.it (A.S.L.); simone.garzon@univr.it (S.G.)
3. Department of Neuroscience, Reproductive Sciences and Dentistry, School of Medicine, University of Naples Federico II, 80131 Naples, Italy; dellacorte.luigi25@gmail.com
* Correspondence: aschiattarella@gmail.com; Tel.: +39-392-165-3275
† Equal contributions (joint first authors).

Received: 30 December 2019; Accepted: 5 February 2020; Published: 7 February 2020

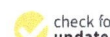

Abstract: Background: Ion channels play a crucial role in many physiological processes. Several subtypes are expressed in the endometrium. Endometriosis is strictly correlated to estrogens and it is evident that expression and functionality of different ion channels are estrogen-dependent, fluctuating between the menstrual phases. However, their relationship with endometriosis is still unclear. Objective: To summarize the available literature data about the role of ion channels in the etiopathogenesis of endometriosis. Methods: A search on PubMed and Medline databases was performed from inception to November 2019. Results: Cystic fibrosis transmembrane conductance regulator (CFTR), transient receptor potentials (TRPs), aquaporins (AQPs), and chloride channel (ClC)-3 expression and activity were analyzed. CFTR expression changed during the menstrual phases and was enhanced in endometriosis samples; its overexpression promoted endometrial cell proliferation, migration, and invasion throughout nuclear factor kappa-light-chain-enhancer of activated B cells-urokinase plasminogen activator receptor (NFκB-uPAR) signaling pathway. No connection between TRPs and the pathogenesis of endometriosis was found. AQP5 activity was estrogen-increased and, through phosphatidylinositol-3-kinase and protein kinase B (PI3K/AKT), helped in vivo implantation of ectopic endometrium. In vitro, AQP9 participated in extracellular signal-regulated kinases/p38 mitogen-activated protein kinase (ERK/p38 MAPK) pathway and helped migration and invasion stimulating matrix metalloproteinase (MMP)2 and MMP9. ClC-3 was also overexpressed in ectopic endometrium and upregulated MMP9. Conclusion: Available evidence suggests a pivotal role of CFTR, AQPs, and ClC-3 in endometriosis etiopathogenesis. However, data obtained are not sufficient to establish a direct role of ion channels in the etiology of the disease. Further studies are needed to clarify this relationship.

Keywords: endometriosis; ion channels; etiology; pathogenesis; CFTR; aquaporin; chloride channels

1. Introduction

Endometriosis, defined as the presence of endometrial-like tissue outside the uterine cavity, is an estrogen-dependent benign disease that affects about 10% of reproductive-age women [1–4]. Of women affected by this pathology, 30%–50% suffer from pelvic pain and/or infertility [3,5–7]. Laparoscopy is considered the gold standard for the diagnosis and treatment of ectopic endometrial-like implants [3,8], however, 40% of treated women refer to a recurrence of the symptoms within five years [9–12], especially without post-operative pharmacological treatments [2,13,14]. Furthermore, endometriosis symptoms are often associated with a significant impairment in psychological wellbeing [15,16], that has also a substantial impact on the quality of life [17,18]. Several different theories have been developed in order to justify the etiopathology of endometriosis; although the theory of retrograde menstruation [19,20], developed by Sampson, was widely accepted several years ago, to date, accumulating evidence suggests a key role of genetics, epigenetics, and immune mechanisms for the onset and progression of the disease [21–24].

Ion channels are a heterogeneous group of transmembrane proteins that permit ions to flow across cell or organelle membranes [25–27]. When ions flow through channels, changes in membrane potential, intracellular pH, second-messenger pathways and intra-extracellular gradients are observed [28–30]. Those characteristics make ion channels crucial for the physiological homeostasis of neuronal signal transmission, as well as myofiber contraction, regulation of extra and intracellular volume, acid-base balance [31], and activation or inhibition of epithelial secretion [32]. At the same time, many pathways and physiological processes lead to strict regulation of their expression and functionality [26,33,34]. A wide spectrum of hormones, including progesterone, estradiol (E2), and growth factors, are known to act as modulators of the cellular expression of different ion channels [35,36]. Moreover, the open/close gating is dynamic; indeed, it can be switched by a variety of factors, including potential membrane changes, mechanical stimuli, temperature, and chemical substances, which allows ion channels to detect changes in the intracellular and extracellular environment and activate or deactivate secondary messengers for several signaling pathways [37,38]. Ion channels also play a significant role in balancing cell proliferation, apoptosis, and migration, which are fundamentally related to cancer development [39]. A significant number of different ion channels have been discovered in the endometrium, both in the epithelium and stroma of humans and animals [25]. Several studies have addressed the presence and altered function of ion channels in both eutopic and ectopic endometrium [40–43], suggesting that their overexpression may play an important role in the pathogenesis of endometriosis [1,44–47]. On that basis, our review aims to summarize these available pieces of evidence and discuss whether ion channels could be crucial in the migration and invasion of ectopic endometrial cells.

2. Materials and Methods

We performed a literature search on the MEDLINE database (accessed through PubMed) for articles written in English and published from inception to November 2019, in order to assess the search question "Does a relation between ion channels and etiopathogenesis of endometriosis exist?" The following Medical Subject Headings (MeSH) terms were used to screen and identify studies: "Endometriosis" (Unique ID: D004715), "ion channels" (Unique ID: D007473), "etiology" (Unique ID: Q000209).

Articles were excluded according to the following criteria: (a) articles were not written in English, (b) were published as conference papers or abstract only, and (c) studies including information that overlapped other publications. In the case of overlapping studies, we retrieved the most recent and/or most comprehensive manuscript. In our search, only articles concerning ion channels, with the exclusion of other genes or proteins, were included. The selection criteria for this narrative review included original articles (randomized and non-randomized clinical trials, including prospective observational studies, retrospective cohort studies, and case-control studies) and review articles regarding the potential role of ion channels on endometriosis development.

Articles that met the inclusion criteria were carefully read, and, when appropriate, further articles retrieved from their references were also reviewed in order to include other critical studies that might have been missed in the initial search. A total amount of eighty-eight references were thus used in this review. We presented here a narrative synthesis of the available evidence about the topic.

3. Cystic Fibrosis Transmembrane Conductance Regulator (CFTR) and Endometriosis

Cystic fibrosis transmembrane conductance regulator (CFTR) is a cyclic adenosine monophosphate (cAMP)-activated Cl⁻ and HCO_3^- ion transporting channel, ubiquitously expressed in the epithelial cells of several tissues [48]. CFTR is essential in the regulation of epithelial fluid secretion, moving H_2O into the organ lumen through a Cl⁻ efflux [49]. CFTR mutations cause cystic fibrosis, in which defective electrolyte and fluid transport can cause heterogeneous phenotypes of disease in different organs [48,50]. CTFR is expressed in the endometrial epithelium of guinea-pigs and other animals. In human endometrium, CFTR is also widely expressed, and its expression changes in a cyclic manner [43,51]. In cultured glandular cells, it was found to be upregulated by progesterone and downregulated by estradiol [51–53]. The expression and role of CFTR in endometriosis has been evaluated by Huang et al. [45]: in ectopic, endometrial-like samples, quantitative real-time polymerase chain reaction (qPCR) results demonstrated a significantly higher expression of CFTR mRNA and proteins in endometriotic lesions compared to normal endometria. Moreover, a CFTR signaling-mediated mechanism has been hypothesized to play a role in endometrial cell migration. Considering that CFTR-regulated cell migration was not dependent on its function as a channel, but by its interaction with other proteins, the aberrantly high levels of expression of CFTR might also be related to the high numbers of proteins that interact with this molecule.

The involvement of NFκB in acting as an intermediate for the effect of CFTR in endometrial cells, as well as the link between CFTR channel and NFκB, was already well described [48], although their direct relationship is still debated and controversial. Concerning cystic fibrosis, an inverse relationship between the two is well demonstrated; indeed, chronic inflammation of the lung, which is a key element of the disease, is strictly linked to the upregulation of NFκB that is found when CFTR is mutated [54]. In addition to this, the inverse relationship between NFκB and CFTR has also been found in the male reproductive tract, disrupting spermatogenesis in a similar way as in cryptorchidism. Moreover, a robust connection between CFTR and NFκB has also been found in the mouse embryo [55], and other female cancers (i.e. cervical cancer) [45]. Indeed, in human endometrial Ishikawa (ISK) cells, when overexpression of CFTR occurred, an enhanced cell migration with upregulated NFκB p65 and urokinase receptor (uPAR) pathway signaling was observed. Conversely, knockdown of CFTR was linked to inhibition of endometrial cell migration capacity. Furthermore, when curcumin or Bay were used to inhibit NFκB [55], they significantly reduced the expression of uPAR and overall cell migration in the CFTR-overexpressing ISK cells [45,53].

Huang et al. [45] also demonstrated the functional role of CFTR in endometrial cell migration. However, the CFTR-regulated cell migration ability was not correlated to its ion channel function but its expression level. These results suggest that CFTR does not directly act as an ion channel in the development of endometriosis: when a high aberrant expression of CFTR is reached, an abnormally high uPAR expression is achieved too; therefore, this may trigger the motility of endometrial cells, which is crucial for the progression of endometriosis [50].

4. Transient Receptor Potential (TRP) Channels and Endometriosis

Transient receptor potential (TRP) channels are known to be involved in the regulation of cell migration, adhesion, and proliferation, as well as neoangiogenesis [56]. The TRP superfamily consists of the following six subfamilies, which are based on sequence homology: ankyrin-rich (TRPA1), vanilloid (TRPV1-6), canonical (TRPC1-7), melastatin-like (TRPM1-8), polycystin (TRPP2/3/5), and mucolipin (TRPML1-3) [57]. Their localization is ubiquitary, and they can be activated by a wide number of molecules and stimuli [56,58,59]. In endometrial biopsies, TRP expression levels have been reported to be differently down- and upregulated during the different phases of the menstrual cycle [60]. High mRNA levels for TRPC1/4, TRPC6, TRPV2, TRPV4, TRPM4, and TRPM7 and the functional expression of TRPV2, TRPV4, TRPC6, and TRPM7 have been found in primary human endometrial stromal cells (hESC) [60]. Moreover, these channels were previously discovered to be somehow involved in several processes that regarded pathogenesis of endometriosis: TRPC1, TRPC4, and TRPV2 are involved in cell migration; TRPC4 in cell adhesion; and TRPM4, TRPM7, and TRPV2 have a crucial role in cell proliferation [47,61–63]. Persoons et al. [47] evaluated the expression profiles of TRP channels in endometrial biopsies from women with endometriosis taken at different times during the menstrual cycle. According to data analysis, several TRPs (TRPV1, TRPV2, TRPV4, TRPV6, TRPM4, TRPM6, TRPM7, TRPC1, TRPC3, TRPC4, and TRPC6) expression levels were higher than the detection limit. In addition, they reported that, for most of the TRP channels, mRNA levels were rising and falling according to different phases of the menstrual cycle. This difference was particularly significant for TRPM3 and TRPM6 between the follicular-late luteal phase and the early luteal phase of the menstrual cycle. Unlike CFTR channels, currently there is poor evidence about the regulation of TRPs by estrogens or progestogens. Nevertheless, it has been found that TRPV6 expression in ISK cells and normal endometrium could be upregulated by estrogen during the follicular phase [60,64]. In addition, TRPM2 mRNA expression is increased when an estrogen treatment is administered in human endometrium and hESC [64]. When estrogen and progesterone are both administered, TRPC1 mRNA has been found to increase. Furthermore, TRPC6 expression could be upregulated by estrogen in hESC [65]. TRPV2, TRPV4, TRPC1/4, and TRPC6 were expressed in hESC samples retrieved from women affected by endometriosis both at the molecular and functional levels. At the same time, the proliferation and migration assays were not affected by TRP expression, so this element raises further concerns and doubts regarding their role in the pathogenesis of the disease [40,47,60]. In addition, there were no significant differences between the RNA expression pattern of TRP channels comparing endometrial samples from eutopic and ectopic endometria. Although there might be no connection between TRPs and the etiopathogenesis of endometriosis, Bohonyi et al. [40] discovered that the expression levels of TRPA1 and TRPV1 were significantly different between DIE stroma and epithelium, as well as in DIE epithelium, when compared with control samples. Moreover, they found elevated stromal TRPV1 immunopositivity in DIE [40]. Interestingly, these findings correlated with dysmenorrhea and dyschezia severity; indeed, stromal and epithelial TRPA1 and TRPV1 immunoreactivities were directly correlated to the pain experienced by the patient. In synthesis, there might be no connection to the pathogenesis of endometriosis, despite the fact that the functional expression of several TRP channels has been found in the endometrium [47].

5. Aquaporins (AQPs) and Endometriosis

Aquaporins (AQPs) consist of a group of 25–34 kDa hydrophobic integral transmembrane channels [66]. These channels allow the physiologic rapid passive movement of H_2O across the cell membrane in order to facilitate osmotic balance [66]. AQPs are ubiquitary across the human body, although they are based on a specific tissue-selective expression pattern [67]. Furthermore, their functions are of paramount importance in epithelial and endothelial cells, where their roles are clearly involved in fluid balance [68]. Besides their well-known peculiarities, it has been hypothesized that AQPs may be involved actively in cell migration, metabolism, and signal transduction [69]. AQP2, AQP5, AQP8, and AQP9 were usually found in endometrial samples [42,70]. Isoforms 2, 5, and 8 were mainly located in luminal and glandular epithelia, and positive immunostaining analysis of frequency was decreased in ectopic endometrium when compared with the eutopic one. Concerning the different expressions during menstrual phases, AQP2, 5, and 8 were found at a low-frequency rate in early-proliferative phase endometria but a higher frequency was observed in late proliferative and secretory phases [42]. In addition, Jiang et al. [46] found that AQP5 expression in hESC was increased by estradiol in a dose-dependent manner, because of an estrogen-responsive-element in the AQP5 promoter both in mice and in humans. Activating the phosphatidylinositol-3-kinase and protein kinase B (PI3K/AKT) pathway, isoform 5 could promote murine in vivo ectopic implants of endometrial-like cells due, at least in part, to pro-estrogenic enhancement [46]. Moreover, due to a low-frequency rate in late proliferative and secretory phases, AQP5 expression might be influenced by other factors, i.e., progesterone, as well [42,46]. In order to better investigate the role of AQ5 in endometriosis, Choi et al. [44] cultured hESC and transfected small interfering RNA (siRNA) of AQP1 to AQP9. They found that the expression for AQP2 and AQP8 was significantly higher than the other isoforms; moreover, the expression of AQP9 was decreased in the eutopic endometrium of patients with endometriosis when compared with the control group. In addition, when AQP9 was transfected throughout siRNA in hESCs, they found a significantly elevated expression of matrix metalloproteinases (MMPs) 2 and 9, which are essential for endometrial cell proliferation, migration, and invasiveness [71–73]. The MMP-9 gene is detected on chromosome 20q12-13 and is able to code an enzyme that directly participates in the degradation of collagen type IV and gelatin, which are the essential components of the basal membrane. Previous data suggest that the increased proteolytic activity, as well as the concomitant increase in the levels of the metalloproteinases, could be linked to the development of endometriosis. Moreover, a study by Chung et al. [74] found that MMP-9 plays a critical role in the implantation as well as invasion by ectopic endometrial tissue. The expression analysis of MMP-9 detected a significantly higher percentage of expression in ectopic endometrial tissues when compared with eutopic endometrial tissues [75]. Furthermore, MMP-9 was able to promote angiogenesis, which is argued to be a key process in the pathogenesis of endometriosis. Several coding single-nucleotide polymorphisms (SNPs) of MMP-9 were also identified, including MMP-9-1562C/T SNP. In addition to these findings, it has been recently demonstrated that the transcriptional activity of the −1562T allele was higher than the −1562C allele [76]. In synthesis, these polymorphisms may be able to alter the structure of MMP-9, giving the women an increased risk of developing endometriosis. The MMP2 gene can be found on chromosome 16q13-2. It encodes a critical enzyme for the reconstruction of the extracellular matrix (ECM) by targeting gelatin and type IV, V, VII, and X collagens. In order to demonstrate a role for MMP-2 in endometriosis, it has been found that women with endometriosis show increased MMP2 expression compared with healthy controls; meanwhile, the levels of the tissue inhibitors of metalloproteinase-2 (an inhibitor of MMP-2) mRNA were significantly lower. In agreement with these data, MMP-2 mRNA levels were found highly expressed in endometriosis tissues, especially in samples from patients with advanced disease [77]. In addition, Western Blot analysis reported increased expression of active (phosphorylated) extracellular signal-regulated kinases (ERK1/2) and phosphorylated p38 mitogen-activated protein kinase (MAPK). Taken together, these findings may suggest a role of AQP9 in the pathogenesis of endometriosis [44].

6. Chloride Channel-3 (ClC-3) and Endometriosis

Chloride channel-3 (ClC-3) is an ion channel encoded by the gene CLCN3. It belongs to the voltage-gated Cl^2 channel superfamily [78]. It has critical roles regarding cellular electric activity and volume homeostasis, and it is also involved in cellular proliferation, migration, invasiveness, and apoptosis [79,80]. Since similar aspects between endometriosis and cancer are traceable, it has been hypothesized that the expression of ion channels like ClC-3 in endometriotic cells are at higher levels than in healthy cells, with an increased ability for migration and invasion. Indeed, chloride channels were found as crucial for the migration of human glioma cells [81] and the chloride channel-3 (ClC-3) chloride channel was directly involved in cancer cell migration and invasion from different types of cancer, suggesting that ClC-3 can be a key promoter of invasiveness [82–84]. Considering these elements, Guan et al. [85] investigated the role of ClC-3 in ectopic endometrial-like cells in order to evaluate their migration and invasion ability in women affected by endometriosis from an epigenetic perspective [86,87]. These authors found that ClC-3 expression was clearly upregulated in human endometriotic tissue samples. More intriguing, several studies have documented that the presence of chronic inflammation is a critical component of tumor development and progression, including endometriosis. Indeed, it is also well reported that ClC-3 plays a critical role in inflammation when upregulated [87]. Although the underlying mechanisms responsible for overexpression of ClC-3 in endometriosis remains unclear, the relationship between ClC-3 and chronic inflammation has been well elucidated over the last ten years. Several studies describe that ClC-3-dependent Cl^2 efflux contributes to tumor necrosis factor (TNF)-α-induced cell inflammation and, therefore, leads to endothelial cell adhesion [88]. Guan et al. highlighted that the expression of the ClC-3 was significantly overexpressed at both mRNA and protein levels in ectopic lesions when compared with eutopic endometrial samples. At the same time, they suggested that the downregulation of ClC-3 expression was correlated to the inhibition of migration and invasion of hESCs [85]. Nonetheless, a strong positive correlation between ClC-3 and MMP9 was found; indeed, in ectopic hESCs, high levels of both proteins were found, and when ClC-3 was knocked down, MMP9 expression was significantly decreased [85]. Therefore, these findings may suggest that ClC-3, throughout the MMP9 upregulation, is involved in the pathogenesis of endometriotic lesions [85].

7. Conclusions

The development of endometriosis is a process in which the endometrial stromal cells acquire and lose parts of their cellular function in order to gain the ability to proliferate, migrate, and invade outside the uterine cavity. Several keys factors characterize the pathogenesis and lead to heterogeneous phenotypes of the disease. In this process, different ion channels families are potentially related to the etiopathogenesis of endometriosis. CFTR, TRPs, AQPs, and ClC-3 expression and activity have been evaluated in both in vitro and in vivo experiments on ectopic and eutopic endometrium, hESCs, ISK cells, and murine models (for a summary of the findings of this review, refer to Table 1 and Figure 1).

Table 1. The main ion channels involved in the pathogenesis of endometriosis.

Ion Channel	Regulation	Main Pathway	Action	References
CFTR	Upregulation	NFκB-p-65-uPAR	Migration; proliferation	[45]
AQP5	Upregulation	PI3K/AKT—MMP2, MMP9	Implantation	[46]
AQP9	Downregulation	ERK/p38 MAPK - MMP2, MMP9	Migration; implantation	[44]
ClC-3	Upregulation	MMP9	Implantation; inflammation	[85]

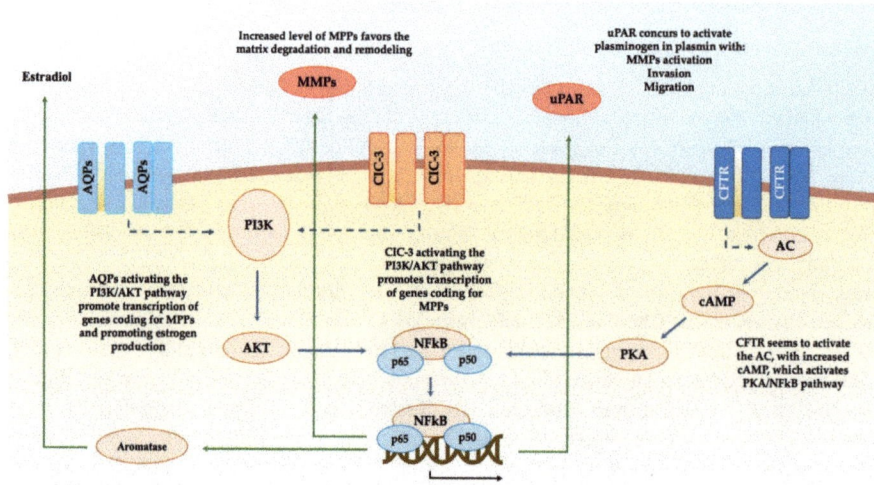

Figure 1. The main pathways involved in the pathogenesis of endometriosis mediated by ion channels. ClC-3: Chloride channel-3. AQPs: aquaporins. CFTR: cystic fibrosis transmembrane conductance regulator. AC: adenylate cyclase. cAMP: cyclical adenosine monophosphate. PKA: protein kinase A. PI3K: phosphatidylinositol-3-kinase. AKT: protein kinase B. MMPs: matrix metalloproteinases. uPAR: urokinase receptor.

CFTR expression was significantly higher in ectopic than eutopic endometrium and has been found to be regulated by estrogen and to fluctuate during the menstrual phases. Additionally, CFTR was able to upregulate the NFκB-p65-uPAR pathway, which orchestrates proliferation, migration, and invasiveness of endometrial cells. Several AQP isoforms were found related to the etiology of endometriosis; in particular, AQP5 was dose-dependently regulated by estrogens and able to activate the PI3K/AKT pathway, promoting implants of ectopic cells in vivo murine models. When AQP9 was down indeed regulated, the endometrial stromal cells' migration and implantation index was enhanced by the upregulation of MMP2 and MMP9 throughout ERK/p38 MAPK signaling. ClC-3 achieved the same upregulation of MMP9 in hESCs, and, at the same time, a more significant cell migration and invasion activity were related to overexpression of ClC-3 in ectopic lesions. Taken together, these data suggest a potentially pivotal role of ion channels such as CFTR, AQPs, and ClC-3 in the complex and multifactorial pathogenesis of endometriosis. These families are able to activate several pathways and promote the capacity of endometrial cells to proliferate, migrate, and implant outside the uterus. Nevertheless, data available so far are still scarce and do not allow a firm conclusion about the topic to be drawn. For this reason, we take this opportunity to solicit further research to better understand the role of ion channels in the onset and progression of endometriosis and elucidate whether they might be considered potential targets for diagnosis and therapy.

Author Contributions: Conceptualization, A.S.L. and S.G.; methodology, L.C. and L.D.C.; data curation, R.A.; writing—original draft preparation, A.S.L. and G.R.; writing—review and editing, M.L.V., A.S., and F.L.; project administration, P.D.F. All authors have read and agree to the published version of the manuscript.

Funding: This research received no external funding.

Conflicts of Interest: The authors declare no conflict of interest.

Abbreviations

DIE	Deep infiltrating endometriosis
Wnt	Wingless-related integration site gene cluster
Hox	Homeobox genes
CFTR	Cystic fibrosis transmembrane conductance regulator
TRP	Transient receptor potential
AQP	Aquaporin
ClC	Chloride channel
NFκB	Nuclear factor kappa-light-chain-enhancer of activated B cells
uPAR	Urokinase plasminogen activator receptor
PI3K	Phosphatidylinositol-3-Kinase
AKT	Protein kinase B
ERK	Extracellular signal-regulated kinases
MAPK	Mitogen-activated protein kinases
MMP	Matrix metalloproteinase
MeSH	Medical subject headings
E2	Estradiol
qPCR	Quantitative real-time polymerase chain reaction
ISK	Human endometrial Ishikawa cell
hESC	Human endometrial stromal cell
siRNA	small interfering RNA
ECM	Extracellular matrix
SNP	Single-nucleotide polymorphism
TNF-α	Tumor necrosis factor α

References

1. Laganà, A.S.; Garzon, S.; Götte, M.; Viganò, P.; Franchi, M.; Ghezzi, F.; Martin, D.C. The Pathogenesis of Endometriosis: Molecular and Cell Biology Insights. *Int. J. Mol. Sci.* **2019**, *20*, 5615. [CrossRef] [PubMed]
2. Laganà, A.S.; Vitale, S.G.; Salmeri, F.M.; Triolo, O.; Ban Frangež, H.; Vrtačnik-Bokal, E.; Stojanovska, L.; Apostolopoulos, V.; Granese, R.; Sofo, V. Unus pro omnibus, omnes pro uno: A novel, evidence-based, unifying theory for the pathogenesis of endometriosis. *Med. Hypotheses* **2017**, *103*, 10–20. [CrossRef] [PubMed]
3. Peiris, A.N.; Chaljub, E.; Medlock, D. Endometriosis. *JAMA* **2018**, *320*, 2608. [CrossRef] [PubMed]
4. Falcone, T.; Flyckt, R. Clinical Management of Endometriosis. *Obstet. Gynecol.* **2018**, *131*, 557–571. [CrossRef] [PubMed]
5. Apostolopoulos, N.V.; Alexandraki, K.I.; Gorry, A.; Coker, A. Association between chronic pelvic pain symptoms and the presence of endometriosis. *Arch. Gynecol. Obstet.* **2015**, *293*, 439–445. [CrossRef]
6. Šalamun, V.; Verdenik, I.; Laganà, A.S.; Vrtačnik-Bokal, E. Should we consider integrated approach for endometriosis-associated infertility as gold standard management? Rationale and results from a large cohort analysis. *Arch. Gynecol. Obstet.* **2017**, *297*, 613–621. [CrossRef]
7. Terzic, M.; Aimagambetova, G.; Garzon, S.; Bapayeva, G.; Ukybassova, T.; Terzic, S.; Norton, M.; Lagana, A.S. Ovulation induction in infertile women with endometriotic ovarian cysts: Current evidence and potential pitfalls. *Minerva Med.* **2019**. [CrossRef]
8. Donnez, J. Endometriosis: Enigmatic in the pathogenesis and controversial in its therapy. *Fertil. Steril.* **2012**, *98*, 509–510. [CrossRef]
9. Bedaiwy, M.A.; Abdel-Aleem, M.A.; Miketa, A.; Falcone, T. Endometriosis: A critical appraisal of the advances and the controversies of a challenging health problem. *Minerva Ginecol.* **2009**, *61*, 285–298.
10. Donnez, J. Introduction: From pathogenesis to therapy, deep endometriosis remains a source of controversy. *Fertil. Steril.* **2017**, *108*, 869–871. [CrossRef]
11. Mele, D.; De Franciscis, P.; Cosenza, C.; Riemma, G.; D'eufemia, M.D.; Schettino, M.T.; Morlando, M.; Schiattarella, A. Surgical management of endometrioma for ovarian safety. *Ital. J. Gynaecol. Obstet.* **2019**, *31*, 49–55. [CrossRef]
12. Siciliano, R.A.; Mazzeo, M.F.; Spada, V.; Facchiano, A.; D'acierno, A.; Stocchero, M.; De Franciscis, P.; Colacurci, N.; Sannolo, N.; Miraglia, N. Rapid peptidomic profiling of peritoneal fluid by MALDI-TOF mass spectrometry for the identification of biomarkers of endometriosis. *Gynecol. Endocrinol.* **2014**, *30*, 872–876. [CrossRef]
13. Bozdag, G. Recurrence of Endometriosis: Risk Factors, Mechanisms and Biomarkers. *Womens Health* **2015**, *11*, 693–699. [CrossRef] [PubMed]
14. Sansone, A.; De Rosa, N.; Giampaolino, P.; Guida, M.; Laganà, A.S.; Di Carlo, C. Effects of etonogestrel implant on quality of life, sexual function, and pelvic pain in women suffering from endometriosis: Results from a multicenter, prospective, observational study. *Arch. Gynecol. Obstet.* **2018**, *298*, 731–736. [CrossRef]
15. Márki, G.; Bokor, A.; Rigó, J.; Rigó, A. Physical pain and emotion regulation as the main predictive factors of health-related quality of life in women living with endometriosis. *Hum. Reprod.* **2017**, *32*, 1432–1438. [CrossRef] [PubMed]
16. La Rosa, V.L.; De Franciscis, P.; Barra, F.; Schiattarella, A.; Tropea, A.; Tesarik, J.; Shah, M.; Kahramanoglu, I.; Marques Cerentini, T.; Ponta, M.; et al. Sexuality in women with endometriosis: A critical narrative review. *Minerva Med.* **2019**. [CrossRef]
17. Soliman, A.M.; Coyne, K.S.; Zaiser, E.; Castelli-Haley, J.; Fuldeore, M.J. The burden of endometriosis symptoms on health-related quality of life in women in the United States: A cross-sectional study. *J. Psychosom. Obstet. Gynaecol.* **2017**, *38*, 238–248. [CrossRef]
18. La Rosa, V.L.; De Franciscis, P.; Barra, F.; Schiattarella, A.; Török, P.; Shah, M.; Karaman, E.; Marques Cerentini, T.; Di Guardo, F.; Gullo, G.; et al. Quality of life in women with endometriosis: A narrative overview. *Minerva Med.* **2019**. [CrossRef]
19. Burney, R.O.; Giudice, L.C. Pathogenesis and pathophysiology of endometriosis. *Fertil. Steril.* **2012**, *98*, 511–519. [CrossRef]
20. Rock, J.A.; Markham, S.M. Pathogenesis of endometriosis. *Lancet* **1992**, *340*, 1264–1267. [CrossRef]

21. Vetvicka, V.; Laganà, A.S.; Salmeri, F.M.; Triolo, O.; Palmara, V.I.; Vitale, S.G.; Sofo, V.; Králíčková, M. Regulation of apoptotic pathways during endometriosis: From the molecular basis to the future perspectives. *Arch. Gynecol. Obstet.* **2016**, *294*, 897–904. [CrossRef] [PubMed]
22. Simonelli, A.; Guadagni, R.; De Franciscis, P.; Colacurci, N.; Pieri, M.; Basilicata, P.; Pedata, P.; Lamberti, M.; Sannolo, N.; Miraglia, N. Environmental and occupational exposure to bisphenol A and endometriosis: Urinary and peritoneal fluid concentration levels. *Int. Arch. Occup. Environ. Health* **2017**, *90*, 49–61. [CrossRef] [PubMed]
23. Maniglio, P.; Ricciardi, E.; Laganà, A.S.; Triolo, O.; Caserta, D. Epigenetic modifications of primordial reproductive tract: A common etiologic pathway for Mayer-Rokitansky-Kuster-Hauser Syndrome and endometriosis? *Med. Hypotheses* **2016**, *90*, 4–5. [CrossRef] [PubMed]
24. Laganà, A.S.; Salmeri, F.M.; Ban Frangež, H.; Ghezzi, F.; Vrtačnik-Bokal, E.; Granese, R. Evaluation of M1 and M2 macrophages in ovarian endometriomas from women affected by endometriosis at different stages of the disease. *Gynecol. Endocrinol.* **2019**, 1–4. [CrossRef] [PubMed]
25. Ruan, Y.C.; Chen, H.; Chan, H.C. Ion channels in the endometrium: Regulation of endometrial receptivity and embryo implantation. *Hum. Reprod. Update* **2014**, *20*, 517–529. [CrossRef]
26. Goldstein, S.A.N. Ion channels: Structural basis for function and disease. *Semin. Perinatol.* **1996**, *20*, 520–530. [CrossRef]
27. Bagal, S.K.; Brown, A.D.; Cox, P.J.; Omoto, K.; Owen, R.M.; Pryde, D.C.; Sidders, B.; Skerratt, S.E.; Stevens, E.B.; Storer, R.I.; et al. Ion Channels as Therapeutic Targets: A Drug Discovery Perspective. *J. Med. Chem.* **2012**, *56*, 593–624. [CrossRef]
28. Li, J.; Liang, X.; Chen, Z. Improving the embryo implantation via novel molecular targets. *Curr. Drug Targets* **2013**, *14*, 864–871. [CrossRef]
29. Mathie, A. Ion channels as novel therapeutic targets in the treatment of pain. *J. Pharm. Pharmacol.* **2010**, *62*, 1089–1095. [CrossRef]
30. Ashcroft, F.M. From molecule to malady. *Nature* **2006**, *440*, 440–447. [CrossRef]
31. Davidson, L.M.; Coward, K. Molecular mechanisms of membrane interaction at implantation. *Birth Defects Res. C Embryo Today Rev.* **2016**, *108*, 19–32. [CrossRef] [PubMed]
32. Zhang, D.; Tan, Y.-J.; Qu, F.; Sheng, J.-Z.; Huang, H.-F. Functions of water channels in male and female reproductive systems. *Mol. Aspects Med.* **2012**, *33*, 676–690. [CrossRef] [PubMed]
33. Zhang, Y.; Ding, S.; Shen, Q.; Wu, J.; Zhu, X. The expression and regulation of aquaporins in placenta and fetal membranes. *Front. Biosci.* **2012**, *17*, 2371–2382. [CrossRef] [PubMed]
34. Leanza, L.; Managò, A.; Zoratti, M.; Gulbins, E.; Szabo, I. Pharmacological targeting of ion channels for cancer therapy: In vivo evidences. *Biochim. Biophys. Acta-Mol. Cell Res.* **2016**, *1863*, 1385–1397. [CrossRef] [PubMed]
35. Deng, Z.; Peng, S.; Zheng, Y.; Yang, X.; Zhang, H.; Tan, Q.; Liang, X.; Gao, H.; Li, Y.; Huang, Y.; et al. Estradiol activates chloride channels via estrogen receptor-α in the cell membranes of osteoblasts. *Am. J. Physiol. Cell Physiol.* **2017**, *313*, C162–C172. [CrossRef]
36. Chabbert-Buffeta, N. Neuroendocrine effects of progesterone. *Steroids* **2000**, *65*, 613–620. [CrossRef]
37. Vega-Vela, N.E.; Osorio, D.; Avila-Rodriguez, M.; Gonzalez, J.; García-Segura, L.M.; Echeverria, V.; Barreto, G.E. L-Type Calcium Channels Modulation by Estradiol. *Mol. Neurobiol.* **2017**, *54*, 4996–5007. [CrossRef]
38. Arnadóttir, J.; Chalfie, M. Eukaryotic mechanosensitive channels. *Annu. Rev. Biophys.* **2010**, *39*, 111–137. [CrossRef]
39. Cuddapah, V.A.; Sontheimer, H. Ion channels and transporters [corrected] in cancer. 2. Ion channels and the control of cancer cell migration. *Am. J. Physiol. Cell Physiol.* **2011**, *301*, C541–C549. [CrossRef]
40. Bohonyi, N.; Pohóczky, K.; Szalontai, B.; Perkecz, A.; Kovács, K.; Kajtár, B.; Orbán, L.; Varga, T.; Szegedi, S.; Bódis, J.; et al. Local upregulation of transient receptor potential ankyrin 1 and transient receptor potential vanilloid 1 ion channels in rectosigmoid deep infiltrating endometriosis. *Mol. Pain* **2017**, *13*. [CrossRef]
41. Greaves, E.; Grieve, K.; Horne, A.W.; Saunders, P.T.K. Elevated peritoneal expression and estrogen regulation of nociceptive ion channels in endometriosis. *J. Clin. Endocrinol. Metab.* **2014**, *99*, E1738–E1743. [CrossRef]
42. Jiang, X.-X.; Wu, R.-J.; Xu, K.-H.; Zhou, C.-Y.; Guo, X.-Y.; Sun, Y.-L.; Lin, J. Immunohistochemical detection of aquaporin expression in eutopic and ectopic endometria from women with endometriomas. *Fertil. Steril.* **2010**, *94*, 1229–1234. [CrossRef]

43. Zheng, X.-Y.; Chen, G.-A.; Wang, H.-Y. Expression of cystic fibrosis transmembrane conductance regulator in human endometrium. *Hum. Reprod.* **2004**, *19*, 2933–2941. [CrossRef] [PubMed]
44. Choi, Y.S.; Park, J.H.; Yoon, J.-K.; Yoon, J.S.; Kim, J.S.; Lee, J.H.; Yun, B.H.; Park, J.H.; Seo, S.K.; Cho, S.; et al. Potential roles of aquaporin 9 in the pathogenesis of endometriosis. *MHR Basic Sci. Reprod. Med.* **2019**, *25*, 373–384. [CrossRef] [PubMed]
45. Huang, W.; Jin, A.; Zhang, J.; Wang, C.; Tsang, L.L.; Cai, Z.; Zhou, X.; Chen, H.; Chan, H.C. Upregulation of CFTR in patients with endometriosis and its involvement in NFκB-uPAR dependent cell migration. *Oncotarget* **2017**, *8*, 66951–66959. [CrossRef] [PubMed]
46. Jiang, X.X.; Fei, X.W.; Zhao, L.; Ye, X.L.; Xin, L.B.; Qu, Y.; Xu, K.H.; Wu, R.J.; Lin, J. Aquaporin 5 Plays a Role in Estrogen-Induced Ectopic Implantation of Endometrial Stromal Cells in Endometriosis. *PLoS ONE* **2015**, *10*. [CrossRef]
47. Persoons, E.; Hennes, A.; De Clercq, K.; Van Bree, R.; Vriens, G.; Dorien, F.O.; Peterse, D.; Vanhie, A.; Meuleman, C.; Voets, T.; et al. Functional Expression of TRP Ion Channels in Endometrial Stromal Cells of Endometriosis Patients. *Int. J. Mol. Sci.* **2018**, *19*, 2467. [CrossRef]
48. Gillen, A.E.; Harris, A. Transcriptional regulation of CFTR gene expression. *Front. Biosci.* **2012**, *4*, 587–592. [CrossRef]
49. Vetter, A.J.; Karamyshev, A.L.; Patrick, A.E.; Hudson, H.; Thomas, P.J. N-Alpha-Acetyltransferases and Regulation of CFTR Expression. *PLoS ONE* **2016**, *11*. [CrossRef]
50. Sweezey, N.B.; Gauthier, C.; Gagnon, S.; Ferretti, E.; Kopelman, H. Progesterone and estradiol inhibit CFTR-mediated ion transport by pancreatic epithelial cells. *Am. J. Physiol. Liver Physiol.* **1996**, *271*, G747–G754. [CrossRef]
51. Mularoni, A.; Adessi, G.L.; Arbez-Gindre, F.; Agnani, G.; Nicollier, M. Competitive RT-PCR to quantify CFTR mRNA in human endometrium. *Clin. Chem.* **1996**, *42*, 1765–1769. [CrossRef] [PubMed]
52. Song, Y.; Wang, Q.; Huang, W.; Xiao, L.; Shen, L.; Xu, W. NF κB expression increases and CFTR and MUC1 expression decreases in the endometrium of infertile patients with hydrosalpinx: A comparative study. *Reprod. Biol. Endocrinol.* **2012**, *10*, 86. [CrossRef] [PubMed]
53. Yang, J.Z.; Ajonuma, L.C.; Tsang, L.L.; Lam, S.Y.; Rowlands, D.K.; Ho, L.S.; Zhou, C.X.; Chung, Y.W.; Chan, H.C. Differential expression and localization of CFTR and ENaC in mouse endometrium during pre-implantation. *Cell Biol. Int.* **2004**, *28*, 433–439. [CrossRef] [PubMed]
54. Knorre, A.; Wagner, M.; Schaefer, H.-E.; Colledge, W.H.; Pahl, H.L. DeltaF508-CFTR causes constitutive NF-kappaB activation through an ER-overload response in cystic fibrosis lungs. *Biol. Chem.* **2002**, *383*, 271–282. [CrossRef] [PubMed]
55. Lu, Y.C.; Chen, H.; Fok, K.L.; Tsang, L.L.; Yu, M.K.; Zhang, X.H.; Chen, J.; Jiang, X.; Chung, Y.W.; Ma, A.C.H.; et al. CFTR mediates bicarbonate-dependent activation of miR-125b in preimplantation embryo development. *Cell Res.* **2012**, *22*, 1453–1466. [CrossRef] [PubMed]
56. Dietrich, A. Transient Receptor Potential (TRP) Channels in Health and Disease. *Cells* **2019**, *8*, 413. [CrossRef]
57. Voets, T.; Vriens, J.; Vennekens, R. Targeting TRP Channels—Valuable Alternatives to Combat Pain, Lower Urinary Tract Disorders, and Type 2 Diabetes? *Trends Pharmacol. Sci.* **2019**, *40*, 669–683. [CrossRef]
58. Lamas, J.A.; Rueda-Ruzafa, L.; Herrera-Pérez, S. Ion Channels and Thermosensitivity: TRP, TREK, or Both? *Int. J. Mol. Sci.* **2019**, *20*, 2371. [CrossRef]
59. Takayama, Y.; Derouiche, S.; Maruyama, K.; Tominaga, M. Emerging Perspectives on Pain Management by Modulation of TRP Channels and ANO1. *Int. J. Mol. Sci.* **2019**, *20*, 3411. [CrossRef]
60. De Clercq, K.; Held, K.; Van Bree, R.; Meuleman, C.; Peeraer, K.; Tomassetti, C.; Voets, T.; D'Hooghe, T.; Vriens, J. Functional expression of transient receptor potential channels in human endometrial stromal cells during the luteal phase of the menstrual cycle. *Hum. Reprod.* **2015**, *30*, 1421–1436. [CrossRef]
61. Bödding, M. TRP proteins and cancer. *Cell. Signal.* **2007**, *19*, 617–624. [CrossRef] [PubMed]
62. Fels, B.; Bulk, E.; Pethő, Z.; Schwab, A. The Role of TRP Channels in the Metastatic Cascade. *Pharmaceuticals* **2018**, *11*, 48. [CrossRef]
63. Smani, T.; Gómez, L.J.; Regodon, S.; Woodard, G.E.; Siegfried, G.; Khatib, A.-M.; Rosado, J.A. TRP Channels in Angiogenesis and Other Endothelial Functions. *Front. Physiol.* **2018**, *9*, 1731. [CrossRef] [PubMed]
64. Hiroi, H.; Momoeda, M.; Watanabe, T.; Ito, M.; Ikeda, K.; Tsutsumi, R.; Hosokawa, Y.; Koizumi, M.; Zenri, F.; Muramatsu, M.; et al. Expression and regulation of transient receptor potential cation channel, subfamily M, member 2 (TRPM2) in human endometrium. *Mol. Cell. Endocrinol.* **2013**, *365*, 146–152. [CrossRef] [PubMed]

65. Kawarabayashi, Y.; Hai, L.; Honda, A.; Horiuchi, S.; Tsujioka, H.; Ichikawa, J.; Inoue, R. Critical role of TRPC1-mediated Ca^{2+} entry in decidualization of human endometrial stromal cells. *Mol. Endocrinol.* **2012**, *26*, 846–858. [CrossRef] [PubMed]
66. Takata, K.; Matsuzaki, T.; Tajika, Y. Aquaporins: Water channel proteins of the cell membrane. *Prog. Histochem. Cytochem.* **2004**, *39*, 1–83. [CrossRef]
67. King, L.S.; Agre, P. Pathophysiology of the Aquaporin Water Channels. *Annu. Rev. Physiol.* **1996**, *58*, 619–648. [CrossRef]
68. Mobasheri, A.; Wray, S.; Marples, D. Distribution of AQP2 and AQP3 water channels in human tissue microarrays. *J. Mol. Histol.* **2005**, *36*, 1–14. [CrossRef]
69. Meli, R.; Pirozzi, C.; Pelagalli, A. New Perspectives on the Potential Role of Aquaporins (AQPs) in the Physiology of Inflammation. *Front. Physiol.* **2018**, *9*, 101. [CrossRef]
70. He, R.-H.; Sheng, J.-Z.; Luo, Q.; Jin, F.; Wang, B.; Qian, Y.-L.; Zhou, C.-Y.; Sheng, X.; Huang, H.-F. Aquaporin-2 expression in human endometrium correlates with serum ovarian steroid hormones. *Life Sci.* **2006**, *79*, 423–429. [CrossRef]
71. Bostanci Durmus, A.; Dincer Cengiz, S.; Yılmaz, H.; Candar, T.; Gursoy, A.Y.; Sinem Caglar, G. The levels of matrix metalloproteinase-9 and neutrophil gelatinase-associated lipocalin in different stages of endometriosis. *J. Obstet. Gynaecol.* **2019**, *39*, 991–995. [CrossRef] [PubMed]
72. Szymanowski, K.; Mikołajczyk, M.; Wirstlein, P.; Dera-Szymanowska, A. Matrix metalloproteinase-2 (MMP-2), MMP-9, tissue inhibitor of matrix metalloproteinases (TIMP-1) and transforming growth factor-β2 (TGF-β2) expression in eutopic endometrium of women with peritoneal endometriosis. *Ann. Agric. Environ. Med.* **2016**, *23*, 649–653. [CrossRef] [PubMed]
73. Zhang, L.; Xiong, W.; Xiong, Y.; Liu, H.; Li, N.; Du, Y.; Liu, Y. Intracellular Wnt/Beta-Catenin Signaling Underlying 17beta-Estradiol-Induced Matrix Metalloproteinase 9 Expression in Human Endometriosis1. *Biol. Reprod.* **2016**, *94*. [CrossRef] [PubMed]
74. Chung, H.-W.; Wen, Y.; Chun, S.-H.; Nezhat, C.; Woo, B.-H.; Lake Polan, M. Matrix metalloproteinase-9 and tissue inhibitor of metalloproteinase-3 mRNA expression in ectopic and eutopic endometrium in women with endometriosis: A rationale for endometriotic invasiveness. *Fertil. Steril.* **2001**, *75*, 152–159. [CrossRef]
75. Collette, T.; Maheux, R.; Mailloux, J.; Akoum, A. Increased expression of matrix metalloproteinase-9 in the eutopic endometrial tissue of women with endometriosis. *Hum. Reprod.* **2006**, *21*, 3059–3067. [CrossRef]
76. Xin, L.; Hou, Q.; Xiong, Q.I.; Ding, X. Association between matrix metalloproteinase-2 and matrix metalloproteinase-9 polymorphisms and endometriosis: A systematic review and meta-analysis. *Biomed. Rep.* **2015**, *3*, 559–565. [CrossRef]
77. Weigel, M.T.; Krämer, J.; Schem, C.; Wenners, A.; Alkatout, I.; Jonat, W.; Maass, N.; Mundhenke, C. Differential expression of MMP-2, MMP-9 and PCNA in endometriosis and endometrial carcinoma. *Eur. J. Obstet. Gynecol. Reprod. Biol.* **2012**, *160*, 74–78. [CrossRef]
78. Hara-Chikuma, M.; Yang, B.; Sonawane, N.D.; Sasaki, S.; Uchida, S.; Verkman, A.S. ClC-3 Chloride Channels Facilitate Endosomal Acidification and Chloride Accumulation. *J. Biol. Chem.* **2004**, *280*, 1241–1247. [CrossRef]
79. Li, M.; Wu, D.B.; Wang, J. Effects of volume-activated chloride channels on the invasion and migration of human endometrial cancer cells. *Eur. J. Gynaecol. Oncol.* **2013**, *34*, 60–64.
80. Mao, J.; Chen, L.; Xu, B.; Wang, L.; Wang, W.; Li, M.; Zheng, M.; Li, H.; Guo, J.; Li, W.; et al. Volume-activated chloride channels contribute to cell-cycle-dependent regulation of HeLa cell migration. *Biochem. Pharmacol.* **2009**, *77*, 159–168. [CrossRef]
81. Ransom, C.B.; O'Neal, J.T.; Sontheimer, H. Volume-activated chloride currents contribute to the resting conductance and invasive migration of human glioma cells. *J. Neurosci.* **2001**, *21*, 7674–7683. [CrossRef] [PubMed]
82. Mao, J.; Chen, L.; Xu, B.; Wang, L.; Li, H.; Guo, J.; Li, W.; Nie, S.; Jacob, T.J.C.; Wang, L. Suppression of ClC-3 channel expression reduces migration of nasopharyngeal carcinoma cells. *Biochem. Pharmacol.* **2008**, *75*, 1706–1716. [CrossRef] [PubMed]
83. Xu, B.; Jin, X.; Min, L.; Li, Q.; Deng, L.; Wu, H.; Lin, G.; Chen, L.; Zhang, H.; Li, C.; et al. Chloride channel-3 promotes tumor metastasis by regulating membrane ruffling and is associated with poor survival. *Oncotarget* **2015**, *6*, 2434–2450. [CrossRef] [PubMed]

84. Mao, J.; Yuan, J.; Wang, L.; Zhang, H.; Jin, X.; Zhu, J.; Li, H.; Xu, B.; Chen, L. Tamoxifen inhibits migration of estrogen receptor-negative hepatocellular carcinoma cells by blocking the swelling-activated chloride current. *J. Cell. Physiol.* **2013**, *228*, 991–1001. [CrossRef] [PubMed]
85. Guan, Y.; Huang, Y.; Wu, J.; Deng, Z.; Wang, Y.; Lai, Z.; Wang, H.; Sun, X.; Zhu, Y.; Du, M.; et al. Overexpression of chloride channel-3 is associated with the increased migration and invasion ability of ectopic endometrial cells from patients with endometriosis. *Hum. Reprod.* **2016**, *31*, 986–998. [CrossRef] [PubMed]
86. Lee, B.; Du, H.; Taylor, H.S. Experimental murine endometriosis induces DNA methylation and altered gene expression in eutopic endometrium. *Biol. Reprod.* **2009**, *80*, 79–85. [CrossRef] [PubMed]
87. Volk, A.P.D.; Heise, C.K.; Hougen, J.L.; Artman, C.M.; Volk, K.A.; Wessels, D.; Soll, D.R.; Nauseef, W.M.; Lamb, F.S.; Moreland, J.G. ClC-3 and IClswell are required for normal neutrophil chemotaxis and shape change. *J. Biol. Chem.* **2008**, *283*, 34315–34326. [CrossRef]
88. Yang, H.; Huang, L.-Y.; Zeng, D.-Y.; Huang, E.-W.; Liang, S.-J.; Tang, Y.-B.; Su, Y.-X.; Tao, J.; Shang, F.; Wu, Q.-Q.; et al. Decrease of intracellular chloride concentration promotes endothelial cell inflammation by activating nuclear factor-κB pathway. *Hypertens* **2012**, *60*, 1287–1293. [CrossRef]

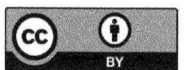

© 2020 by the authors. Licensee MDPI, Basel, Switzerland. This article is an open access article distributed under the terms and conditions of the Creative Commons Attribution (CC BY) license (http://creativecommons.org/licenses/by/4.0/).

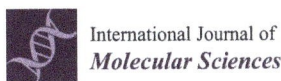

Article

Impaired Expression of Ectonucleotidases in Ectopic and Eutopic Endometrial Tissue Is in Favor of ATP Accumulation in the Tissue Microenvironment in Endometriosis

Carla Trapero [1,2], August Vidal [1,2,3], Maria Eulàlia Fernández-Montolí [2,4], Buenaventura Coroleu [5], Francesc Tresserra [5], Pere Barri [5], Inmaculada Gómez de Aranda [1], Jean Sévigny [6,7], Jordi Ponce [2,4], Xavier Matias-Guiu [2,3] and Mireia Martín-Satué [1,2,*]

[1] Departament de Patologia i Terapèutica Experimental, Facultat de Medicina i Ciències de la Salut, Campus Bellvitge, Universitat de Barcelona, 08907 Barcelona, Spain; ctrapero@idibell.cat (C.T.); avidal@bellvitgehospital.cat (A.V.); igomezdearanda@ub.edu (I.G.d.A.)
[2] Oncobell Program, CIBERONC, Institut d'Investigació Biomèdica de Bellvitge (IDIBELL), 08908 Barcelona, Spain; mefernandez@bellvitgehospital.cat (M.E.F.-M.); jponce@bellvitgehospital.cat (J.P.); fjmatiasguiu.lleida.ics@gencat.cat (X.M.-G.)
[3] Servei d'Anatomia Patològica, Hospital Universitari de Bellvitge, 08907 Barcelona, Spain
[4] Servei de Ginecologia, Hospital Universitari de Bellvitge, 08907 Barcelona, Spain
[5] Salud de la Mujer Dexeus, Hospital Universitari Quiron Dexeus, 08028 Barcelona, Spain; VENCOR@dexeus.com (B.C.); francesc.tresserra@quironsalud.es (F.T.); barper@dexeus.com (P.B.)
[6] Centre de Recherche du CHU de Québec - Université Laval, Québec City, QC G1V 4G2, Canada; jean.sevigny@crchudequebec.ulaval.ca
[7] Départment de Microbiologie-Infectiologie et d'Immunologie, Faculté de Médecine, Université Laval, Quebec City, QC G1V 4G2, Canada
* Correspondence: martinsatue@ub.edu

Received: 16 September 2019; Accepted: 2 November 2019; Published: 6 November 2019

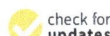

Abstract: Endometriosis is a prevalent disease defined by the presence of endometrial tissue outside the uterus. Adenosine triphosphate (ATP), as a proinflammatory molecule, promotes and helps maintain the inflammatory state of endometriosis. Moreover, ATP has a direct influence on the two main symptoms of endometriosis: infertility and pain. Purinergic signaling, the group of biological responses to extracellular nucleotides such as ATP and nucleosides such as adenosine, is involved in the biology of reproduction and is impaired in pathologies with an inflammatory component such as endometriosis. We have previously demonstrated that ectonucleotidases, the enzymes regulating extracellular ATP levels, are active in non-pathological endometria, with hormone-dependent changes in expression throughout the cycle. In the present study we have focused on the expression of ectonucleotidases by means of immunohistochemistry and in situ activity in eutopic and ectopic endometrial tissue of women with endometriosis, and we compared the results with endometria of women without the disease. We have demonstrated that the axis CD39-CD73 is altered in endometriosis, with loss of CD39 and CD73 expression in deep infiltrating endometriosis, the most severe, and most recurring, endometriosis subtype. Our results indicate that this altered expression of ectonucleotidases in endometriosis boosts ATP accumulation in the tissue microenvironment. An important finding is the identification of the nucleotide pyrophophatase/phosphodiesterase 3 (NPP3) as a new histopathological marker of the disease since we have demonstrated its expression in the stroma only in endometriosis, in both eutopic and ectopic tissue. Therefore, targeting the proteins directly involved in ATP breakdown could be an appropriate approach to consider in the treatment of endometriosis.

Keywords: endometriosis; endometrium; uterus; purinergic signaling; ATP

1. Introduction

Endometriosis is a chronic gynecological estrogen-dependent disease characterized by the presence of endometrial tissue, both glands and stroma, outside the uterus. There are multiple possible locations for this ectopic tissue which may be grouped into three endometriosis subtypes: peritoneal, ovarian, with ovarian cysts called endometriomas, and deeply infiltrative. It is a debilitating disorder affecting around 10% of women of reproductive age [1], with pelvic pain and infertility as the two main symptoms. The etiology and physiopathology of this disease remain unknown and there are no clinical biomarkers; in consequence, there is no cure and a long delay in the diagnosis. Studies focused on the discovery of diagnostic tools for endometriosis to help to design effective treatments that preserve fertility are of great interest.

Inflammation is necessary for the establishment and maintenance of endometrial cells in ectopic locations [2–5]. Purinergic signaling, the group of biological effects mediated by extracellular nucleotides, such as adenosine triphosphate (ATP), and nucleosides, such as adenosine, is involved in a wide range of physiological and pathological inflammatory conditions [6]. Extracellular ATP is mostly a proinflammatory molecule released during tissue stress situations, such as necrosis or apoptosis, hypoxia, and inflammation. Purinergic signaling is also studied in the context of human reproduction [7–11]; for instance, ATP is involved in the initiation and maintenance of myometrium and oviduct contractions. It increases the oviductal ciliary beat frequency [12] and contributes to the regulation of the uterine fluid microenvironment [9]. Moreover, adenosine, an ATP hydrolysis product, is necessary for sperm capacitation [10]. ATP is also a pain-related molecule, and some of the pharmacological treatments used to relieve pain in endometriosis do indeed affect ATP levels or their effects. Moreover, extracellular ATP and its derivative adenosine influence cell migration, proliferation and survival—three necessary events for the establishment of ectopic endometrial foci.

Extracellular ATP and adenosine levels are controlled by the ecto-nucleotidases, which are broadly expressed enzymes that, acting alone or sequentially, hydrolyze ATP into adenosine. There are four families of ectonucleotidases: (i) the ecto-nucleoside triphosphate diphosphohydrolase (E-NTPDase) family, also known as CD39 family, which hydrolyzes the ATP, and adenosine diphosphate (ADP), to adenosine monophosphate (AMP); (ii) the ecto-nucleotide pyrophophatase/phosphodiesterase (E-NPP) family, which mainly hydrolyzes ATP to AMP; (iii) the 5'-nucleotidase (5'-NT) (known as CD73) that dephosphorylates AMP to adenosine; and, (iv) the alkaline phosphatases family that hydrolyzes nucleoside triphosphates and diphosphates to monophosphates [6]. Adenosine deaminase (ADA) inactivates adenosine. This is a soluble enzyme often associated with CD26/dipeptidyl peptidase IV, expressed at the cell membrane [13]. Ectonucleotidases and CD26 are well characterized in human cyclic and postmenopausal endometria, showing differences in its expression and distribution throughout the cycle [8,14]. The presence of ectonucleotidases in the contents of endometrioma had previously been described [15,16] but no studies had yet to be conducted on eutopic and ectopic endometrial tissue from women with endometriosis.

With the present study, we aimed to characterize the expression of ectonucleotidases in the eutopic and ectopic endometrial tissue of women with endometriosis and compare it with the eutopic endometrium of women without this pathology. We believe that assessing the participation of these proteins directly involved in ATP breakdown in endometriosis could contribute to facilitating the diagnosis and ameliorating the treatment status of this pathology.

2. Results

Protein expression of NTPDase1 (CD39 from here on), NTPDase2, NTPDase3, NPP3, 5'-NT (CD73 from here on), and CD26 was detected in the eutopic and ectopic endometrial tissue of women with endometriosis. Results are compared with endometria from women without the disease whose data was previously published [8,14]. Staining distribution and intensity scores were recorded for each protein by double blinded observation. In situ nucleotidase activity, in the presence or absence of specific inhibitors, was also detected. The most relevant findings in eutopic endometria and endometrial lesions are described for each protein hereafter, and compiled in detail in Tables 1 and 2. The proportion of positive tissues stained in the immunolabeling assays is commented on in the text and compiled in Appendix A (Table A1).

Table 1. Summary of the ectoenzyme expression in the eutopic endometrium from women with endometriosis.

	NTPDase1 (CD39)	NTPDase2	NTPDase3	NPP3	5′-NT (CD73)	CD26
Proliferative endometrium						
Surface epithelium	-	+++	+	++	++	-
Glandular epithelium						
Functional layer	-	+++	++	++	+++	++/- [1]
Basal layer	-	+++	+	+	+++	+++
Endometrial stromal cells	-	+++	-	+++	++	-
Spiral arteries	+++	-	-	+	-	-
Secretory endometrium						
Surface epithelium	-	+++	+/- [1]	+++	+++	+
Glandular epithelium						
Functional layer	-	+++	+++	+++	++	+++
Basal layer	-	+++	+++	+++	+++	++
Endometrial stromal cells	-	+++	-	+	++	-
Spiral arteries	+++	-	-	+	-	-
Atrophic endometrium						
Surface epithelium	-	+++	-	+	+	++/- [1]
Glandular epithelium	-	+++	-	++	++	-
Endometrial stromal cells	++	+++	-	++	-	-
Vessels	++	-	-	+	-	-

Semi-quantitative analysis independently evaluated by two observers. Label is recorded as: (-) negative, (+) weak, (++) moderate, (+++) strong. [1] 50% of tissues studied had each of these staining intensities.

Table 2. Summary of the ectoenzyme expression in the ectopic endometrial tissue (peritoneal, ovarian, and deep infiltrative lesions) from women with endometriosis.

	NTPDase1 (CD39)	NTPDase2	NTPDase3	NPP3	5′-NT (CD73)	CD26
Peritoneal endometriosis						
Endometrial epithelial cells	-	+++	+	+++	+++	+++
Endometrial stromal cells	+++	++	-	++	++	-
Vessels of the lesion	+++	-	-	-	-	-
Ovarian endometriosis						
Endometrial epithelial cells	-	+++	+++	+++	+++	+++
Endometrial stromal cells	++	-	-	+	-	-
Vessels of the lesion	+++	-	-	-	-	-
Deep endometriosis						
Endometrial epithelial cells	-	+++	-	++	+++	+++
Endometrial stromal cells	-	++	-	+	-	-
Vessels of the lesion	-	-	-	-	-	-

Semi-quantitative analysis independently evaluated by two observers. Label is recorded as: (-) negative, (+) weak, (++) moderate, (+++) strong.

2.1. CD39 Expression in the Eutopic and Ectopic Endometrial Tissues

CD39 staining was detected in stromal cells and in endothelial cells from blood vessels of endometria from women without endometriosis (Figure 1), coinciding with previously published findings [8]. In the eutopic cyclic endometria from women with endometriosis, CD39 label in the stroma was absent in 65% of cases although it was always present in endothelial cells (Figure 1). However, atrophic endometria from women with endometriosis maintained the CD39 expression in the stromal component (Figure S1).

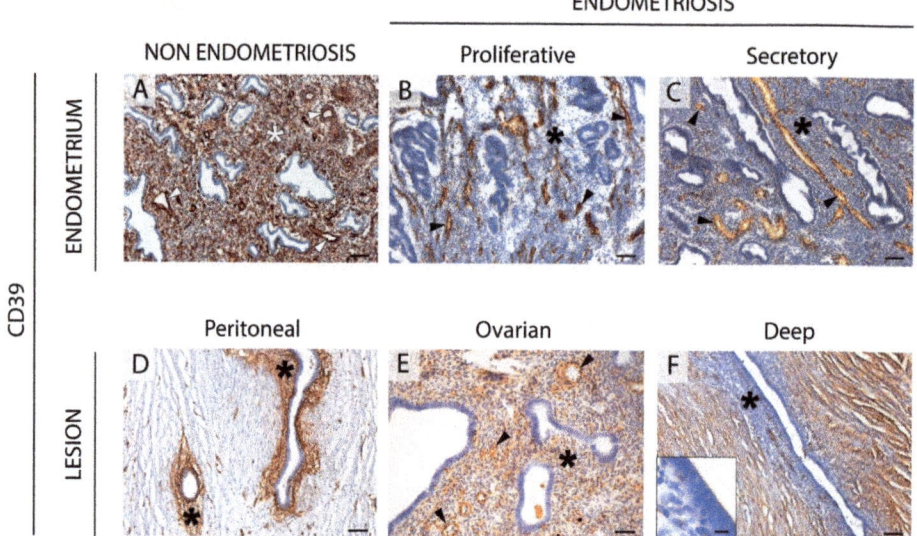

Figure 1. Immunolocalization of CD39 in eutopic (**A–C**) and ectopic (**D–F**) endometrial tissue. CD39 was expressed in blood vessels (arrowheads) of eutopic endometria from women without (NON ENDOMETRIOSIS, (**A**) or with endometriosis (ENDOMETRIOSIS, (**B**,**C**), and in peritoneal (**D**), ovarian (**E**), and deep infiltrating (**F**) lesions. CD39 was immunodetected in the stroma (asterisk) of endometrium of women without the disease (**A**), but not in endometria of women with endometriosis (**B**,**C**). Stroma is also labelled in the peritoneal (**D**) and ovarian (**E**) ectopic tissues of women with endometriosis. Inset in (**F**) is a detail of a deep lesion (oviductal infiltrating nodule) showing the absence of CD39 in the endometrial stroma. Scale bars are 100 μm (**A–F**) and 10 μm (**F** inset).

In endometriotic lesions, CD39 was immunodetected with strong labeling in the stroma of the peritoneal (86% of cases) and ovarian (59%) lesions, but not in the deep ones, where this label was only in 36% of the samples. Moreover, 54% of deeply infiltrative lesions lost the expression of CD39 in blood vessels. ADPase activity was seen at the same locations where the protein was immunodetected. The activity was inhibited by the E-NTPDase inhibitor POM 1 (Figure 2).

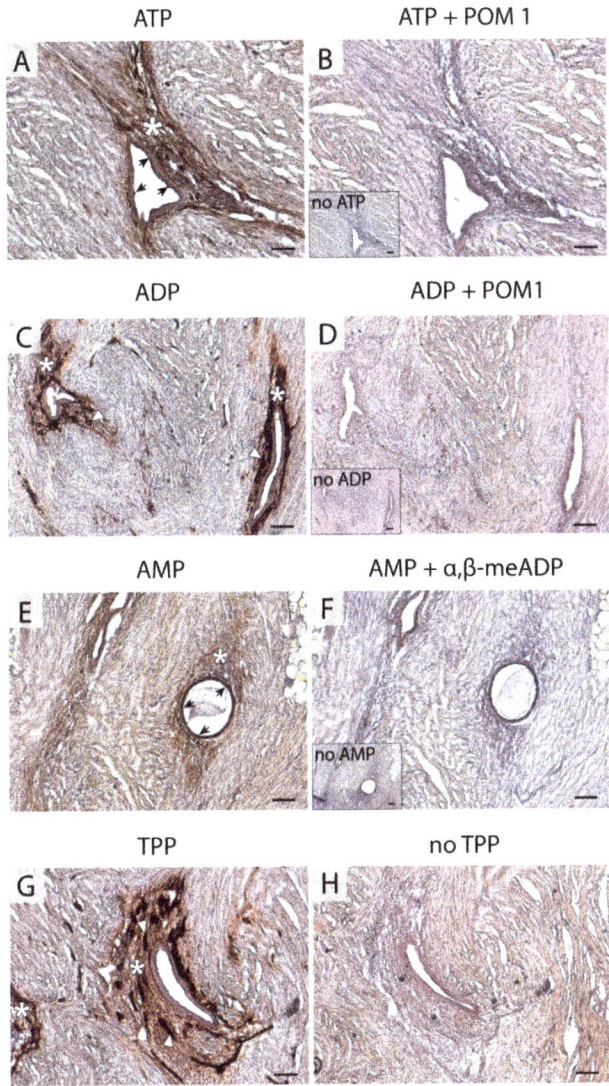

Figure 2. Nucleotidase in situ histochemistry in superficial peritoneal endometriosis lesions. Dark brown deposits correspond to enzyme activity. ATPase activity was detected in the epithelial cells (arrows) and stroma (asterisk) of the lesion (A). ADPase activity was strongly detected in the stroma (asterisks) of the lesion and, remarkably, in blood vessels (arrowheads) (C). ATPase and ADPase activities were abrogated in the presence of the NTPDase inhibitor POM 1 (B,D, respectively). In situ AMPase activity was detected in the epithelial (arrows) and stromal (asterisk) components of the lesion (E). The AMPase was inhibited in the presence of α,β-meADP (F). Insets in (B,D,F) correspond to the activity experiments performed in the absence of substrate (no ATP, no ADP, and no AMP, respectively). TPPase activity was distributed in the stroma (asterisks), including the blood vessels (arrowheads) of lesions (G). As a control, TPPase activity was also performed without substrate (no TPP, H). Scale bars are 100 µm.

2.2. NTPDase2 Expression in the Eutopic and Ectopic Endometrial Tissues

NTPDase2 label in endometria of women with endometriosis was found in basal stroma and cilia of epithelial ciliated cells (Figure 3), coinciding with the recently described expression in non-pathological endometria [14]. All types of ectopic lesions displayed cilia staining, except three deeply infiltrative lesions localized in oviducts that did not display NTPDase2 staining in the cilia. However, the rest of the deep lesions with another ectopic location showed NTPDase2 labeling in their ciliated cells. Stroma was labeled in peritoneal (100% of the cases) and deep lesions (65%), but much less so in ovarian lesions (37%). In situ ATPase activity was detected in the same locations where NTPDase2 was expressed, and it was inhibited by the E-NTPDase inhibitor POM 1 (Figure 2).

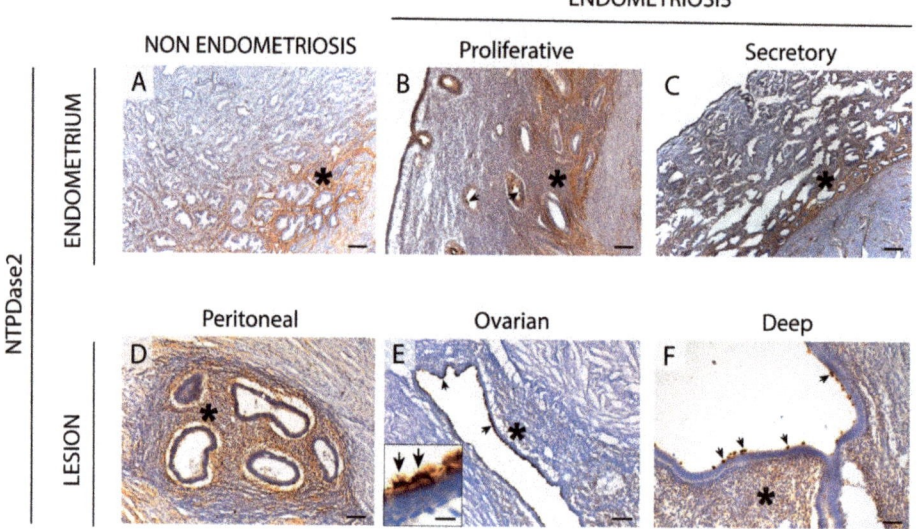

Figure 3. Immunolocalization of NTPDase2 in the eutopic (**A–C**) and ectopic (**D–F**) endometrial tissue. NTPDase2 was detected in the stroma of the basal layer (asterisks) in cyclic endometria from women without (**A**) and with (**B,C**) endometriosis. It was also present in the stromal component (asterisks) of the superficial peritoneal (**D**) and deep infiltrating lesions (**F**, vaginal nodule). NTPDase2 was also found in eutopic and ectopic epithelial ciliated cells in the cilia (arrows) (detail in the inset in **E**). Scale bars are 200 µm (**A,C**), 100 µm (**B,D–F**), and 10 µm (inset in **E**).

Interestingly, we observed the NTPDase2 label in the connective tissue that surrounds the lesions clearly defining the limits of the ectopically located endometrial tissue in a large number of cases (Figure S2).

Perivascular NTPDase2+ cells were also found in eutopic and ectopic endometrial tissue. We confirmed that these cells were also positive for the endometrial mesenchymal stem cell (eMSC) marker Sushi Domain Containing 2 (SUSD2). Double immunolabeling for NTPDase2 and SUSD2 revealed that both proteins were expressed by the same perivascular cells (Figure S3). This coincides with recently published results in non-pathological endometria [14]. Nevertheless, NTPDase2+ SUSD2+ perivascular cells were not present in all the endometriotic lesions.

2.3. NTPDase3 Expression in the Eutopic and Ectopic Endometrial Tissues

In endometrium, NTPDase3 was immunolocalized apically in the epithelial glandular cells. The expression varied during the cycle, being maximal in the secretory phase, as previously described for non-pathological endometria [8]. Ciliated cells were also apically labeled with the label accumulated at the base of the cilia (Figure 4). In addition, NTPDase3 was not detected in atrophic endometria in endometriosis (Figure S1) while it is expressed in atrophic endometria of women without the disease.

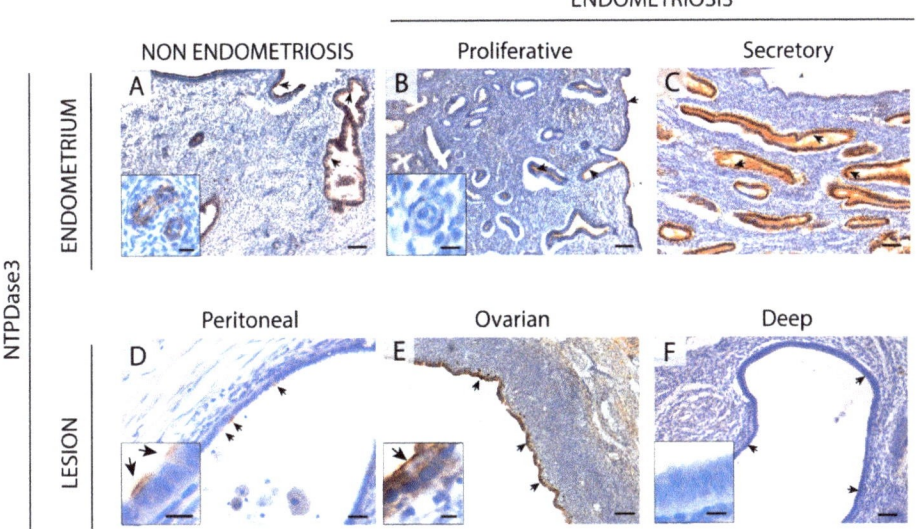

Figure 4. Immunolocalization of NTPDase3 in the eutopic (**A–C**) and ectopic (**D–F**) endometrial tissue. NTPDase3 was immunodetected in ciliated and non-ciliated cells of cyclic endometrium from women without (**A**) and those with (**B,C**) endometriosis (arrows), with changes in expression along the menstrual cycle, reaching a maximum at the secretory phase (**C**). Moreover, NTPDase3 was present in the endothelial cells of spiral arteries of women without endometriosis (inset in **A**) but not in the cyclic endometria from women with the disease (inset in **B**). In ectopic endometrial tissue, NTPDase3 was weakly expressed in the epithelial cells (arrows) of peritoneal lesions (**D**) and highly expressed in the epithelium (arrows) of the ovarian endometriomas (**E**). NTPDase3 was absent in the deep infiltrating lesions (**F**, vaginal nodule) (arrows). Insets in images (**D–F**) are details of the epithelium of the three different ectopic lesions. Scale bars are 100 μm (**A–F**), 20 μm (inset in **A**), and 10 μm (insets in **B,D–F**).

The only, but not negligible, difference between endometria from women with and those without endometriosis is the lack of NTPDase3 staining in spiral arteries in endometriosis. It was previously reported that NTPDase3 was a marker of spiral arteries, displaying a perivascular smooth muscle actin (SMA)+ labeling [8].

In endometriotic lesions, NTPDase3 expression was found in the epithelial component. And while in ovarian lesions labeling was intense, in deep infiltrating lesions labeling was sparse and it was only present in 44% of lesions (Figure 4).

2.4. NPP3 Expression in the Eutopic and Ectopic Endometrial Tissues

NPP3 was expressed in epithelial cells of endometria from women with endometriosis with changes in expression throughout the cycle, being maximal in the secretory phase, similar to the features described in a non-endometriosis condition [8].

Remarkably, de novo NPP3 expression was seen in the stroma of endometrial tissue, both eutopic (including atrophic) and ectopic, from women with endometriosis (Figure 5 and Figure S1). Thiamine pyrophosphatase (TPPase) in situ activity, a functional assay for E-NPPs, was also seen in the stroma of eutopic endometrium and endometriotic lesions (Figure 2).

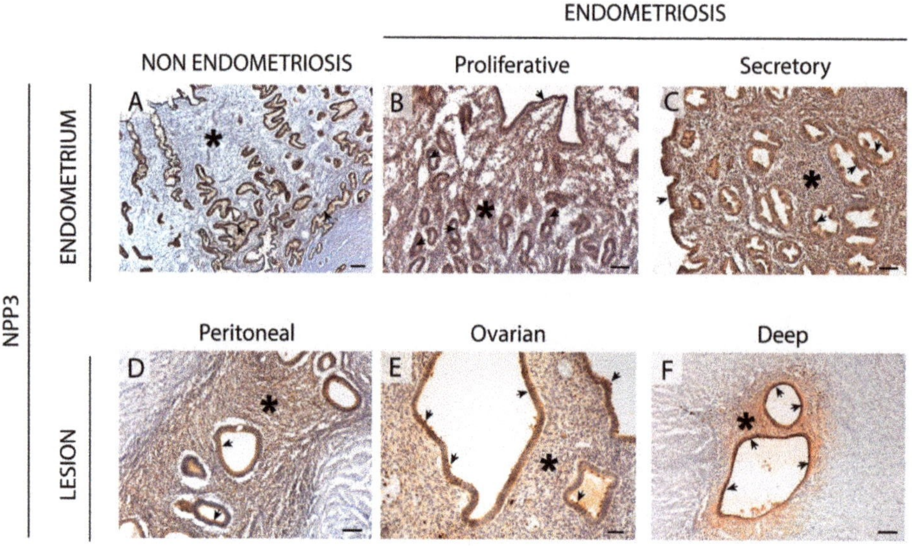

Figure 5. Immunolocalization of NPP3 in the eutopic (**A–C**) and ectopic (**D–F**) endometrial tissue. NPP3 is present in the luminal and glandular epithelial cells of endometrium from women without (**A**) or with (**B,C**) endometriosis (arrows), with changes in expression along the menstrual cycle, reaching a maximum at the secretory phase (**C**). NPP3 was expressed by the stroma (asterisks) only in endometriosis condition, including eutopic endometrium (**B,C**), and ectopic lesions: peritoneal (**D**), ovarian (**E**), and deep infiltrating (**F**, intestinal nodule). NPP3 is also present in the endometrial epithelial cells of lesions (arrows). Scale bars are 200 μm (**A**) and 100 μm (**B–F**).

2.5. CD73 Expression in the Eutopic and Ectopic Endometrial Tissues

CD73 was expressed in ciliated cells from the surface epithelium. The label is apical and comprised the entire length of the cilia. CD73 was also immunodetected in glands.

Moreover, CD73 was detected in the stromal cells in both proliferative and secretory phases, mainly in the functional layer. CD73 was, however, absent in the stromal cells of the atrophic endometria from women with endometriosis, in contrast to the atrophic endometria of women without endometriosis (Figure 6). The ectopic endometrial tissue also displayed CD73 epithelial label; however, the endometriotic lesions with stromal CD73 label decreased in relation to the severity of the lesion. In fact, 71% of peritoneal lesions presented CD73 in the endometrial stromal cells versus 48% of the ovarian endometriomas and 22% of deep infiltrating lesions.

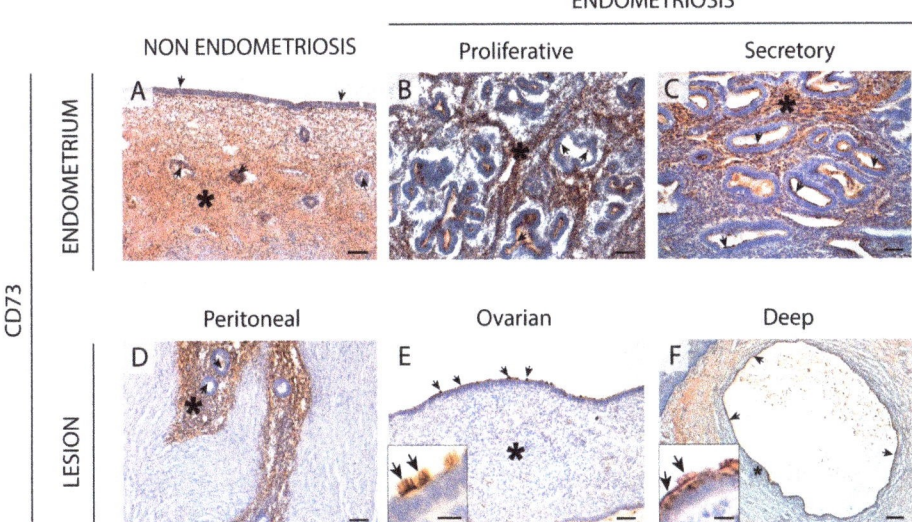

Figure 6. Immunolocalization of CD73 in the eutopic (**A–C**) and ectopic (**D–F**) endometrial tissue. CD73 was detected in the stroma (asterisks) of the cyclic endometrium from women without (**A**) or with (**B,C**) endometriosis and in the superficial peritoneal lesions (**D**). CD73 labelling was absent in the stroma (asterisks) of the ovarian (**E**) and deep infiltrating lesions (**F**, vaginal nodule). CD73 was also present in the ciliated and non-ciliated epithelial cells in the eutopic and ectopic endometrial tissue (arrows). Insets in images E and F correspond to the epithelium of ovarian and deep lesions, respectively. Scale bars are 100 µm (**A,B,D**), 50 µm (**C,E**), 10 µm (**E** inset), 200 µm (**F**), and 15 µm (**F** inset).

In situ AMPase activity was detected in the same locations where CD73 was expressed and it was inhibited by the specific inhibitor α, β-methylene-ADP (α, β-meADP) (Figure 2).

2.6. Enzyme Dipeptidyl Peptidase IV/CD26 Expression in the Eutopic and Ectopic Endometrial Tissues

CD26 was immunodetected in endometria from women with and without endometriosis. CD26 was only detected in the epithelial cells of endometrium with the already described changes in the level of expression throughout the cycle (Figure 7). CD26 staining was very weak in atrophic endometria, and only 33% of cases presented CD26 labeling in the glandular epithelium (Figure S1).

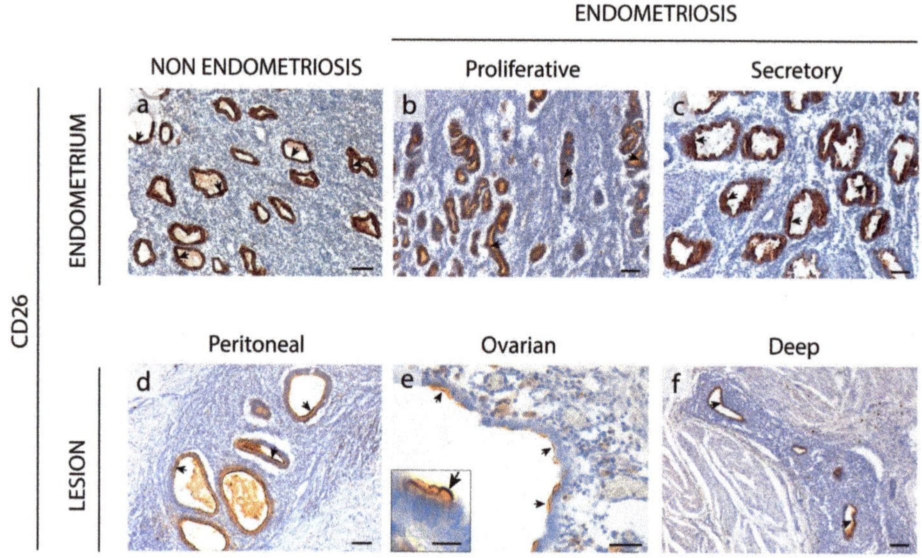

Figure 7. Immunolocalization of CD26 in the eutopic (**a–c**) and ectopic (**d–f**) endometrial tissue. CD26 was detected in epithelial cells (arrows) of the cyclic endometria of women without (**a**) or with (**b,c**) endometriosis. CD26 was also expressed by the endometrial epithelial cells (arrows) of peritoneal (**d**), ovarian (**e**), and deep infiltrating lesions (**F**, vesical nodule). Inset in (**e**) shows a detail of the CD26 labelling at the apical membrane of epithelial non-ciliated cells of an ovarian lesion. Scale bars are 100 µm (**a–d,f**), 50 µm (**e**), and 10 µm (**e** inset).

CD26 was expressed in the epithelial component of all types of endometriotic lesions (Figure 7).

3. Discussion

Purinergic signaling plays a role in reproduction, and changes in its elements have been described in the pathology of endometriosis. Extracellular ATP may be involved in two of the major symptoms of endometriosis, which are infertility and pain [9,15,16]. In the present study we characterized the expression in eutopic and ectopic endometrial tissue of different ectonucleotidases involved in the regulation of ATP levels in tissue microenvironment. We have compared the results with those previously published in non-pathological endometria [8,14]. Tissue distribution in endometriosis coincides with the control condition except in the case of NPP3 which is present in stroma only in endometriosis. Ciliated cells of endometria display the same expression pattern as in control fallopian tubes. Changes in expression and activity are consistently recorded, the greatest being in the stroma (Figure 8). These findings provide information to elucidate the cellular and molecular mechanism as well as the etiology and the progression of the disease, which might help to identify new diagnostic and therapeutic targets.

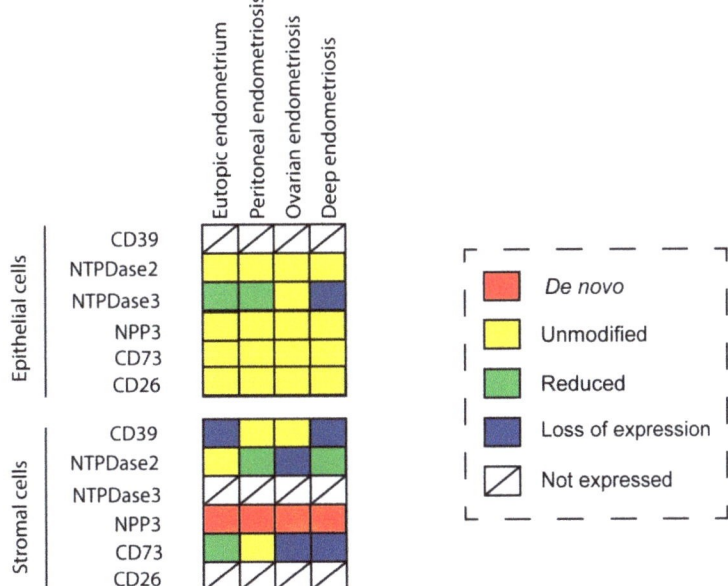

Figure 8. Color representation of changes of ectonucleotidase expression in the eutopic and ectopic endometrial tissue in endometriosis in comparison to the endometria of women without endometriosis. De novo, in red, indicates that this is the first time the label is detected in this cell type; unmodified; in yellow, indicates no changes in label between endometriosis and non-endometriosis; reduced, in green, indicates that the label is diminished in the endometriosis condition; loss of expression, in blue, indicates lack of expression in endometriosis; not expressed indicates that the label is never reported in this particular cell type in any condition.

The CD39-adenosinergic axis, with CD39 and CD73 acting sequentially to hydrolyze ATP to adenosine, is considered the main duo responsible for metabolizing extracellular ATP, generating an immunosuppressive adenosine-rich microenvironment in physiological and pathophysiological conditions [17]. In endometrium, the expression pattern of these ectonucleotidases and their changes throughout the cycle are well studied. Under physiological conditions, endometrial stromal cells express both CD39 and CD73. While CD39 expression is constant throughout the cycle, CD73 fluctuates [8,18], thus determining variations in adenosine level in the microenvironment. In the present study we note that eutopic endometrium of women with endometriosis displays the same already known expression pattern of CD73 but mostly loses CD39 stromal expression. A plausible consequence of the concomitant unbalanced ATP hydrolysis is the accumulation of extracellular ATP in the endometrial stromal microenvironment. This might well play a role in the generation and maintenance of the chronic inflammatory state of endometria of women with endometriosis. Moreover, extracellular ATP is closely related to various immune and inflammatory factors that are known to be involved in the infertility of women with endometriosis, by reducing the quality of gametes and their rates of transport and implantation, and by increasing the pregnancy loss rate [19].

This situation could explain the de novo stromal expression of NPP3 in endometriosis throughout the cycle and in atrophic endometrium, as a cellular tool to offset the loss of ATPase activity due to the lack of CD39. However, NPP3 action would not be sufficient to replace ATPase activity because NPP3 has a lower affinity for ATP than CD39 [6]; moreover stromal NPP3 expression is not coordinated with CD73 expression throughout the cycle.

Changes in the CD39-CD73 pathway were also found in endometriotic lesions. Our findings indicate that the changes in ATP hydrolysis resulting from CD39 and CD73 activity are related to the severity of endometriosis since their expression is lost in deep infiltrating lesions. These changes of expression would lead to an extracellular ATP accumulation that would in turn promote the secretion of cytokines and growth factors into the ectopic milieu, with a concomitant increase in survival and growth rates of endometrial cells [20,21]. Unfortunately, the exact function of extracellular ATP in endometriosis is not clear. While ATP signaling seems to be closely related to the origin and progression of endometriosis, intramuscular injection of ATP in a rat model of endometriosis was found to reduce the size of the ectopic induced lesions [22]. Our results are in line with previous studies that showed differing expression of the protein ATPase Na+/K+ Transporting Family Member Beta 4 (ATP1B4) between patients with and without endometriosis, in favor of a decrease of the hydrolysis of ATP in the endometriosis patients [23,24]. The authors stated that ATP was clearly related with the formation and development of endometriosis disease. Moreover, pain is a characteristic symptom of endometriosis, and ATP is a pain factor mainly acting through the purinoreceptor P2X3 that has also been studied in endometriosis. P2X3 has been found in the epithelial and some stromal cells of eutopic and ectopic endometrial tissue as well as on sensory nerve fibers in endometriotic lesions. Its expression levels correlate with the severity of pain in women with endometriosis [25]. Moreover, the use of A-317491, a selective P2X3 receptor antagonist, relieved pain with a prolonged antinociceptive effect in rats [26], and the receptor is thus a target for the pharmacological approach of endometriosis pain relief. Therefore, the increased levels of extracellular ATP might well be related to the endometriosis-associated pain. These results parallel the difference in CD73 and CD39 expression between the three entities of endometriosis, where the most extreme change has been detected in the deep infiltrating lesions, an important indicator of the severity of pain in endometriosis [27]. Additionally, the downregulation of CD73 has been described in poorly differentiated and advanced-stage endometrial carcinoma. Adenosine generated by the activity of CD73 located in the areas of cell-cell contacts regulates cell-cell adhesions by the regulation of the primary component of filopodia (F-actin). In fact, cell migration and invasion in high-grade and advanced-stage endometrial carcinomas is dependent on the loss of the adenosine generated by CD73 [28]. According to Sampson's theory of retrograde menstruation, endometrial tissue detached during menses has to travel through the fallopian tubes to the ectopic site of implantation, such as the ovarian surface or the peritoneal wall, and must then invade and adhere to the self-tissue of the new localization, proliferating and evading the immune response to form the endometriotic lesion [29]. For this reason, the loss of CD73 in the two most severe entities of endometriosis, ovarian and deep endometriosis, as well as its implication in the inflammatory state of endometriosis, might also play a role in the migration and invasive properties of ectopic cells needed to generate the lesion.

An important finding is the identification of NPP3 label as a new histopathological marker of the disease since we have demonstrated its expression and activity in the stroma only in endometriosis, in both eutopic and ectopic tissues. NPP3 has already been identified in endometrial epithelial cells, a fact that is also confirmed in the case of endometriosis without any variation. A previous study by our group also demonstrated the presence of NPP3 in the contents of endometriomas although the levels did not differ from those of the simple ovarian cysts used as controls and therefore its presence was not exclusive of endometriosis [16]. The relevance of the study reported here is its presence in eutopic endometria which discriminates between endometriosis and non-endometriosis conditions, which might allow its use as a histopathological diagnostic tool. To our knowledge, NPP3 has been identified in epithelial cell types, in cells of the immune system, mainly mast cells, and in tumor cells with an epithelial or myeloid origin [8,30–34]. The specific detection of NPP3 in the endometrial stromal cells of eutopic endometria and in all three entities of endometriosis can be used as a histopathologic marker of endometriosis disease. In addition to its role in the control of extracellular ATP levels, NPP3 might well play a role in the invasive capacity of the stromal endometrial cells in endometriosis since it is known that overexpression of NPP3 in murine fibroblasts stimulates the motility and the invasiveness of these cells [35]. Our finding of de novo NPP3 in stromal cells, with greater expression in the functional layer which is shed during menses, and the relation of NPP3 with the cell motility and invasion, suggest involvement of NPP3 in the formation and progression of endometriotic lesions based on the retrograde menstruation theory [29]. Besides the importance of NPP3 as histopathological marker, additional studies are needed to determine the precise role of NPP3 in the pathogenesis and progression of endometriosis. It might well be a new target for pharmacological therapy of endometriosis. Indeed, targeting NPP3 is feasible since phase 1 trials using an antibody drug conjugate targeting this protein have been completed in patients with advanced metastatic renal cell carcinoma with promising antitumor results [36].

We found NTPDase2 expression in the same cell types and structures as in the non-endometriosis condition. Moreover, NTPDase2 was expressed by perivascular cells in some lesions with colocalization with the eMSCs marker SUSD2. Functional studies are needed to determinate whether NTPDase2+ SUSD2+ cells are eMSCs as in the eutopic endometrium. Retrograde shedding of stem cells into the pelvic cavity without immune clearance is thought to be lesion-initiating. Therefore, it would be of interest to compare lesions containing the NTPDase2+ SUSD2+ cell population with lesions without it.

NTPDase3 was described in epithelial cells and spiral arteries in healthy endometria. In fact, NTPDase3 has been considered a spiral artery marker [8]. But we did not find NTPDase3 labeling in spiral arteries of women with endometriosis. Spiral artery remodeling plays a central role in establishing and maintaining a normal pregnancy, and impaired remodeling is involved in common pregnancy disorders. This might be also one of the mechanisms underlying the decreased pregnancy rates in women with endometriosis. It is important to highlight the loss of NTPDase3 in the epithelial cells of deep infiltrating lesions. Although NTPDase3 has been little explored in pathological conditions, a decrease in *ntpdase3* expression has been described during the induction of mouse bladder cancer, suggesting its participation in cancer establishment and progression [37]. This result, together with the loss of NTPDase3 in the epithelial cells of the most severe form of endometriosis, provides further evidence of the need to study its role in the pathophysiology of endometriosis and cancer.

CD26 or dipeptidyl peptidase IV (DPPIV) is a membrane glycoprotein that binds, among other peptides, the ectoenzyme ADA in humans. It is involved in the protection of the tissue against local inflammation and in intracellular signaling. CD26 has been described as a cancer stem cell marker and tumor suppressor protein in certain types of cancer. By contrast, CD26 overexpression promotes cell proliferation, invasion, and tumorigenesis in endometrial carcinoma cells [38]. In endometriosis, Tan et al. [39] described the increase of endometrial stromal cell migration and invasion in part by reduced expression of CD26 under hypoxia conditions and also by CD26 inhibition. Other studies performed in tissue, including ours, have not matched these in vitro results with cell culture since we were not able to detect CD26 in endometrial stroma, but only in epithelial glandular cells. This might be due to the differing behavior of cells in vitro or even to technical reasons. Here, we show high expression of CD26 in the epithelial cells of eutopic endometrium and in ectopic tissue. The difference with the endometrial expression in women without endometriosis is that CD26 expression in endometriosis is constant throughout the cycle. It would be interesting to see whether the high expression of CD26 in ectopic epithelial cells has a similar effect to that of endometrial carcinoma cells on cell migration and invasion ability. In relation to the ATP metabolism, knowing the levels of ADA, the soluble enzyme that hydrolyses the extracellular adenosine to control the immunosuppressive milieu, is key to understanding what is happening in endometriosis. In a previous study, high levels of ADA were found in the contents of ovarian endometriomas [16]. We were, however, unable to detect ADA by immunostaining due to the technical limitations of the antibodies available, and we cannot be certain whether high levels of CD26 in tissue is related to an increase in ADA activity.

The changes in the expression of the ectonucleotidases described here in eutopic and ectopic endometrium argue for extracellular ATP accumulation. The greatest loss of ectonucleotidase expression was found in the deep infiltrating endometriosis, the most severe endometriosis subtype [40,41]. Our results, together with the role of ATP in pain [25,42], lend support to the involvement of ectonucleotidase expression changes with the severity of endometriosis. Moreover, our results reinforce the relevance of the stroma and tissue microenvironment in the etiopathology and progression of endometriosis disease. Future studies on the role of purinergic signaling in endometriosis are needed to identify biomarkers of the disease and to develop new therapeutic strategies that would allow for earlier detection and respect for the reproductive wishes of women with endometriosis. However, unlike in cancer, where ectonucleotidase blockade is a therapeutic tool, in endometriosis the use of inhibitors of ectonucleotidases does not seem to represent an appropriate strategy. On the contrary, increasing the ATPase activity would combat the eventual ATP accumulation of endometrial microenvironment. In line with this, the use of A-317491, an antagonist of the ATP receptor P2X3, relieves pain in endometriosis [26]. Administration of soluble CD39 is known to be safe and is well studied in the context of cardiovascular diseases where it is known to prevent thrombus formation (reviewed in [43]).

4. Materials and Methods

4.1. Samples

The ethical principles of this study adhere to the Helsinki Declaration, and all the procedures were approved by the ethics committee for clinical investigation of Bellvitge Hospital (project identification code PR090/15, Acta 21/16, 12/2016). All the patients included gave written informed consent. Fifty-seven patients with endometriotic lesions (ectopic endometrial tissue) were recruited for the study by the Gynecology Service of Bellvitge Hospital (Barcelona, Spain) between March 2016 and July 2019, and by the Gynecology Service of Dexeus Institute (Barcelona, Spain) between October 2016 and March 2018. Thirty-four endometrium samples were obtained by the Gynecology Service of Bellvitge Hospital from women without endometriosis or endometrial malignancy as a control group (including 10 proliferative, 4 secretory, and 20 atrophic endometria; age mean of patients = 55.03 years, standard derivation = 11.83).

Human endometrial samples from women with endometriosis ($n = 25$) were obtained from hysterectomy specimens without endometrial malignancy at the pathology services of Bellvitge Hospital and Dexeus Hospital. Peritoneal endometriosis ($n = 7$), ovarian endometriosis ($n = 27$), and/or deep endometriosis ($n = 28$) were surgically removed in the gynecology services of the same hospitals. Demographic description of the samples from the women with endometriosis are summarized in Table 3. Endometrial dating was carried out by the pathology services.

Table 3. Demographics of patients with endometriosis.

Type of Endometrium	Number of Cases	Age (years) ± Standard Deviation	Average (Range)
Proliferative	12	44.33 ± 3.11	39–51
Secretory	10	45.00 ± 5.21	38–53
Atrophic	3	43.00 ± 4.00	39–47
Type of Lesion			
Peritoneal	7	40.29 ± 4.96	35–46
Ovarian	27	43.42 ± 8.36	23–57
Deep	21	38.00 ± 5.73	27–47

Excised tissue samples were fixed with 4% paraformaldehyde, cryoprotected by introducing them into a 30% (w/v) sucrose solution at 4 °C for 24 h, and then embedded in O.C.T freezing media (Tissue-Tek®; Sakura Finetk, Zoeterwoude, Netherlands). Fifteen μm sections were obtained using a Cryostat Leica CM1950 (Leica, Wetzlar, Germany). Sections were put onto poly-L-lysine coated glass slides and stored at −20 °C until use. Routine haematoxylin and eosin staining was performed.

4.2. Antibodies

Primary antibodies used in this study are listed in Table 4. Secondary antibodies used for immunohistochemistry were horseradish peroxidase (HRP)-conjugated goat anti-mouse (EnVision™ + System; DAKO, Carpinteria, CA, USA) and HRP-conjugated goat anti-rabbit (EnVision™ + System).

Table 4. List of primary antibodies used for immunolabeling experiments.

Antibody Specificity	Name/Clone	Source	Supplier	Dilution
NTPDase1 (CD39)	BU-61	Mouse	Ancell (188-820)	1:500
NTPDase2	-	Rabbit	Enzo (ALX-215-045)	1:100
NTPDase2	H9s	Mouse	http://ectonucleotidases-ab.com	1:400
NTPDase3	B_3S_{10}	Mouse	http://ectonucleotidases-ab.com	1:500
NPP3	NP4D6	Mouse	Abcam (ab90754)	1:100
5'-nucleotidase (CD73)	4G4	Mouse	Abcam (ab81720)	1:50
CD26	202-36	Mouse	Abcam (ab3154)	1:100
CD26	202-36	Mouse	NovusBio (NBP2-44571)	1:100
SUSD2	-	Rabbit	Abcam (ab121214)	1:400

Secondary antibodies used for immunofluorescence assays were Alexa Fluor 488 goat anti-mouse and Alexa Fluor 647 goat anti-rabbit (Thermo Fisher Scientific, Rockford, Illinois, USA). Secondary antibodies were used at 1:500 and dilutions were made in PBS.

4.3. Immunolabeling Experiments

Slices were washed twice with PBS to remove the O.C.T freezing media and then pre-incubated for 1 h at room temperature (RT) with PBS containing 20% normal goat serum (NGS, Gibco, Paisley, UK), 0.2% Triton and 0.2% gelatin (Merck, Darmstadt, Germany). For immunohistochemistry experiments a previous blocking of endogenous peroxidase activity was performed with 10% methanol (v/v) and 2% H2O2 (v/v) in PBS for 30 min. Slices were then incubated overnight (O/N) at 4 °C with the primary antibodies (listed in Table 2) diluted in PBS. After three washes in PBS, tissue sections were incubated with the appropriate secondary antibodies for 1 h at RT, except HRP-goat anti-mouse and HRP-goat anti-rabbit, which were incubated for 30 min at RT. Secondary antibodies alone were routinely included as controls for the experiments.

For immunohistochemistry, the peroxidase reaction was performed in a solution containing 0.6 mg/mL 3, 3'-diaminobenzidine substrate (DAB; D-5637, Sigma-Aldrich, Saint Louis, MO, USA) and 0.5 µL/mL H2O2 in PBS for 10 min, and stopped with PBS. Nuclei were counterstained with haematoxylin and slides were then dehydrated and mounted with DPX mounting medium. Samples were observed under light Nikon Eclipse E200 and photographed under a light Leica DMD 108 microscope. In fluorescence assays, for nuclei labeling, slides were mounted with aqueous mounting medium with DAPI (ProLong™ Gold antifade reagent with DAPI, Life Technologies, Paisley, UK). Samples were then observed and photographed under a Zeiss LSM 880 Confocal Laser Scanning Microscope. Fluorescence images were processed with the software ZEN 2.3 SP1 (Zeiss, Oberkochen, Germany).

Immunohistochemical staining was independently evaluated by two observers. Staining distribution was recorded. Label intensity was scored as negative (-), weak (+), intermediate (++), or strongly positive (+++).

4.4. In situ ATPase, ADPase, AMPase, and TPPase Activity Experiments

A protocol based on the Wachstein/Meisel lead phosphate method was used [8,11,44,45]. The sections were washed twice with 50 mM Tris-maleate buffer pH 7.4 and pre-incubated for 30 min at RT with 50 mM Tris-maleate buffer pH 7.4 containing 2 mM $MgCl_2$ and 0.25 mM sucrose. The enzymatic reaction was carried out by incubating tissue sections for 1 h at 37 °C with 50 mM

Tris-maleate buffer pH 7.4 supplemented with 0.25 mM sucrose, 2 mM MgCl$_2$, 5 mM MnCl$_2$, 3 % Dextran, 2 mM Pb(NO$_3$)$_2$, and 2 mM CaCl$_2$. All experiments were performed in the presence of 2.5 mM levamisole, as an inhibitor of alkaline phosphatase (AP) activity, and in the presence of 1 mM AMP, ADP, ATP, or TPP as a substrate. TPP is a false substrate, which can be cleaved by the pyrophosphatase activity of E-NPPs. Control assays were performed in the absence of nucleotide. For E-NTPDase inhibition experiments, 1 mM POM 1 was added to pre-incubation and enzymatic reaction buffers. For CD73 inhibition experiments, 1 mM α, β-meADP was added to pre-incubation and enzymatic reaction buffers. The reaction was revealed by incubation with 1% (NH$_4$)$_2$S (v/v) for exactly 1 min. Nuclei were counterstained with haematoxylin. Samples were mounted with aqueous mounting medium (FluoromountTM, Sigma-Aldrich), observed under a light Nikon Eclipse E200 microscope, and photographed under a light Leica DMD 108 microscope.

4.5. Statistical Analysis

The predictive analytics software IBM SPSS Statistics v22 (IBM Corp., Armonk, NY, USA) was used for the creation of frequency tables with the distribution of ectonucleotidases in each endometrial component as well as the label intensity score in each case.

5. Conclusions

In the present study, we examined the presence of ectonucleotidases in eutopic and ectopic endometrial tissue in endometriosis. The main changes in expression and activity were found in the stromal compartment. We observed loss of the main route of ATP hydrolysis, the CD39-CD73 axis, in deep infiltrating endometriosis, the most severe endometriosis subtype. These findings point to ATP accumulation in the endometrial tissue microenvironment in endometriosis as possibly contributing to the two main symptoms of the disease: pain and infertility. Remarkably, we noted that immunodetection of NPP3 in endometrial stroma is exclusive to the endometriosis condition, and therefore it may well be a histological marker of the disease. Future studies on the role of purinergic signaling in endometriosis are needed to elucidate the underlying cellular and molecular mechanisms and to identify new diagnostic and therapeutic targets.

Supplementary Materials: Supplementary materials can be found at http://www.mdpi.com/1422-0067/20/22/5532/s1. Figure S1. Immunolocalization of CD39 (A), NTPDase2 (B), NTPDase3 (C), NPP3 (D), CD73 (E), and CD26 (F) in atrophic endometria from women with endometriosis. Scale bars are 100 μm (A,C–F) and 200 μm (B). Figure S2. Immunolocalization of NTPDase2 in peritoneal (A), ovarian (B), and deep endometriosis lesions (C). There is NTPDase2 labelling in the connective tissue limiting the lesions (*arrows*). Scale bars are 100 μm (A,C) and 300 μm (B). Figure S3. Confocal fluorescence images of a proliferative endometrium (A–D) of a woman with endometriosis and an ovarian endometrioma (E–H) labeled with the antibodies against NTPDase2 (A,E) and the eMSC marker SUSD2 (B,F). Nuclei were labeled with DAPI (C,G). Merge images (D,H) show the co-localization of NTPDase2 and SUSD2 in perivascular cells in the eutopic and ectopic endometrial tissue. Scale bars are 50 μm (D,H).

Author Contributions: C.T. contributed to the design and execution of the experiments, and contributed to the writing of the paper. A.V., F.T., and X.M.-G. performed the histopathologic diagnostic. I.G.d.A. contributed to conducting the experiments. J.S. generated the antibodies against *ENTPD2* and *ENTPD3*. M.E.F.-M., P.B., B.C., and J.P. visited the women included in the study, made the clinical diagnoses, and performed the surgery to obtain the samples. M.M.-S. conceived the study and contributed to conducting the experiments and to the writing of the paper.

Funding: This study was supported by the Instituto de Salud Carlos III (grant numbers: FIS PI15/00036, PI18/00541), co-funded by FEDER funds/European Regional Development Fund (ERDF)-"a Way to Build Europe"-//FONDOS FEDER "una manera de hacer Europa", and a grant from the Fundación Merck Salud (Ayuda Merck de Investigación 2016-Fertilidad). JS received support from the Canadian Institutes of Health Research (CIHR) and was the recipient of a "Chercheur National" research award from the Fonds de Recherche du Québec – Santé (FRQS).

Acknowledgments: We dedicate this work to the memory of our beloved colleague and friend Lluís de Jover Armengol. We thank CERCA Programme (Generalitat de Catalunya) for institutional support, Tom Yohannan for language editing, and Serveis Científics i Tecnològics (Campus Bellvitge, Universitat de Barcelona) for technical support. We are grateful to the women who donated their samples for the study and to the endometriosis association Endo&Cat for supporting the project.

Conflicts of Interest: The authors declare no conflict of interest. The funders had no role in the design of the study, in the collection, analyses, or interpretation of data, in the writing of the manuscript, or in the decision to publish the results.

Abbreviations

ATP	Adenosine triphosphate
E-NPP	Ecto-nucleotide pyrophophotase/phosphodiesterase
E-NTPDase	Ecto-nucleoside triphosphate diphosphohydrolase
ADP	Adenosine diphosphate
AMP	Adenosine monophosphate
5'-NT	5'-nucleotidase
ADA	Adenosine deaminase
eMSC	Endometrial mesenchymal stem cell
SUSD2	Sushi domain containing 2
SMA	Smooth muscle actin
TPP	Thiamine pyrophosphate
α, β-meADP	α, β-methylene-ADP
ATP1B4	ATPase Na+/K+ Transporting Family Member Beta 4
DPPIV	Dipeptidyl peptidase IV
HRP	Horseradish peroxidase
DAB	3, 3'-diaminobenzidine substrate
AP	Alkaline phosphatase

Appendix A

Table A1. Summary of the number and proportion of tissues labeled with different antibodies.

Samples Stained	NTPDase1 (CD39)	NTPDase2	NTPDase3	NPP3	5'-NT (CD73)	CD26
	Positive Cases/Total of Samples (% of Tissues Stained)					
Eutopic endometrium						
Surface epithelium	1/14 (7.1%)	14/14 (100%)	7/13 (53.8%)	12/13 (92.3%)	9/12 (75%)	7/14 (50%)
Glandular epithelium	1/20 (5%)	20/20 (100%)	16/20 (80%)	18/19 (94.7%)	20/20 (100%)	15/20 (75%)
Endometrial stromal cells	7/20 (35%)	20/20 (100%)	0/20 (0%)	15/19 (78.9%)	12/20 (60%)	0/20 (0%)
Spiral arteries	19/20 (95%)	3/20 (15%)	5/20 (25%)	16/18 (88.9%)	3/20 (15%)	3/19 (15.8%)
Peritoneal endometriosis						
Endometrial epithelial cells	1/7 (14.3%)	7/7 (100%)	7/7 (100%)	7/7 (100%)	5/7 (71.4%)	4/7 (57.1%)
Endometrial stromal cells	6/7 (85.7%)	7/7 (100%)	0/7 (0%)	7/7 (100%)	5/7 (71.4%)	2/7 (28.6%)
Vessels of the lesion	5/7 (71.4%)	0/7 (0%)	0/7 (0%)	0/7 (0%)	1/7 (14.28%)	0/7 (0%)
Ovarian endometriosis						
Endometrial epithelial cells	8/28 (28.6%)	20/28 (71.4%)	16/28 (57.1%)	24/28 (85.7%)	24/28 (85.7%)	19/28 (67.9%)
Endometrial stromal cells	16/27 (59.3%)	10/27 (37%)	3/27 (11.1%)	16/27 (59.3%)	13/27 (48.1%)	2/27 (7.4%)
Vessels of the lesion	23/28 (82.1%)	1/28 (3.6%)	2/28 (7.1%)	8/28 (28.6%)	3/28 (10.7%)	3/28 (10.7%)
Deep endometriosis						
Endometrial epithelial cells	6/28 (21.4%)	23/26 (88.5%)	12/27 (44.4%)	24/28 (85.7%)	17/28 (60.7%)	15/28 (53.6%)
Endometrial stromal cells	9/25 (36%)	17/26 (65.4%)	1/27 (3.7%)	18/27 (66.7%)	6/27 (22.2%)	1/27 (3.7%)
Vessels of the lesion	11/24 (45.8%)	5/25 (20%)	1/27 (3.7%)	7/27 (25.9%)	7/27 (25.9%)	0/27 (0%)

References

1. Ponandai-Srinivasan, S.; Andersson, K.L.; Nister, M.; Saare, M.; Hassan, H.A.; Varghese, S.J.; Peters, M.; Salumets, A.; Gemzell-Danielsson, K.; Lalitkumar, P.G.L. Aberrant expression of genes associated with stemness and cancer in endometria and endometrioma in a subset of women with endometriosis. *Hum. Reprod.* **2018**, *33*, 1924–1938. [CrossRef] [PubMed]
2. Grandi, G.; Mueller, M.D.; Papadia, A.; Kocbek, V.; Bersinger, N.A.; Petraglia, F.; Cagnacci, A.; McKinnon, B. Inflammation influences steroid hormone receptors targeted by progestins in endometrial stromal cells from women with endometriosis. *J. Reprod. Immunol.* **2016**, *117*, 30–38. [CrossRef] [PubMed]

3. Nothnick, W.; Alali, Z. Recent advances in the understanding of endometriosis: The role of inflammatory mediators in disease pathogenesis and treatment. *F1000Research* **2016**, *5*. [CrossRef] [PubMed]
4. Ahn, S.H.; Khalaj, K.; Young, S.L.; Lessey, B.A.; Koti, M.; Tayade, C. Immune-inflammation gene signatures in endometriosis patients. *Fertil. Steril.* **2016**, *106*, 1420–1431. [CrossRef]
5. Zhang, T.; De Carolis, C.; Man, G.C.W.; Wang, C.C. The link between immunity, autoimmunity and endometriosis: A literature update. *Autoimmun. Rev.* **2018**, *17*, 945–955. [CrossRef]
6. Yegutkin, G.G. Enzymes involved in metabolism of extracellular nucleotides and nucleosides: Functional implications and measurement of activities. *Crit. Rev. Biochem. Mol. Biol.* **2014**, *49*, 473–497. [CrossRef]
7. Ziganshin, A.U.; Zaitcev, A.P.; Khasanov, A.A.; Shamsutdinov, A.F.; Burnstock, G. Term-dependency of P2 receptor-mediated contractile responses of isolated human pregnant uterus. *Eur. J. Obstet. Gynecol. Reprod. Biol.* **2006**, *129*, 128–134. [CrossRef]
8. Aliagas, E.; Vidal, A.; Torrejon-Escribano, B.; Taco Mdel, R.; Ponce, J.; de Aranda, I.G.; Sevigny, J.; Condom, E.; Martin-Satue, M. Ecto-nucleotidases distribution in human cyclic and postmenopausic endometrium. *Purinergic Signal.* **2013**, *9*, 227–237. [CrossRef]
9. Burnstock, G. Purinergic signalling in the reproductive system in health and disease. *Purinergic Signal.* **2014**, *10*, 157–187. [CrossRef]
10. Bellezza, I.; Minelli, A. Adenosine in sperm physiology. *Mol. Asp. Med.* **2017**, *55*, 102–109. [CrossRef]
11. Villamonte, M.L.; Torrejon-Escribano, B.; Rodriguez-Martinez, A.; Trapero, C.; Vidal, A.; Gomez de Aranda, I.; Sevigny, J.; Matias-Guiu, X.; Martin-Satue, M. Characterization of ecto-nucleotidases in human oviducts with an improved approach simultaneously identifying protein expression and in situ enzyme activity. *Histochem. Cell Biol.* **2018**, *149*, 269–276. [CrossRef] [PubMed]
12. Barrera, N.P.; Morales, B.; Villalon, M. Plasma and intracellular membrane inositol 1,4,5-trisphosphate receptors mediate the Ca(2+) increase associated with the ATP-induced increase in ciliary beat frequency. *Am. J. Physiol. Cell Physiol.* **2004**, *287*, C1114–C1124. [CrossRef] [PubMed]
13. Yegutkin, G.G. Nucleotide- and nucleoside-converting ectoenzymes: Important modulators of purinergic signalling cascade. *Biochim. Biophys. Acta* **2008**, *1783*, 673–694. [CrossRef] [PubMed]
14. Trapero, C.; Vidal, A.; Rodriguez-Martinez, A.; Sevigny, J.; Ponce, J.; Coroleu, B.; Matias-Guiu, X.; Martin-Satue, M. The ectonucleoside triphosphate diphosphohydrolase-2 (NTPDase2) in human endometrium: A novel marker of basal stroma and mesenchymal stem cells. *Purinergic Signal.* **2019**, *15*, 225–236. [CrossRef] [PubMed]
15. Texido, L.; Romero, C.; Vidal, A.; Garcia-Valero, J.; Fernandez Montoli, M.E.; Baixeras, N.; Condom, E.; Ponce, J.; Garcia-Tejedor, A.; Martin-Satue, M. Ecto-nucleotidases activities in the contents of ovarian endometriomas: Potential biomarkers of endometriosis. *Mediat. Inflamm.* **2014**, *2014*, 120673. [CrossRef]
16. Trapero, C.; Jover, L.; Fernandez-Montoli, M.E.; Garcia-Tejedor, A.; Vidal, A.; Gomez de Aranda, I.; Ponce, J.; Matias-Guiu, X.; Martin-Satue, M. Analysis of the ectoenzymes ADA, ALP, ENPP1, and ENPP3, in the contents of ovarian endometriomas as candidate biomarkers of endometriosis. *Am. J. Reprod. Immunol.* **2018**, *79*. [CrossRef] [PubMed]
17. Bono, M.R.; Fernandez, D.; Flores-Santibanez, F.; Rosemblatt, M.; Sauma, D. CD73 and CD39 ectonucleotidases in T cell differentiation: Beyond immunosuppression. *FEBS Lett.* **2015**, *589*, 3454–3460. [CrossRef]
18. Aliagas, E.; Torrejon-Escribano, B.; Lavoie, E.G.; de Aranda, I.G.; Sevigny, J.; Solsona, C.; Martin-Satue, M. Changes in expression and activity levels of ecto-5′-nucleotidase/CD73 along the mouse female estrous cycle. *Acta Physiol.* **2010**, *199*, 191–197. [CrossRef]
19. Mate, G.; Bernstein, L.R.; Torok, A.L. Endometriosis is a cause of infertility. Does reactive oxygen damage to gametes and embryos play a key role in the pathogenesis of infertility caused by endometriosis? *Front. Endocrinol.* **2018**, *9*, 725. [CrossRef]
20. Ahn, S.H.; Monsanto, S.P.; Miller, C.; Singh, S.S.; Thomas, R.; Tayade, C. Pathophysiology and immune dysfunction in endometriosis. *Biomed. Res. Int.* **2015**, *2015*, 795976. [CrossRef]
21. Faas, M.M.; Saez, T.; de Vos, P. Extracellular ATP and adenosine: The yin and yang in immune responses? *Mol. Asp. Med.* **2017**, *55*, 9–19. [CrossRef] [PubMed]
22. Zhang, C.; Gao, L.; Yi, Y.; Han, H.; Cheng, H.; Ye, X.; Ma, R.; Sun, K.; Cui, H.; Chang, X. Adenosine triphosphate regresses endometrial explants in a rat model of endometriosis. *Reprod. Sci.* **2016**, *23*, 924–930. [CrossRef] [PubMed]

23. Zhang, H.; Niu, Y.; Feng, J.; Guo, H.; Ye, X.; Cui, H. Use of proteomic analysis of endometriosis to identify different protein expression in patients with endometriosis versus normal controls. *Fertil. Steril.* **2006**, *86*, 274–282. [CrossRef] [PubMed]
24. Zhao, Y.; Liu, Y.N.; Li, Y.; Tian, L.; Ye, X.; Cui, H.; Chang, X.H. Identification of biomarkers for endometriosis using clinical proteomics. *Chin. Med. J.* **2015**, *128*, 520–527. [CrossRef] [PubMed]
25. Ding, S.; Zhu, L.; Tian, Y.; Zhu, T.; Huang, X.; Zhang, X. P2X3 receptor involvement in endometriosis pain via ERK signaling pathway. *PLoS ONE* **2017**, *12*, e0184647. [CrossRef]
26. Yuan, M.; Ding, S.; Meng, T.; Lu, B.; Shao, S.; Zhang, X.; Yuan, H.; Hu, F. Effect of A-317491 delivered by glycolipid-like polymer micelles on endometriosis pain. *Int. J. Nanomed.* **2017**, *12*, 8171–8183. [CrossRef]
27. Alimi, Y.; Iwanaga, J.; Loukas, M.; Tubbs, R.S. The clinical anatomy of endometriosis: A review. *Cureus* **2018**, *10*, e3361. [CrossRef]
28. Bowser, J.L.; Blackburn, M.R.; Shipley, G.L.; Molina, J.G.; Dunner, K., Jr.; Broaddus, R.R. Loss of CD73-mediated actin polymerization promotes endometrial tumor progression. *J. Clin. Investig.* **2016**, *126*, 220–238. [CrossRef]
29. Sampson, J. Peritoneal endometriosis due to the menstrual dissemination of endometrial tissue into the peritoneal cavity. *Am. J. Obstet. Gynecol.* **1927**, *14*, 422–469. [CrossRef]
30. Hood, B.L.; Liu, B.; Alkhas, A.; Shoji, Y.; Challa, R.; Wang, G.; Ferguson, S.; Oliver, J.; Mitchell, D.; Bateman, N.W.; et al. Proteomics of the human endometrial glandular epithelium and stroma from the proliferative and secretory phases of the menstrual cycle. *Biol. Reprod.* **2015**, *92*, 106. [CrossRef]
31. Boggavarapu, N.R.; Lalitkumar, S.; Joshua, V.; Kasvandik, S.; Salumets, A.; Lalitkumar, P.G.; Gemzell-Danielsson, K. Compartmentalized gene expression profiling of receptive endometrium reveals progesterone regulated ENPP3 is differentially expressed and secreted in glycosylated form. *Sci. Rep.* **2016**, *6*, 33811. [CrossRef] [PubMed]
32. Donate, F.; Raitano, A.; Morrison, K.; An, Z.; Capo, L.; Avina, H.; Karki, S.; Yang, P.; Ou, J.; Moriya, R.; et al. AGS16F is a novel antibody drug conjugate directed against ENPP3 for the treatment of renal cell carcinoma. *Clin. Cancer Res.* **2016**, *22*, 1989–1999. [CrossRef] [PubMed]
33. Tsai, S.H.; Takeda, K. Regulation of allergic inflammation by the ectoenzyme E-NPP3 (CD203c) on basophils and mast cells. *Semin. Immunopathol.* **2016**, *38*, 571–579. [CrossRef] [PubMed]
34. Chen, Q.; Xin, A.; Qu, R.; Zhang, W.; Li, L.; Chen, J.; Lu, X.; Gu, Y.; Li, J.; Sun, X. Expression of ENPP3 in human cyclic endometrium: A novel molecule involved in embryo implantation. *Reprod. Fertil. Dev.* **2018**, *30*, 1277–1285. [CrossRef]
35. Deissler, H.; Blass-Kampmann, S.; Bruyneel, E.; Mareel, M.; Rajewsky, M.F. Neural cell surface differentiation antigen gp130(RB13-6) induces fibroblasts and glioma cells to express astroglial proteins and invasive properties. *FASEB J.* **1999**, *13*, 657–666. [CrossRef]
36. Thompson, J.A.; Motzer, R.J.; Molina, A.M.; Choueiri, T.K.; Heath, E.I.; Redman, B.G.; Sangha, R.S.; Ernst, D.S.; Pili, R.; Kim, S.K.; et al. Phase I Trials of Anti-ENPP3 Antibody-drug conjugates in advanced refractory renal cell carcinomas. *Clin. Cancer Res.* **2018**, *24*, 4399–4406. [CrossRef]
37. Rockenbach, L.; Braganhol, E.; Dietrich, F.; Figueiro, F.; Pugliese, M.; Edelweiss, M.I.; Morrone, F.B.; Sevigny, J.; Battastini, A.M. NTPDase3 and ecto-5'-nucleotidase/CD73 are differentially expressed during mouse bladder cancer progression. *Purinergic Signal.* **2014**, *10*, 421–430. [CrossRef]
38. Yang, X.; Zhang, X.; Wu, R.; Huang, Q.; Jiang, Y.; Qin, J.; Yao, F.; Jin, G.; Zhang, Y. DPPIV promotes endometrial carcinoma cell proliferation, invasion and tumorigenesis. *Oncotarget* **2017**, *8*, 8679–8692. [CrossRef]
39. Tan, C.W.; Lee, Y.H.; Tan, H.H.; Lau, M.S.; Choolani, M.; Griffith, L.; Chan, J.K. CD26/DPPIV down-regulation in endometrial stromal cell migration in endometriosis. *Fertil. Steril.* **2014**, *102*, 167–177. [CrossRef]
40. Busacca, M.; Chiaffarino, F.; Candiani, M.; Vignali, M.; Bertulessi, C.; Oggioni, G.; Parazzini, F. Determinants of long-term clinically detected recurrence rates of deep, ovarian, and pelvic endometriosis. *Am. J. Obstet. Gynecol.* **2006**, *195*, 426–432. [CrossRef]
41. Koninckx, P.R.; Meuleman, C.; Demeyere, S.; Lesaffre, E.; Cornillie, F.J. Suggestive evidence that pelvic endometriosis is a progressive disease, whereas deeply infiltrating endometriosis is associated with pelvic pain. *Fertil. Steril.* **1991**, *55*, 759–765. [CrossRef]
42. Burnstock, G. Purinergic mechanisms and pain. *Adv. Pharmacol.* **2016**, *75*, 91–137. [CrossRef] [PubMed]
43. Fung, C.Y.; Marcus, A.J.; Broekman, M.J.; Mahaut-Smith, M.P. P2X(1) receptor inhibition and soluble CD39 administration as novel approaches to widen the cardiovascular therapeutic window. *Trends Cardiovasc. Med.* **2009**, *19*, 1–5. [CrossRef] [PubMed]

44. Wachstein, M.; Meisel, E. Histochemistry of hepatic phosphatases of a physiologic pH; with special reference to the demonstration of bile canaliculi. *Am. J. Clin. Pathol.* **1957**, *27*, 13–23. [CrossRef]
45. Martín-Satué, M.; Rodríguez-Martínez, A.; Trapero, C. In situ identification of ectoenzymes involved in the hydrolysis of extracellular nucleotides. In *Immunohistochemistry*; IntechOpen: London, UK, 2019.

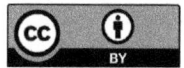

© 2019 by the authors. Licensee MDPI, Basel, Switzerland. This article is an open access article distributed under the terms and conditions of the Creative Commons Attribution (CC BY) license (http://creativecommons.org/licenses/by/4.0/).

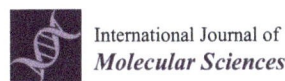

Article

Role of B-Cell Translocation Gene 1 in the Pathogenesis of Endometriosis

Jeong Sook Kim [1], Young Sik Choi [2,3], Ji Hyun Park [4], Jisun Yun [2], Soohyun Kim [4], Jae Hoon Lee [2], Bo Hyon Yun [2,3], Joo Hyun Park [3,4], Seok Kyo Seo [2,3], SiHyun Cho [3,4,*], Hyun-Soo Kim [5,*] and Byung Seok Lee [2,3]

[1] Department of Obstetrics and Gynecology, University of Ulsan College of Medicine, Ulsan University Hospital, Ulsan 44033, Korea
[2] Department of Obstetrics and Gynecology, Severance Hospital, Yonsei University College of Medicine, Seoul 03722, Korea
[3] Institute of Women's Life Medical Science, Yonsei University College of Medicine, Seoul 03722, Korea
[4] Department of Obstetrics and Gynecology, Gangnam Severance Hospital, Yonsei University College of Medicine, Seoul 06273, Korea
[5] Department of Pathology and Translational Genomics, Samsung Medical Center, Sungkyunkwan University School of Medicine, Seoul 06351, Korea
* Correspondence: sihyuncho@yuhs.ac (S.C.); hyun-soo.kim@samsung.com (H.-S.K.)

Received: 22 June 2019; Accepted: 5 July 2019; Published: 9 July 2019

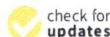

Abstract: Estrogen affects endometrial cellular proliferation by regulating the expression of the *c-myc* gene. B-cell translocation gene 1 (BTG1), a translocation partner of the *c-myc*, is a tumor suppressor gene that promotes apoptosis and negatively regulates cellular proliferation and cell-to-cell adhesion. The aim of this study was to determine the role of BTG1 in the pathogenesis of endometriosis. *BTG1* mRNA and protein expression was evaluated in eutopic and ectopic endometrium of 30 patients with endometriosis (endometriosis group), and in eutopic endometrium of 22 patients without endometriosis (control group). The effect of BTG1 downregulation on cellular migration, proliferation, and apoptosis was evaluated using transfection of primarily cultured human endometrial stromal cells (HESCs) with *BTG1* siRNA. *BTG1* mRNA expression level of eutopic and ectopic endometrium of endometriosis group were significantly lower than that of the eutopic endometrium of the control group. Migration and wound healing assays revealed that BTG1 downregulation resulted in a significant increase in migration potential of HESCs, characterized by increased expression of matrix metalloproteinase 2 (MMP2) and MMP9. Downregulation of BTG1 in HESCs significantly reduced Caspase 3 expression, indicating a decrease in apoptotic potential. In conclusion, our data suggest that downregulation of BTG1 plays an important role in the pathogenesis of endometriosis.

Keywords: BTG1; endometriosis; human endometrial stromal cells

1. Introduction

Endometriosis is a commonly occurring gynecological disorder that may cause pelvic pain and infertility [1]. The diagnosis of endometriosis is pathologically confirmed by the ectopic presence of endometrial-like epithelium and stroma. Endometriosis is prevalent in approximately 10% of all reproductive women, 20–30% of women with infertility, and 40–80% of women with chronic pelvic pain, or both [2]. Although several pathogenic theories have been suggested, the exact underlying mechanisms of endometriosis still remains unclear. The long-term management of endometriosis-related symptoms and recurrence after surgery also remains a challenge. Understanding endometrial cellular expression of certain genes and proteins may result in improved diagnosis and treatment of endometriosis.

Cellular proliferation, differentiation, and apoptosis are cell cycle-dependent processes [3]. Disruption of cell cycle regulation results in tumor formation and progression [4]. Estrogen regulates endometrial cellular proliferation by binding to an atypical *cis*-element in *c-myc* promoter [5]. Serum estrogen levels are 5–8 times higher than normal in women with endometriosis [6]. Estrogen receptor-α and *c-myc* are highly expressed in deeply infiltrating endometriotic tissue [7]. Therefore, the *c-myc* gene may play a crucial role in endometriosis.

B-cell translocation gene 1 (*BTG1*) was identified as a translocation partner of the *c-myc* gene in B-cell chronic lymphocytic leukemia [8]. BTG1 belongs to the BTG/TOB family of anti-proliferative proteins that include BTG2, BTG3, TOB1, and TOB2, which regulates cell growth and differentiation [9–11]. BTG1 is primarily expressed in quiescent cells at G_0/G_1 phase of cell cycle, and its level declines as cells enter S phase [12]. Exogenous overexpression of BTG1 reduces proliferation of murine fibroblasts by inducing G1 arrest and/or apoptosis [12]. BTG1 also negatively regulate proliferation of murine microglial cells [13].

BTG1 is also a known tumor suppressor gene that negatively regulates cellular proliferation, cell-to-cell adhesion, migration, and invasion in carcinomas of esophagus, nasopharynx, liver, breast, kidneys and lungs [14–18]. We recently demonstrated that BTG1 expression is significantly reduced in ovarian carcinoma tissues, and that BTG1 silencing in ovarian carcinoma occurs through epigenetic repression [19].

The role of BTG1 in endometrial cellular proliferation and the precise molecular mechanisms of BTG1 function in the pathogenesis of endometriosis remain unclear. In this study, we investigated BTG1 expression in eutopic and ectopic endometrial tissue samples obtained from patients with or without endometriosis. We also analyzed the expression levels of *BTG1* mRNA and protein and several cell cycle-related genes in primarily culture human endometrial stromal cells (HESCs), and examined whether downregulation of BTG1 affects cellular migration, proliferation, and/or apoptosis of HESCs.

2. Results

2.1. Clinical Characteristics

The clinical characteristics of the participants are shown in Table 1. The endometriosis group showed significantly decreased gravidity ($p = 0.034$) and parity ($p = 0.006$) compared to the control group. Patients with endometriosis exhibited lower body mass index than those without endometriosis, even though the difference between the groups was not statistically significant ($p = 0.092$). Serum levels of cancer antigen 125 were significantly higher in the endometriosis group than in the control group ($p = 0.002$). The differences in visual analogue scale (VAS) for pain between the groups were statistically significant. Mean VAS were significantly higher in the endometriosis group (6.57 ± 8.43) than in the control group (1.55 ± 9.88; $p < 0.001$).

Table 1. Patient characteristics.

Characteristic	Endometriosis Group	Control Group	*p*-Value
Number of patients	30	22	
Age (years)	34.93 ± 1.33	37.41 ± 1.78	0.349
Gravidity (frequency)	0.90 ± 0.24	1.91 ± 0.38	0.034 *
Parity (frequency)	0.47 ± 0.16	1.23 ± 0.22	0.006 *
Body mass index (kg/m^2)	20.67 ± 0.34	21.76 ± 0.53	0.092
Cancer antigen 125 (U/mL)	84.06 ± 25.83	18.60 ± 3.17	0.002 *
Visual analogue scale	6.57 ± 0.84	1.55 ± 0.98	<0.001 *

* Statistically significant. Data are expressed as mean ± standard error of mean.

2.2. Expression of BTG1 mRNA and Protein in Eutopic and Ectopic Endometrium of Patients with and without Endometriosis

Eutopic endometrium of the control group (1.95 ± 0.35) displayed significantly higher *BTG1* mRNA expression than both eutopic (1.12 ± 0.14; $p = 0.048$) and ectopic (0.81 ± 0.22; $p = 0.004$) endometrium of the endometriosis group (Figure 1A). In both groups, differences in *BTG1* mRNA expression between proliferative and secretory phases were not statistically significant, although the endometriosis groups exhibited lower expression levels than the control group in both the proliferative and secretory endometrial tissue samples (Table 2).

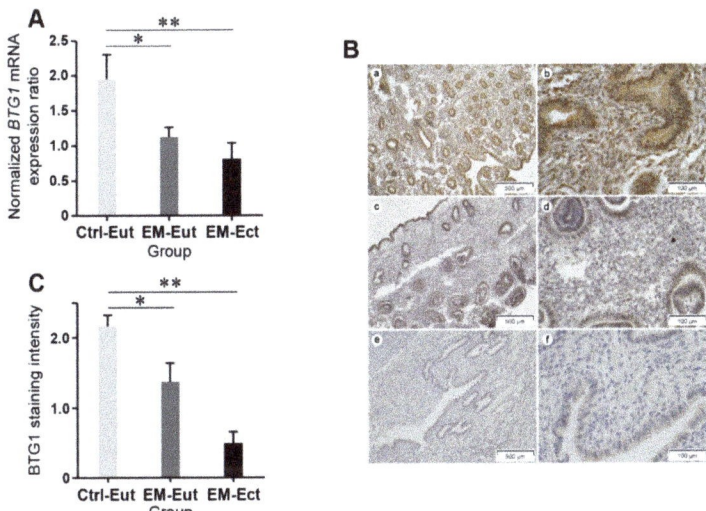

Figure 1. *BTG1* mRNA expression in eutopic and ectopic endometrial tissue samples obtained from patients with or without endometriosis. (**A**) Differences in *BTG1* mRNA expression levels among 3 groups: eutopic endometrium of the control group (Ctrl-Eut) and the endometriosis group (EM-Eut) and ectopic endometrium (EM-Ect). The expression levels of *BTG1* mRNA are normalized to that of *GAPDH* mRNA. (**B**) BTG1 protein expression in eutopic and ectopic endometrial tissue samples. (a) Eutopic endometrial tissue shows uniform and strong BTG1 immunoreactivity in the glandular and stromal cells (×100). (b) High-power view of image a. The cells in the endometrial glands and stroma exhibit strong BTG1 expression both in the nucleus and cytoplasm (×400). (c) Eutopic endometrial tissue of a patient with endometriosis displays patchy BTG1 expression with variable staining intensity (×100). (d) High-power view of image c. About half of the endometrial glandular epithelium and stromal cells show weak-to-moderate nuclear and cytoplasmic BTG1 immunoreactivity (×400). (e) Ectopic endometrial tissue in a patient with endometriosis (×100). (f) High-power view of image e. BTG1 expression is absent in the ectopic endometrial tissue. A faint nonspecific cytoplasmic staining is observed in the glandular epithelium (×400). (**C**) Differences in BTG1 staining intensity among 3 groups. * $p < 0.05$, ** $p < 0.01$. Error bars represent standard error of mean.

Table 2. *BTG1* mRNA expression in endometrium according to the phase of endometrium.

Phase of Endometrium	Group		*p*-Value
	Endometriosis	Control	
Proliferative phase	1.23 ± 0.21 (*n* = 14)	1.75 ± 0.50 (*n* = 8)	0.570
Secretory phase	1.03 ± 0.20 (*n* = 15)	1.88 ± 0.60 (*n* = 10)	0.091

Data are expressed as mean ± standard error of mean.

Using immunohistochemistry, we investigated BTG1 protein expression in eutopic and ectopic endometrial tissue samples in patients with and without endometriosis. Representative photomicrographs showing BTG1 immunoreactivity are shown in Figure 1B. Eutopic endometrial tissue of the control group showed strong BTG1 immunoreactivity in the endometrial glands and stroma. BTG1 was localized in both the nucleus and the cytoplasm of glandular epithelial and stromal cells. In contrast, BTG1 immunostaining was patchy and markedly reduced in the eutopic endometrium of the endometriosis group. About half of the glandular epithelial and stromal cells showed mild-to-moderate staining intensity. BTG1 staining intensity in eutopic and ectopic endometrium of the endometriosis group was markedly decreased compared with that in the eutopic endometrial tissue samples of the control group (Figure 1C). BTG1 was almost absent in the endometrial-type glands and stroma, although a faint nonspecific cytoplasmic staining was observed in the glandular epithelium. The BTG1 immunostaining results were in agreement with the mRNA expression data.

2.3. Effect of BTG1 Downregulation on Migration Potential of HESCs

We observed that the expression levels of BTG1 was reduced in endometriosis. Therefore, we speculated that downregulation of BTG1 may have effects on the migration of HESCs. We confirmed a reduction in BTG1 expression after *BTG1* siRNA transfection of HESCs (Figure 2A), and then examined the mRNA expression levels of *MMP2* and *MMP9*, which encode matrix metalloproteinase 2 (MMP2) and MMP9, respectively. They are well-known indicators for cell migration [20–23], and previous studies have shown that expression of MMP2 and/or MMP9 were elevated in endometriosis [24–26]. RT-PCR revealed that *BTG1* siRNA-transfected cells exhibited 1.18- and 1,94-fold increases in *MMP2* and *MMP9* mRNA expression levels compared to vehicle-treated control cells, with marginal significance ($p = 0.059$ and $p = 0.089$, respectively; Figure 2B). In line with this finding, the expression levels of MMP2 and MMP9 proteins were significantly increased in the transfected cells compared with the control cells (Figure 2C), indicating that BTG1 downregulation in HESCs induces an increase in their migration potential.

We further performed migration (Figure 2D) and wound healing (Figure 2E) assays. Compared to the control cells (4.40 ± 0.49), a significantly higher number of migrating cells was observed in the transfected cells (41.80 ± 1.07; $p < 0.001$). Wound healing assay revealed that scratched areas filled up with more HESCs in the transfected cells compared with the control cells ($p = 0.005$). Taken together, our observations suggest that BTG1 suppresses migration potential of in HESC.

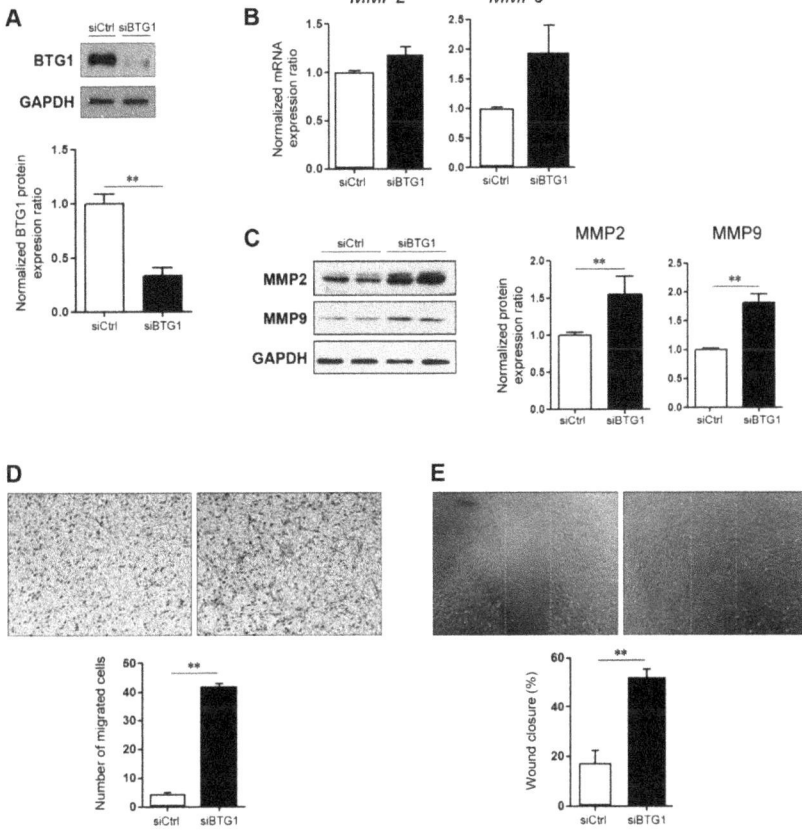

Figure 2. Effect of BTG1 downregulation on migration potential in HESCs. (**A**) Marked reduction in BTG1 protein expression after *BTG1* siRNA transfection. (**B**) The increases in the expression levels of *MMP2* and *MMP9* mRNA after BTG1 downregulation. (**C,D**) The significant increases in (C) the expression levels of MMP2 and MMP9 protein and (D) the number of migrated HESCs after BTG1 downregulation (×100). (**E**) Significantly higher rate of wound closure in the *BTG1* siRNA-transfected cells (×100). ** $p < 0.01$. Error bars represent standard error of mean.

2.4. Effect of BTG1 Downregulation on Apoptotic Potential and Proliferative Activity of HESCs

To investigate the role of BTG1 in apoptosis of HESCs, the mRNA expression levels of *Caspase 3*, *Caspase 8*, *Fas*, and *FasL* were measured in HESCs transfected with *BTG1* siRNA or treated with vehicle control (Figure 3A). Among them, *Caspase 3* mRNA expression was significantly affected by BTG1 downregulation. The transfected cells showed a 0.78-fold decrease in the expression level of *Caspase 3* mRNA compared to the control cells ($p = 0.029$). To validate this finding, we evaluated the expression levels of pro- and anti-apoptotic proteins including Caspase 3, cleaved Caspase 3, Bax, and Bcl-2 (Figure 3B). BTG1 downregulation reduced the expression levels of pro-apoptotic factors (cleaved Caspase 3 and Bcl-2) and elevated the expression level of anti-apoptotic factor (Bax). *Fas* mRNA and protein expression appeared to be increased in the transfected cells, the alterations were not statistically significant. Flow cytometry analysis (Figure 4A) revealed that the percentage of Annexin V-positive cells decreased significantly after transfection (6.34 ± 0.34 versus 4.69 ± 0.07%; $p = 0.008$). In addition, MTT assay (Figure 4B) revealed that relative cell proliferation of HESCs was increased significantly after BTG1 downregulation. These findings indicate that downregulation of BTG1 in HESCs induced a decrease in apoptotic potential and an increase in cellular proliferation.

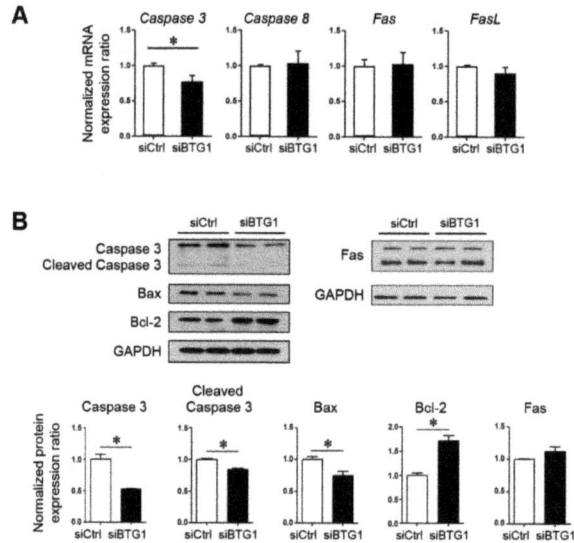

Figure 3. Effect of BTG1 downregulation on the expression of apoptosis-related proteins in HESCs. (**A**) mRNA expression levels of *Caspase 3*, *Caspase 8*, *Fas*, and *FasL* after *BTG1* siRNA transfection. (**B**) Protein expression levels of Caspase 3, cleaved Caspase 3, Bax, Bcl-2, and Fas. * $p < 0.05$. Error bars represent standard error of mean.

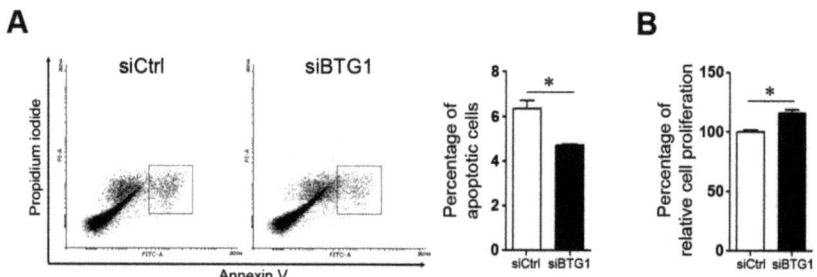

Figure 4. Effect of BTG1 downregulation on apoptotic potential and proliferative activity of HESCs. (**A**) Flow cytometry analysis showing decreased apoptotic potential of HESCs after BTG1 downregulation. A significant decrease in the percentage of apoptosis cells is observed in the *BTG1* siRNA-transfected cells. (**B**) MTT assay showing a significant increase in the percentage of relative cell proliferation after BTG1 downregulation. * $p < 0.05$. Error bars represent standard error of mean.

3. Discussion

Although *BTG1* is a known anti-proliferative gene, the role of BTG1 in the pathophysiology of endometriosis has remained unclear. In this study, we observed that BTG1 expression was significantly reduced in ectopic and eutopic endometrial tissues of patients with endometriosis. Downregulation of BTG1 increased proliferative activity and migration potential of HESCs, and decreased their apoptotic potential. Our observations suggest that reduced expression of BTG1 facilitates proliferation and migration of HESCs and suppresses their apoptosis, resulting in the progression of endometriosis.

MMPs are enzymes that degrade extracellular matrix proteins and are important for the tissue remodeling process [27]. MMP2 (gelatinase A) and MMP9 (gelatinase B) degrade type IV collagen and fibronectin [20]. Previous studies reported that MMP2 expression is increased along with other proteases in the late secretory endometrium [23], and that the expression level of MMP9 is elevated in patients with endometriosis, suggesting that their endometrial tissue is inherently more invasive [22]. In this study, we demonstrated that downregulation of BTG1 in HESCs resulted in elevated MMP2 and MMP9 expression levels, suggesting that BTG1 negatively regulates endometrial cell migration.

The apoptotic signaling is classified into two major pathways: extrinsic or cytoplasmic and intrinsic pathways. The extrinsic pathway is regulated by the Fas death receptor, and the intrinsic pathway is regulated by the Bcl-2 family of proteins [28,29]. The ratio of anti-apoptotic Bcl-2 to pro-apoptotic Bax is a critical factor for the intrinsic pathway. Hetero-dimerization of Bcl-2 with Bax, which inhibits apoptosis, is controlled by a family of cysteinyl proteases called caspases [30–32]. In this study, we showed that cellular apoptosis was reduced after downregulation of BTG1 in HESCs. The expression levels of *Caspase 3* mRNA were significantly reduced after BTG1 downregulation, whereas there were no significant alterations in mRNA expression levels of *Caspase 8*, *Fas*, or *FasL*. The *BTG1* siRNA-transfected HESCs also displayed decreased Bax expression and increased Bcl-2 expression. A previous study documented that overexpression of BTG1 induces apoptosis of breast carcinoma cells, accompanied by a decline in the Bcl-2 level and an increase in the Bax and Caspase 3 levels [18]. Our data suggest that BTG1 regulates cellular apoptosis via the intrinsic pathway in HESCs, thus affecting the pathogenesis of endometriosis.

There are a few limitations in this study. First, we conducted a pilot study using a relatively small number of the endometriosis subjects. Nevertheless, a significant reduction in BTG1 expression was observed in ectopic and eutopic endometrium of patients with endometriosis. Second, the control group did not include disease-free subjects. Since surgical resection of nonpathological ovarian or endometrial tissues from healthy patients raises ethical implications, we inevitably used tissue samples obtained from patients with ovarian mature teratoma, ovarian serous cystadenoma, or paratubal cyst. These benign ovarian lesions are not associated with ovarian endometriosis or endometrial pathology. Third, the majority of patients had moderate-to-severe endometriosis; therefore, we failed to investigate the association between BTG1 expression status and the severity of endometriosis. Fourth, we did not observe any expression of BTG1 in the Ishikawa cell line before and after BTG1 downregulation. We additionally measured MMP2 and MMP9 expression levels in Ishikawa cell line, but there was no difference in the expression levels (Figure 5). Since BTG1 is a tumor suppressor and the Ishikawa cell line is derived from endometrial carcinoma, lack of BTG1 expression was an expected finding.

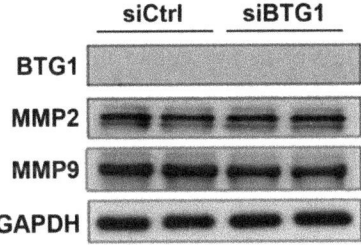

Figure 5. Effect of BTG1 downregulation on the protein expression levels of BTG1, MMP2 and MMP9 in Ishikawa cell line.

In conclusion, we demonstrated that downregulation of BTG1 could play an important role in the progression of endometriosis. We observed that BTG1 expression was significantly reduced in ectopic and eutopic endometrial tissues of patients with endometriosis. BTG1 downregulation via siRNA transfection increased migration potential and proliferative activity of HESCs, and decreased their apoptotic potential.

4. Materials and Methods

4.1. Patients and Tissue Samples

This study (3-2015-0250, 23 November 2015) was reviewed and approved by the Institutional Review Board of Gangnam Severance Hospital (Seoul, Korea). Between 1 June 2015 and 31 July 2015, 54 women who underwent laparoscopy for various gynecological conditions (pelvic mass, pelvic pain, endometriosis, and infertility) were enrolled after obtaining their written informed consent. Thirty-two and 22 patients participated in the endometriosis and control groups, respectively. Their ages ranged from 19 to 45 years. Patients with postmenopausal symptoms, previous hormone or gonadotropin-releasing hormone agonist use, uterine adenomyosis, endometrial lesion (polyp, hyperplasia, or malignancy), infectious disease, acute or chronic inflammatory disease, autoimmune disease, and cardiovascular disease were excluded.

All probable endometriotic lesions were surgically resected and sent to the pathology department for histopathological examination. Patients were assigned to the endometriosis group only after pathological confirmation of endometriosis. The extent of endometriosis was determined according to the revised American Society for Reproductive Medicine Classification of endometriosis [33]. Among 32 patients with peritoneal and/or ovarian endometriosis, 30 patients exhibited a moderate-to-severe form of endometriosis, while the remaining 2 patients had a mild form of the disease. The presence and intensity of endometriosis-related pain, including dysmenorrhea, deep dyspareunia, and/or non-menstrual pelvic pain, were assessed using VAS [34].

Fifteen of the 22 patients who participated in the control group were diagnosed as having mature cystic teratoma, and the remaining 7 patients had serous cystadenoma (5 patients) or paratubal cyst (2 patients). These benign ovarian lesions were not associated with ovarian endometriosis or endometrial pathology. Since surgical resection of nonpathological ovarian or endometrial tissues from healthy patients raises ethical implications, the control group did not include disease-free subjects. Endometrial tissue samples were obtained using a Pipelle catheter.

4.2. Culture of Primary Endometrial Stromal Cells and Ishikawa Cell Line

We cultured primary endothelial stromal cells as previously described [35]. Endometrial tissue was finely minced and the cells were dispersed by incubation in Hanks Balanced Salt Solution containing 4-(2-hydroxyethyl)-1-piperazineethanesulfonic acid (2 mmol/mL), 1% penicillin/streptomycin, and collagenase (1 mg/mL, 15 U/mg) for 60 min at 37 °C with agitation and pipetting. The cells were centrifuged and cell pellets were washed, suspended in Dulbecco's modified Eagle's medium:Ham F12 (1:Z1) solution containing 10% fetal bovine serum and 1% penicillin/streptomycin, passed through a 40-μm cell strainer (Corning Inc., Corning, NY, USA), and plated on commercially available 75 cm^2 tissue culture Falcon flasks (BD Biosciences, San Jose, CA, USA). We used cultured HESCs at 3–5 passages for analysis. We cultured the Ishikawa cell line in Minimum Essential Media (Invitrogen, Carlsbad, CA, USA) containing 2.0 mmol/L 1-glutamine and Earl salts, supplemented with 10% fetal bovine serum, 1% sodium pyruvate, and 1% penicillin/streptomycin.

4.3. Cell Transfection

Cells were seeded in 6-well plates, cultured to 70–80% confluence, and transfected with *BTG1* siRNA or control siRNA-A (Santa Cruz, Dallas, TX, USA) using Lipofectamine 3000 (Invitrogen) according to the manufacturer's recommendations at a final concentration of 50 nM. The transfected cells were harvested after 48 h.

4.4. RNA Isolation and Quantitative Real-Time Polymerase Chain Reaction (qRT-PCR)

To measure *BTG1* mRNA levels, total RNAs were isolated from cultured cells using the RNeasy Mini Kit (Qiagen Inc., Valencia, CA, USA). RNA sample concentrations were analyzed using a Nanodrop 2000 spectrophotometer (Thermo Fisher Scientific, Waltham, MA, USA). The Superscript III kit (Invitrogen) was used to synthesize cDNA using 1 µg of total RNA primed with oligo(dT). PCR was performed in a C1000 Thermal Cycler (Bio-Rad Laboratories, Hercules, CA, USA). The synthesized cDNA products were stored at −20 °C. qPCR was performed with 2 µL of synthesized cDNA as template using a 7300 Real-Time PCR System (Applied Biosystems, Foster City, CA, USA). Real-time PCR was performed using the Power SYBR Green PCR master mix (Applied Biosystems). The reaction mixture included the cDNA template, forward and reverse primers, ribonuclease-free water, and the SYBR Green PCR master mix at a final reaction volume of 20 µL. Reactions were performed at 95 °C for 5 min, followed by 40 cycles of 95 °C for 30 s, 60 °C for 30 s, 72 °C for 1 min, and a final extension at 72 °C for 5 min. Threshold cycle (Ct) values and melting curves were calculated using the 7300 Real-time PCR system software (Applied Biosystems). Each reaction was performed in triplicates. If not specified, the mRNA levels in each sample were normalized to those of *GAPDH*. Primer sequences for *BTG1*, *Caspase 3*, *Caspase 8*, *Fas*, *FasL*, *MMP2*, *MMP9* and *GAPDH* are shown in Table 3. The product amount was calibrated to the internal control reference using the ∆∆Ct analysis [36].

Table 3. Primer sequences used.

Gene		Sequence
BTG1	Forward	CAA GGG ATC GGG TTA CCG TTG T
	Reverse	AGC CAT CCT CTC CAA TTC TGT AGG
Caspase 3	Forward	GGA AGC GAA TCA ATG GAC TCT GG
	Reverse	GCA TCG ACA TCT GTA CCA GAC C
Caspase 8	Forward	CCA GAG ACT CCA GGA AAA GAG A
	Reverse	GAT AGA GCA TGA CCC TGT AGG C
Fas	Forward	AGC TTG GTC TAG AGT GAA AA
	Reverse	GAG GCA GAA TCA TGA GAT AT
FasL	Forward	CAG CTC TTC CAC CTG CAG AAG G
	Reverse	AGA TTC CTC AAA ATT GAT CAG AGA GAG
MMP2	Forward	ACC GCG ACA AGA AGT ATG GC
	Reverse	CCA CTT GCG GTC ATC ATC GT
MMP9	Forward	CGA TGA CGA GTT GTG GTC CC
	Reverse	TCG TAG TTG GCC GTG GTA CT
GAPDH	Forward	ACC ACA GTC CAT GCC ATC AC
	Reverse	TCC ACC ACC CTG TTG CTG TA

4.5. Immunohistochemistry

BTG1 protein expression was assessed by immunohistochemistry using the Bond Polymer Intense Detection System (Leica Biosystems, Newcastle upon Tyne, UK) according to the manufacturer's recommendations. Surgically resected tissues were fixed in 10% neutral buffered formalin for 12–24 h. The tissues were then sectioned, processed with an automatic tissue processor, and embedded in paraffin blocks. A rotary microtome was used to cut 4-µm thick sections from each formalin-fixed, paraffin-embedded tissue block. Deparaffinization was performed using Bond Dewax Solution (Leica Biosystems). Antigen retrieval was performed using Bond Epitope Retrieval Solution (Leica Biosystems) for 30 min at 100 °C. Endogenous peroxidases were quenched with hydrogen peroxide for 5 min. Sections were incubated with anti-rabbit antibody against BTG1 (1:100, polyclonal, Abcam, Cambridge, MA, USA) for 15 min at ambient temperature. Biotin-free polymeric horseradish peroxidase-linker antibody conjugate system and Bond-maX automatic slide stainer (Leica Biosystems) were used. Visualization was performed using 1 mM 3,3'-diaminobenzidine, 50 mM Tris-hydrogen chloride buffer (pH 7.6), and 0.006% hydrogen peroxide. The sections were counterstained with hematoxylin. Positive and negative control samples were included with each reaction to minimize inter-assay variation. Normal colonic tissue was used as positive control. The negative control was prepared by replacing the primary antibody with non-immune serum; no detectable staining was evident. The staining intensity of BTG1 was assessed on a scale of 0–3, with 0 indicating negative staining; 1, weak; 2, moderate; and 3, strong.

4.6. Protein Extraction and Western Blot Analysis

We prepared protein extracts using a radio-immunoprecipitation assay buffer containing protease and a phosphatase inhibitor cocktail (Thermo Fisher Scientific). We determined the concentrations of total cell lysates using Pierce BCA protein assay kit (Thermo Fisher Scientific). We mixed 20 µg of total protein with 5× sample buffer, and then heated at 95 °C for 5 min. Samples were loaded on 12% sodium dodecyl sulfate-polyacrylamide gels and transferred to a polyvinylidene fluoride membrane (EMD Millipore, Burlington, MA, USA) with use of a Transblot apparatus (Bio-Rad Laboratories). Membranes (EMD Millipore) were blocked with 5% non-fat skim milk in Tris-buffered saline solution (10 mmol/L Tris-hydrogen chloride (pH 7.4) and 0.5 mol/L sodium chloride) with 0.1% *v/v* of Tween-20 (TBS-T). The blots were probed with primary antibodies against BTG1 (1:200, Abcam), MMP9 (1:250, Santa Cruz) with TBS-T; MMP2 (1:250, Santa Cruz) with TBS-T, Caspase 3 (1:1,000, Cell Signaling Technology, Danvers, MA, USA) with TBS plus 5% skim milk, Bax (1:500, Santa Cruz) with TBS plus 5% skim milk, Bcl-2 (1:1000, Cell Signaling Technology) with TBS plus 5% skim milk, and GAPDH (1:1000, Santa Cruz) with TBS plus 5% skim milk. They were then incubated in horseradish peroxidase-conjugated secondary antibodies (1:2000, Thermo Fisher Scientific). Proteins were detected using enhanced chemiluminescence (Santa Cruz). The experiment was repeated three times and the data shown are representative.

4.7. Migration and Wound Healing Assay

We performed migration assay for BTG1-transfected cells using 8-mm-pore polycarbonate membranes (EMD Millipore) within 24-well plates. Freshly treated by trypsin and washed cells were suspended in 200 mL of serum-free medium and positioned in the top chamber of each insert (5×10^4 cells/well); 600 mL of medium containing 10% fetal bovine serum was added into the lower chambers. Cells were fixed and stained with hematoxylin after incubation for 24 h at 37 °C in a 5% carbon dioxide humidified incubator. Cells in the inner chamber were removed using a cotton swab and the cells that were attached to the bottom side of the membrane were counted and imaged using an inverted microscope (Olympus, Tokyo, Japan) at 200× magnification over ten random fields in each well. For the wound healing assay, HESCs were transfected with control or *BTG1* siRNA for 48 h. The transfected cells were seeded using Dulbecco's modified Eagle's medium/F12 (1:1) with 10% fetal bovine serum and antibiotics and cultured in 24-well plates incubated at 37 °C with 5% carbon dioxide for 24 h. A linear wound (scratch) was generated using a sterile 100 µL pipette tip and debris was washed twice with phosphate-buffered saline. Cells were grown in culture for 18–24 h at 37 °C with 5% carbon dioxide. The scratched areas in each well were imaged using the EVOS inverted microscope (Advanced Microscopy Group, Mill Creek, WA, USA) to calculate the migration ability of *BTG1*-knockdown cells using ImageJ Version 1.51, a Java-based image processing program developed at the National Institutes of Health (Bethesda, MD, USA) [37]. The experiments were repeated four times.

4.8. Flow Cytometry

Cells were seeded in 6-well plates, incubated with indicated concentrations of chemical for 24 or 48 h, and transfected for 48 h. Cells were washed twice with phosphate-buffered saline; and suspended in 400 mL of binding buffer. Cells were stained with 5 mL Annexin V-fluorescein isothiocyanate (FITC) and 4 mL propidium iodide and incubated at room temperature for 10 min using Annexin V-FITC Apoptosis Detection Kit (BD Biosciences). The stained cells were quantified by flow cytometry using the FACS Canto II system (BD Biosciences) and the data were analyzed using DIVA software (version 8.0; BD Biosciences).

4.9. MTT Assay

Cytotoxicity was performed using the CellTiter 96 Non-Radioactive Cell Proliferation Assay (MTT) kit as manufacturer's recommendations (Promega, Madison, WI, USA). Briefly, 1×10^4 HESCs/well were seeded onto 96 well plates and incubated for 24 hr. After removal of supernatant, the plates were incubated with mixed solution (new media 100 μL and MTT solution 10 μL) for 4 h at 37 °C in a carbon dioxide incubator. Solubilization and stop solution mixture was added. The dark blue formazan product was quantified using a microplate reader at 570 nm (with a 690 nm reference filter; Molecular Device, Sunnyvale, CA, USA).

4.10. Statistical Analysis

All data were assessed for normal distribution using the Kolmogorov-Smirnov test or the Shapiro-Wilk test. The Student *t*-test or the Mann-Whitney U test was used for comparisons. One-way analysis of variance was performed in conjunction with the Tukey's post-hoc test to evaluate differences among groups. Statistical analyses were performed using SPSS for Windows, Version 16.0 (SPSS Inc., Chicago, IL, USA).

Author Contributions: All authors (J.S.K., Y.S.C., J.H.P. (Ji Hyun Park), J.Y., S.K., J.H.L., B.H.Y., J.H.P. (Joo Hyun Park), S.K.S., S.C., H.-S.K. and B.S.L.) were responsible for: acquisition of data, or analysis and interpretation of data, final approval of the version to be published. Additionally, J.S.K., Y.S.C., S.C. and H.-S.K. were responsible for substantial contributions to conception and design and drafting the manuscript. Especially, S.C. and H.-S.K. were responsible for revising the manuscript critically for important intellectual content.

Funding: This research was supported by the Basic Science Research Program through the National Research Foundation of Korea (NRF) funded by the Ministry of Education (2016R1D1A1B03934875 and 2016R1D1A1B03935584).

Acknowledgments: We thank all other members, who were not listed here, in the department for their contribution of active discussions.

Conflicts of Interest: The authors have no conflict of interest to declare.

References

1. Zegers-Hochschild, F.; Adamson, G.D.; Dyer, S.; Racowsky, C.; de Mouzon, J.; Sokol, R.; Rienzi, L.; Sunde, A.; Schmidt, L.; Cooke, I.D.; et al. The International Glossary on Infertility and Fertility Care, 2017. *Hum. Reprod.* **2017**, *32*, 1786–1801. [CrossRef] [PubMed]
2. Giudice, L.C.; Kao, L.C. Endometriosis. *Lancet* **2004**, *364*, 1789–1799. [CrossRef]
3. Agathocleous, M.; Harris, W.A. Metabolism in physiological cell proliferation and differentiation. *Trends Cell Biol.* **2013**, *23*, 484–492. [CrossRef] [PubMed]
4. Shibata, D.; Aaltonen, L.A. Genetic predisposition and somatic diversification in tumor development and progression. *Adv. Cancer Res.* **2001**, *80*, 83–114. [PubMed]
5. Bulun, S.E. Endometriosis. *N. Engl. J. Med.* **2009**, *360*, 268–279. [CrossRef] [PubMed]
6. Huhtinen, K.; Desai, R.; Stahle, M.; Salminen, A.; Handelsman, D.J.; Perheentupa, A.; Poutanen, M. Endometrial and endometriotic concentrations of estrone and estradiol are determined by local metabolism rather than circulating levels. *J. Clin. Endocrinol. Metab.* **2012**, *97*, 4228–4235. [CrossRef] [PubMed]
7. Vinci, G.; Arkwright, S.; Audebourg, A.; Radenen, B.; Chapron, C.; Borghese, B.; Dousset, B.; Mehats, C.; Vaiman, D.; Vacher-Lavenu, M.C.; et al. Correlation Between the Clinical Parameters and Tissue Phenotype in Patients Affected by Deep-Infiltrating Endometriosis. *Reprod. Sci.* **2016**, *23*, 1258–1268. [CrossRef] [PubMed]
8. Waanders, E.; Scheijen, B.; van der Meer, L.T.; van Reijmersdal, S.V.; van Emst, L.; Kroeze, Y.; Sonneveld, E.; Hoogerbrugge, P.M.; van Kessel, A.G.; van Leeuwen, F.N.; et al. The origin and nature of tightly clustered BTG1 deletions in precursor B-cell acute lymphoblastic leukemia support a model of multiclonal evolution. *PLoS Genet.* **2012**, *8*, e1002533. [CrossRef] [PubMed]
9. Berthet, C.; Guehenneux, F.; Revol, V.; Samarut, C.; Lukaszewicz, A.; Dehay, C.; Dumontet, C.; Magaud, J.P.; Rouault, J.P. Interaction of PRMT1 with BTG/TOB proteins in cell signalling: Molecular analysis and functional aspects. *Genes Cells Devoted Mol. Cell. Mech.* **2002**, *7*, 29–39. [CrossRef]

10. Doidge, R.; Mittal, S.; Aslam, A.; Winkler, G.S. The anti-proliferative activity of BTG/TOB proteins is mediated via the Caf1a (CNOT7) and Caf1b (CNOT8) deadenylase subunits of the Ccr4-not complex. *PLoS ONE* **2012**, *7*, e51331. [CrossRef]

11. Rouault, J.P.; Rimokh, R.; Tessa, C.; Paranhos, G.; Ffrench, M.; Duret, L.; Garoccio, M.; Germain, D.; Samarut, J.; Magaud, J.P. BTG1, a member of a new family of antiproliferative genes. *Embo J.* **1992**, *11*, 1663–1670. [CrossRef] [PubMed]

12. Corjay, M.H.; Kearney, M.A.; Munzer, D.A.; Diamond, S.M.; Stoltenborg, J.K. Antiproliferative gene BTG1 is highly expressed in apoptotic cells in macrophage-rich areas of advanced lesions in Watanabe heritable hyperlipidemic rabbit and human. *Lab. Investig. A J. Tech. Methods Pathol.* **1998**, *78*, 847–858.

13. Lee, H.; Cha, S.; Lee, M.S.; Cho, G.J.; Choi, W.S.; Suk, K. Role of antiproliferative B cell translocation gene-1 as an apoptotic sensitizer in activation-induced cell death of brain microglia. *J. Immunol.* **2003**, *171*, 5802–5811. [CrossRef] [PubMed]

14. Sun, G.G.; Wang, Y.D.; Cheng, Y.J.; Hu, W.N. BTG1 underexpression is an independent prognostic marker in esophageal squamous cell carcinoma. *Tumour Biol. J. Int. Soc. Oncodev. Biol. Med.* **2014**, *35*, 9707–9716. [CrossRef] [PubMed]

15. Sun, G.G.; Lu, Y.F.; Cheng, Y.J.; Hu, W.N. The expression of BTG1 is downregulated in NSCLC and possibly associated with tumor metastasis. *Tumour Biol. J. Int. Soc. Oncodev. Biol. Med.* **2014**, *35*, 2949–2957. [CrossRef] [PubMed]

16. Sun, G.G.; Wang, Y.D.; Cheng, Y.J.; Hu, W.N. The expression of BTG1 is downregulated in nasopharyngeal carcinoma and possibly associated with tumour metastasis. *Mol. Biol. Rep.* **2014**, *41*, 5979–5988. [CrossRef] [PubMed]

17. Liu, C.; Tao, T.; Xu, B.; Lu, K.; Zhang, L.; Jiang, L.; Chen, S.; Liu, D.; Zhang, X.; Cao, N.; et al. BTG1 potentiates apoptosis and suppresses proliferation in renal cell carcinoma by interacting with PRMT1. *Oncol. Lett.* **2015**, *10*, 619–624. [CrossRef] [PubMed]

18. Zhu, R.; Zou, S.T.; Wan, J.M.; Li, W.; Li, X.L.; Zhu, W. BTG1 inhibits breast cancer cell growth through induction of cell cycle arrest and apoptosis. *Oncol. Rep.* **2013**, *30*, 2137–2144. [CrossRef] [PubMed]

19. Kim, J.Y.; Do, S.I.; Bae, G.E.; Kim, H.S. B-cell translocation gene 1 is downregulated by promoter methylation in ovarian carcinoma. *J. Cancer* **2017**, *8*, 2669–2675. [CrossRef] [PubMed]

20. Aznavoorian, S.; Murphy, A.N.; Stetler-Stevenson, W.G.; Liotta, L.A. Molecular aspects of tumor cell invasion and metastasis. *Cancer* **1993**, *71*, 1368–1383. [CrossRef]

21. Di Nezza, L.A.; Misajon, A.; Zhang, J.; Jobling, T.; Quinn, M.A.; Ostor, A.G.; Nie, G.; Lopata, A.; Salamonsen, L.A. Presence of active gelatinases in endometrial carcinoma and correlation of matrix metalloproteinase expression with increasing tumor grade and invasion. *Cancer* **2002**, *94*, 1466–1475. [CrossRef]

22. Shaco-Levy, R.; Sharabi, S.; Benharroch, D.; Piura, B.; Sion-Vardy, N. Matrix metalloproteinases 2 and 9, E-cadherin, and beta-catenin expression in endometriosis, low-grade endometrial carcinoma and non-neoplastic eutopic endometrium. *Eur. J. Obstet. Gynecol. Reprod. Biol.* **2008**, *139*, 226–232. [CrossRef] [PubMed]

23. Talbi, S.; Hamilton, A.E.; Vo, K.C.; Tulac, S.; Overgaard, M.T.; Dosiou, C.; Le Shay, N.; Nezhat, C.N.; Kempson, R.; Lessey, B.A.; et al. Molecular phenotyping of human endometrium distinguishes menstrual cycle phases and underlying biological processes in normo-ovulatory women. *Endocrinology* **2006**, *147*, 1097–1121. [CrossRef] [PubMed]

24. Weigel, M.T.; Kramer, J.; Schem, C.; Wenners, A.; Alkatout, I.; Jonat, W.; Maass, N.; Mundhenke, C. Differential expression of MMP-2, MMP-9 and PCNA in endometriosis and endometrial carcinoma. *Eur. J. Obstet. Gynecol. Reprod. Biol.* **2012**, *160*, 74–78. [CrossRef]

25. Liu, H.; Wang, J.; Wang, H.; Tang, N.; Li, Y.; Zhang, Y.; Hao, T. Correlation between matrix metalloproteinase-9 and endometriosis. *Int. J. Clin. Exp. Pathol.* **2015**, *8*, 13399–13404.

26. Collette, T.; Maheux, R.; Mailloux, J.; Akoum, A. Increased expression of matrix metalloproteinase-9 in the eutopic endometrial tissue of women with endometriosis. *Hum. Reprod.* **2006**, *21*, 3059–3067. [CrossRef]

27. Emonard, H.; Grimaud, J.A. Matrix metalloproteinases. A review. *Cell. Mol. Biol.* **1990**, *36*, 131–153. [PubMed]

28. Nahta, R.; Esteva, F.J. Bcl-2 antisense oligonucleotides: A potential novel strategy for the treatment of breast cancer. *Semin. Oncol.* **2003**, *30*, 143–149. [CrossRef]

29. Ghobrial, I.M.; Witzig, T.E.; Adjei, A.A. Targeting apoptosis pathways in cancer therapy. *CA A Cancer J. Clin.* **2005**, *55*, 178–194. [CrossRef]
30. Cohen, G.M. Caspases: The executioners of apoptosis. *Biochem. J.* **1997**, *326 Pt 1*, 1–16. [CrossRef]
31. Thornberry, N.A.; Lazebnik, Y. Caspases: Enemies within. *Science* **1998**, *281*, 1312–1316. [CrossRef] [PubMed]
32. Kymionis, G.D.; Dimitrakakis, C.E.; Konstadoulakis, M.M.; Arzimanoglou, I.; Leandros, E.; Chalkiadakis, G.; Keramopoulos, A.; Michalas, S. Can expression of apoptosis genes, bcl-2 and bax, predict survival and responsiveness to chemotherapy in node-negative breast cancer patients? *J. Surg. Res.* **2001**, *99*, 161–168. [CrossRef] [PubMed]
33. Canis, M.; Donnez, J.G.; Guzick, D.S.; Halme, J.K.; Rock, J.A.; Schenken, R.S.; Vernon, M.W. Revised American Society for Reproductive Medicine classification of endometriosis: 1996. *Fertil. Steril.* **1997**, *67*, 817–821.
34. Bourdel, N.; Alves, J.; Pickering, G.; Ramilo, I.; Roman, H.; Canis, M. Systematic review of endometriosis pain assessment: How to choose a scale? *Hum. Reprod. Update* **2015**, *21*, 136–152. [CrossRef] [PubMed]
35. Cho, S.; Mutlu, L.; Zhou, Y.; Taylor, H.S. Aromatase inhibitor regulates let-7 expression and let-7f-induced cell migration in endometrial cells from women with endometriosis. *Fertil. Steril.* **2016**, *106*, 673–680. [CrossRef] [PubMed]
36. Cho, S.; Ahn, Y.S.; Choi, Y.S.; Seo, S.K.; Nam, A.; Kim, H.Y.; Kim, J.H.; Park, K.H.; Cho, D.J.; Lee, B.S. Endometrial osteopontin mRNA expression and plasma osteopontin levels are increased in patients with endometriosis. *Am. J. Reprod. Immunol.* **2009**, *61*, 286–293. [CrossRef] [PubMed]
37. Grewal, S.; Carver, J.G.; Ridley, A.J.; Mardon, H.J. Implantation of the human embryo requires Rac1-dependent endometrial stromal cell migration. *Proc. Natl. Acad. Sci. USA* **2008**, *105*, 16189–16194. [CrossRef] [PubMed]

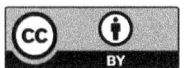

© 2019 by the authors. Licensee MDPI, Basel, Switzerland. This article is an open access article distributed under the terms and conditions of the Creative Commons Attribution (CC BY) license (http://creativecommons.org/licenses/by/4.0/).

MDPI
St. Alban-Anlage 66
4052 Basel
Switzerland
Tel. +41 61 683 77 34
Fax +41 61 302 89 18
www.mdpi.com

International Journal of Molecular Sciences Editorial Office
E-mail: ijms@mdpi.com
www.mdpi.com/journal/ijms

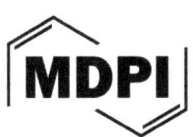

www.ingramcontent.com/pod-product-compliance
Lightning Source LLC
LaVergne TN
LVHW070624100526
838202LV00012B/716